INSTANT VETERINARY DRUG INDEX
(Biologics and Pharmaceutics)

INSTANT VETERINARY DRUG INDEX
(Biologics and Pharmaceutics)

Compiled by:

Y.P.S. Dabas

B.Sc., B.V.Sc. & A.H., M.V.Sc., Ph.D. (Pantnagar)
Professor
Veterinary & Animal Husbandry Extension
College of Veterinary Sciences
G.B. Pant Univ. of Agri. & Tech.
Pantnagar-263145, (U.S. Nagar) U.P.

Har Pal Singh

B.Sc., B.V.Sc. & A.H., M.V.Sc., Ph.D. (Illinois)
Professor
Veterinary Surgery
College of Veterinary Sciences
G.B. Pant Univ. of Agri. & Tech.
Pantnagar-263145, (U.S. Nagar) U.P.

S.N. Maurya

B.V.Sc. & A.H., M.V.Sc., Ph.D. (Illinois)
Professor
Veterinary Gynaecology & Obstetrics
College of Veterinary Sciences
G.B. Pant Univ. of Agri. & Tech.
Pantnagar-263145, (U.S. Nagar) U.P.

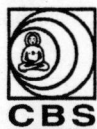

CBS

CBS Publishers & Distributors Pvt. Ltd.

New Delhi • Bengaluru • Chennai • Kochi • Kolkata • Mumbai
Hyderabad • Uttarakhand • Nagpur • Patna • Pune • Jharkhand

Instant Veterinary Drug Index

ISBN: 978-81-239-2690-2

First CBS Reprint: 2015
Reprint: 2019

Published by **Satish Kumar Jain** and produced by **Varun Jain** for
CBS Publishers & Distributors Pvt. Ltd.,
4819/XI Prahlad Street, 24 Ansari Road, Daryaganj, New Delhi - 110002
delhi@cbspd.com, cbspubs@airtelmail.in • www.cbspd.com
Ph.: 23289259, 23266861, 23266867 • Fax: 011-23243014

Corporate Office: 204 FIE, Industrial Area, Patparganj, Delhi - 110 092
Ph: 49344934 • Fax: 011-49344935
E-mail: publishing@cbspd.com • publicity@cbspd.com

Branches:
- *Bengaluru:* 2975, 17th Cross, K.R. Road, Bansankari 2nd Stage,
  Bengaluru - 70 • Ph: +91-80-26771678/79 • Fax: +91-80-26771680
  E-mail: cbsbng@gmail.com, bangalore@cbspd.com
- *Chennai:* No. 7, Subbaraya Street, Shenoy Nagar, Chennai - 600030
  Ph: +91-44-26681266, 26680620 • Fax: +91-44-42032115
  E-mail: chennai@cbspd.com
- *Kochi:* Ashana House, 39/1904, A.M. Thomas Road, Valanjambalam,
  Ernakulum, Kochi • Ph: +91-484-4059061-65
  Fax: +91-484-4059065 • E-mail: cochin@cbspd.com
- *Kolkata:* 6-B, Ground Floor, Rameshwar Shaw Road, Kolkata - 700014
  Ph: +91-33-22891126/7/8 • E-mail: kolkata@cbspd.com
- *Mumbai:* 83-C, Dr. E. Moses Road, Worli, Mumbai - 400018
  Ph: +91-9833017933, 022-24902340/41 • E-mail: mumbai@cbspd.com

Representatives:
- Hyderabad: 0-9885175004
- Patna: 0-9334159340
- Jharkhand: 0-9811541605
- Nagpur: 0-9021734563
- Pune: 0-9623451994
- Uttarakhand: 0-9716462459

Printed at:
Neekunj Print Process, Delhi (India)

PREFACE

The growing awareness of the importance of prevention and treatment of diseases in animals and poultry has put extra demand on veterinary pharmaceuticals and biologicals etc. As a consequence recent years have seen a tremendous spurt in the production of veterinary biologicals and pharmaceuticals and a large number of renowned drug companies, hitherto, producing drugs for human use only, have entered into production of drugs for veterinary use.

The number of veterinary pharmaceutical products and companies producing them have gone so high that it has virtually become impossible for the present day veterinarian especially the practicing veterinarian and students to keep track of new companies entering the market and additions of drugs now and then.

Efforts, therefore, have been made in this publication to present useful information, on about 75 pharmaceutical companies, 1000 propriety and non-propriety products with their composition, indications and dosage and about 80 biological products and sera etc. in the form of a compendium for ready reference of veterinary clinicians and students.

The book consists of two broad sections viz veterinary biologicals and pharmaceutics. Complete information on vaccines and sera, veterinary preparations with therapeutic and brand name index, alphabetical index of pharmaceutical drugs, product information and alphabetical index of pharmaceutical companies etc. has been covered under the two heads. A separate section on medical products found useful and commonly used in veterinary practice has also been added.

Every effort has been made to ensure the accuracy of the information given and make it exhaustive to be useful.

We wish to acknowledge the help of all who have contributed in the preparation of this compendium.

Authors also record their thanks to M/s International Book Distributing Co., Lucknow for bringing out the quality publication.

Pantnagar.   Authors

Dated : 30-1-99

CONTENTS

VETERINARY BIOLOGICS

VACCINES AND SERA

(a)	Dog Vaccine:	Canine distemper, Canine hepatitis, Leptospirosis, Adenovirus, Parainfluenza, Anti-rabies, Canine Parvo virus and Canine Corona virus vaccines.
(b)	Livestock Vaccine:	Anthrax vaccine, Black Quarter vaccine, Brucella abortus vaccine, Foot and Mouth Disease vaccine, H.S. vaccine, Rinderpest vaccine, Theileriosis vaccine, Enterotoxemia vaccine, Sheep pox vaccine, Swine fever vaccine, Anti-rabic vaccine (post-bite).
(c)	Poultry Vaccine:	Avian Encephalomyelitis vaccine, Infectious Bronchitis vaccine, Egg Drop Syndrome '76', Fowl Cholera vaccine, Fowl Pox vaccine, Infectious Bursal disease vaccine, Infectious Coryza vaccine, Laryngotracheitis vaccine, Marek's disease vaccine, New Castle disease vaccine.
(d)	Sera:	Anti-anthrax serum, Anti-B.Q. serum, H.S. Anti-serum, Anti-R.P. serum, Anti-Snake venum serum, Tetanus anti-toxin, Tetanus toxoid.

DOG VACCINES

There are several major diseases responsible for higher mortality in pups and dogs. It is essential when you take a pup into your home, get the protection of vaccine against the major killing diseases. The diseases of dogs which can be prevented by the vaccination include: canine distemper, canine hepatitis, leptospirosis, canine parvo disease, rabies and canine corona virus.

Bitches which have high antibody levels as a result of regular vaccinations, pass on the protection to their puppies through milk. This resistance falls below the level needed for protection at the time when pups have been weaned and at that time vaccination in pups should be performed. For giving full protection in early life, the young weanling pups must be vaccinated against canine distemper, canine parvo virus disease, canine corona virus. Pups should be given a course of two or more injections. Because in early life the residual maternal antibodies may disturb the formation of active immunity, second injection around 4-5 weeks after first injection is essential for effective vaccination. Usually booster injections are essential against all the diseases every year to top up the immunity to a safe level.

It is also advisable to keep your pups away from infection. Young pup is most vulnerable to infection and hence must be kept inside the house, except for relieving and that too at a safe place. If already there is another dog, make sure it is fully vaccinated.

It is important that pups/dogs are healthy when vaccinated. Accordingly, deworm your pet prior to vaccination. Now a days most of the vaccines are combined injections protecting dog against several diseases. Some of the following vaccines can be used.

CANINE DISTEMPER, CANINE HEPATITIS, LEPTOSPIROSIS, ADENO VIRUS AND PARAINFLUENZA VACCINES

There are several brands of vaccines available which protect the pups/dogs against canine distemper, canine hepatitis, leptospirosis (L. canicola and L. icterohaemorrhagiae), adenovirus type-2, and parainfluenza. Some of them are single vaccines and some combined one.

    (a) Canine distemper vaccine (I.V.R.I., Izatnagar)
    (b) Canine distemper vaccine (Bio-Med, Ghaziabad)
    (c) Quadrivalent vaccine (Canine distemper, canine hepatitis and two strains of leptospira)
        (i) Candur-DHL (Hoechst India Ltd.)
        (ii) Canilep-DHL (Glaxo India Ltd.)
        (iii) Nobi Vac-DHL (Intercare Ltd.)
        (iv) Caniffa (Serum Institute of India)

First vaccination is recommended at the age of 7-9 weeks and second vaccination at 12-14 weeks of age, either by intramuscular or subcutaneous route. If the vaccination is carried out after the 12th week of age, one vaccination will generally be sufficient. The effective immunity is established in 1-2 weeks after vaccination and lasts for 1-2 years in case of distemper and hepatitis and for 1 year in case of leptospirosis. Annual revaccination is recommended.

    (d) Nobi-Vac DHPPI (Intercare) (Canine distember, Hepatitis, Parvo virus and Parainfluenza)
    (e) Nobi Vac DH+RL (Intercare)-Canine distember, hepatitis, rabies, leptospirosis

(f)   Nobi Vac-L (Intercare) - Leptospirosis

(g)   Duramune DA$_2$ LP + PV (Fort Dodge), Adenomune-7 (Tech America) -7-in-1 (Smith Kline Beechem): Canine distemper, canine hepatitis, adeno virus type-2, para influenza, parvo virus and leptospira (2 strains) one ml s/c or i/m in puppies of age between 9-14 weeks, repeat every 4 weeks until 16 weeks of age. Annual revaccination is recommended.

(h)   Duramune (8 in 1) (Fort Dodge) – protects dogs against corono virus along with above 7 diseases.

(i)   Injection of "attenuated measles virus" can also protect the pup against canine distemper.

ANTI-RABIES VACCINES

Several brands of anti-rabic vaccines are available in market. Some of them are as follows:

(a)   Rabies vaccine (I.V.R.I, Izatnagar)

Freeze dried vaccine is reconstituted with 3 ml distilled water for deep intramuscular injection.

·(b)   Rabies vaccine 'LEP' Flury strain (Bio-Med, Ghaziabad) is reconstituted in 2 ml distilled water for deep intramuscular injection.

(c)   Rabisin (Serum Institute of India) – one ml s/c or i/m

(d)   Rabguard-TC (Smithkline Beechem) one ml s/c or i/m

(e)   Raksharab (Indian Immunologicals) – one ml s/c

(f)   Nobi vac-R (Intercare Ltd.)

(g)   Dura-Rab (Tech America) – one ml i/m
    (i)   Dura-Rab-1 (One year immunity)
    (ii) Dura-Rab-3 (Three-year immunity)

(h)   Annumune (Fort Dodge)

(i)   Candur-R (Hoechst India Ltd.)

(j)   Rabdomun (Cadila Health Care)

First injection for all the vaccines can be given at the age of 4 weeks in pups. If pups were born to vaccinated bitches, the vaccination can be postponed until the 11th week i.e. after elimination of the maternal antibodies. Although all the above vaccines provide three years immunity but it is recommended to follow annual revaccination due to endemic nature of rabies in India.

(k)   Rabipur (Hoechst India Ltd.): Protective pre-exposure vaccination against rabies consists of one injection intramuscularly on each of days 0, 28 and 56 or if immediate prophylaxis appears necessary on days 0, 7 and 21. Reinforce vaccinations after one year.

(l)   Penta Dog (Serum Institute of India): Pentavalent vaccine (distemper, canine hepatitis, leptospiral infection and rabies), consists of two vaccines (Biviro-vax-Distemper and canine hepatitis; Leptorab-rabies and leptospiral vaccine) which are mixed at the time of use. One ml s/c or i/m at the age of 7 weeks or older in pups. Second injection after 4 weeks of the first injection but not before 11 weeks of age. Annual vaccination is recommended.

CANINE PARVO VIRUS VACCINES

(a)   Vanguard CPV

(b)   Parvocine (Tech America)

(c)   Duramune DA$_2$ LP + PV

(d)   Adenomune-7

(e)   Duramune DA$_2$ PP + CVK
Nobi Vac Puppy DP (Intercare)
Nobi Vac Parvo-c (Intercare)
Nobi Vac DHPPI (Intercare)
Inject 1 ml of vaccine by i/m or s/c route. First vaccination at 9-12 weeks and above.
Second dose at 15-16 weeks of age in pups and above.

–   Non-vaccinated pregnant bitches – 4 weeks before and 2 weeks before parturition (with Parvocine).

–   Vaccinated pregnant bitches – 3 weeks before parturition (with Parvocine).

–   Non-vaccinated adult dogs – 2 doses, 1 to 4 weeks apart.

Vaccination Schedule of Dog

	Disease	Vaccine	Age of Vaccination	Period of Immunity
1.	Canine Distemper Canine Hepatitis Leptospirosis	Candur DHL, Canilep DHL Caniffa, Penta dog, Nobi Vac DHL, DHPPI, Adenomune-7, Duramune DA$_2$ LP + PV	Ist Vaccination 7-9 weeks of age IInd Vaccination 4 weeks after Ist Vaccination	1 to 2 years Yearly vaccination recommended
2.	Canine parvo virus Disease	Parvocine, Vanguard-CPV, Adenomune-7, Duramune DA$_2$ LP+PV, Nobi Vac Pavro-c, Nobi Vac Puppy DP	Ist Vaccination 9-12 weeks of age. IInd vaccination 15-16 weeks of age Pregnant bitch: i) Non-vaccinated—4 weeks before and 2 weeks before parturition ii) Vaccinated –3 weeks before parturition Non-vaccinated adult dog 2 doses, 1-4 weeks apart	One year
3.	Parainfluenza	Adenomune-7, Duramune DA$_2$LP+PV	9-12 weeks of age Repeat every 4 weeks until 16 weeks of age	Annual revaccination is recommended
4.	Adenovirus type-2	Adenomune-7 Duramune (7-in-1) Duramune (8-in-1)	9-14 weeks of age. Repeat every 4 weeks until 16 weeks of age	nnual revaccination is recommended
5.	Rabies	Rabies vaccine, Rabisin, Nobi-Vac. R., Pentadog, Rabguard TC, Raksharab, Durarab, Rabipur, Annumune, Candur-R, Rabdomune, Nobi Vac DH +RL	Ist Vaccination – 3 months of age. Booster dose – 6 months after first vaccination	1 to 3 years, but yearly vaccination required
6.	Corona Virus	Duramune CVK Duramune PC Puppyshot Duramune (8-in-1)	6 weeks onward, repeat every 4th week till the age of 12 weeks or more	1 year

Note:

i) Deworm your pet prior to vaccination.

ii) Immunize only healthy pets.

iii) Maintain about 15 days interval between two vaccines.

Vaccinating the bitch against parvo disease before mating or during pregnancy (with Parvocine) can protect her puppies by passing anti-bodies to them through her milk. A temporary dose of the same vaccine can be given to the litter at weaning and a permanent dose at 12 weeks of age.

Yearly vaccination should be performed particularly in contaminated kennels. Revaccination is recommended prior to placing dogs in kennels, dog show or where increased exposure is likely. Immunize healthy animals only.

CANINE CORONA VIRUS VACCINES

(a)   Duramune CV-K (Fort Dodge) – Canine corona virus vaccine.

(b)   Duramune PC (Fot Dodge) – Canine corona virus and parvo virus vaccine.

(c)   Puppyshot Duramune (8-in-1) (Fort Dodge) – Canine distemper, canine hepatitis, adeno virus type 2, parainfluenza, leptospira, parvo virus and corona virus vaccine.

Canine corona virus vaccination can be initiated at 6 weeks of age, repeat at every 4 weeks till the age of 12 weeks or more and booster vaccination should be performed annually.

LIVESTOCK VACCINES

ANTHRAX VACCINES

Anthrax spore vaccine (Live):I.V.R.I., Izatnagar; B.P. Section, Lucknow; Institute of Veterinary Preventive Medicine–Ranipet (Chennai); Livestock Research Station, Patna; Veterinary Biological and Research Institute, Hyderabad; BAIF.

The vaccine is a suspension of live spores of an uncapsulated avirulent strain of *Bacillus anthracis* in 50% glycerine saline.

Cattle, buffaloes, horses, camels: 1 ml s/c

Sheep, goat: 0.5 ml s/c

Immunity is established in about 10 days and remains upto 1 year. Vaccinated animals may have a mild local and febrile reaction lasting for 2-3 days. Storage upto 3 months at 2-5°C temp.

BLACK QUARTER VACCINES

(i) (a) BAIF Black Quarter vaccine: contain antigenic strain of *Clostridium chauvoei* inactivated by formaldehyde and adjuvanted by Aluminox.

Cattle and buffaloes: – 2ml s/c, revaccinate annually. Calves: – 2 ml s/c after completion of 6 months age and revaccinated annually.

(b) BAIF HS and B.Q. vaccine : 4 ml s/c

(ii) Black Quarter vaccine (Polyvalent) I.V.R.I.: – The vaccine is a mixture of *Cl. chauvoei* and *Cl. septicum* atoxic by formaldehyde, effective against B.Q. and malignant oedema in ruminants.

Cattle and buffaloes : – 5-10 ml s/c

Sheep and goat :– 2-3 ml s/c

Second vaccination at the same dose rate may be carried at 10 days after first vaccination in case where a high degree of immunity is required. Annual revaccination before the onset of rainy season recommended. Can be stored upto 6 months at 2-5°C temp.

(iii)   Black Quarter vaccine, Haryana Veterinary Vaccine Institute, Hissar:

        Cattle and buffaloes : 5 ml s/c

        Sheep and goat   : 2-3 ml s/c

        Immunity remains for 1 year. Animal to be revaccinated annually before the onset of rainy season. Can be stored at refrigerator temp for 2 years.

Other Sources of B.Q. Vaccines:

- Biological Products Section, Lucknow.
- Institute of Veterinary Biological Products, Pune.
- Institute of Veterinary Preventive Medicine, Ranipet (Chennai).
- Karnataka Serum Institute, Hebbal (Bangalore).
- Livestock Research Station, Patna.
- M.P. Vaccine and Research Institute, Mhow.
- Punjab Veterinary Vaccine Institute, P.A.U., Ludhiana.
- Regional Veterinary and Biological Unit, Veterinary Hospital, Jaipur.
- Veterinary Biological and Research Institute, Hyderabad.
- Bio-Med, Ghaziabad.

BRUCELLA ABORTUS VACCINES

(i)   Brucella abortus (strain-19) Live vaccine : I.V.R.I.

(ii)   BAIF Brucella abortus C-19 Live vaccine: BAIF
contains living culture of *Brucella abortus* strain-19 of low virulence.

Female calves (6-9 months of age): 5 ml s/c (I.V.R.I.)

Female calves (3-6 months of age): 5 ml s/c (BAIF)

Young male calves can be vaccinated but they should be castrated after about one month following vaccination.

    Immunity is durable and satisfactory over the first or two pregnancies but may diminish gradually in successive pregnancies. Storage at 2-5°C. Since the keeping quality of the vaccine is low it should be used within 10 days of its despatch.

FOOT AND MOUTH DISEASE VACCINES

(i)   FMD Polyvalent vaccine : I.V.R.I.: contains FMD virus type 0, A, C and Asia 1.

        Cattle and buffaloes : 10 ml s/c

        Sheep and goat   : 5 ml s/c

Calves below one month of age, 5 ml followed by second vaccination after 21 days. These calves should be given 10 ml at 5-6 months of age followed by 10 ml at one year of age and repeated with 10 ml annually.

        Immunity last for 9-12 months.

In highly susceptible and exotic animals 6 monthly vaccination may be done.

(ii)   FMD vaccine (Hoechst): contains four virus type 0, A-22,C and Asia-1.

        Cattle, buffaloes and calves : 10 ml s/c

        Sheep and goat   : 5 ml s/c

When an adult animal is vaccinated first time, booster dose should be given after 2-3 months; in 4-6 months old calves booster 6 months later. In 6 weeks old calves booster at 4 months of age and in calves of 4 weeks and below booster must be given in 6 weeks, after initial vaccination.

Revaccinate the animals at 6, 9 or 12 monthly intervals. It is advisable to vaccinate exotic and high graded cross bred animals 2-3 times a year.

(iii) (a)   BAIF FMD vaccine (Quadrivalent) : contains O, A, C and Asia-1 virus type.

Cattle, buffaloes and calves : 10 ml s/c

Sheep and goats : 5 ml s/c

In calves (6-8 weeks old) booster vaccination should be given at 4 months of age and then 6 months later and when adult animal is vaccinated first time booster 3-4 months later. In young animals (4-6 months) booster 6 months later. Revaccinate the animals at 6, 9 or 12 months interval.

(b)   BAIF FMD Vaccine (Monovalent): contains virus type A-22. Cattle, buffaloes, Calves, sheep and goat: 2 ml s/c
Vaccination schedule same as for quadrivalent vaccine.

(iv)   Raksha FMD Vaccine (Indian Immunologicals) : contains virus type O, A, Asia-1 and A-22.

Cattle, buffaloes and calves :- 3 ml s/c

Sheep and goat : 1 ml s/c

Primary vaccination at 4 months of age, booster 2-4 weeks after primary vaccination and revaccination should be performed every 6th month thereafter.

HAEMORRHAGIC SEPTICAEMIA VACCINES

(i)   H.S. Adjuvant vaccine: (I.V.R.I.): Vaccine is a homogenous suspension of formalized agar washed *Pasteurella multocida* in liquid paraffin and lanolin.

Cattle, buffaloes upto 300 lbs b.wt : 2 ml I.M.

Above 300 lbs b.wt : 3 ml I.M.

Sheep and goat : 2 ml I.M.

Immunity is established in about 21 days and remains up to 1 year.

(ii)   H.S. Alum precipitated vaccine (B.P. Section, Lucknow : 5 to 10 ml s/c. Immunity is established in about 10 days and lasts for a period of six months.

(iii)   BAIF H.S. Vaccine (a) Adjuvant : Adjuvanted with Aluminox. Cattle, buffaloes and calves (6 months or above) : 2 ml s/c. Every year before monsoon.

(iii)   (b) BAIF H.S. and B.Q. Combined Vaccine: Combined inactivated antigens of *P. multocida* and *Cl. chauvoei* adjuvanted with Aluminox. 4 ml s/c. Revaccinate annually.

(iv)   H.S. Vaccine (Haryana Veterinary Vaccine Institute, Hissar)

(a)   H.S. Alum ppt. Vaccine: Cattle, buffaloes, sheep, swine:-5 ml s/c

Duration of immunity 6 months. Animals to be vaccinated before the onset of rainy season.

(b)   H.S.Oil Adjuvant vaccine: Cattle, buffaloes, sheep, goat, swine : 3ml IM - Duration of immunity 1 year.

iv)   Raksha H.S. Vaccine (Indian Immunologicals): Adjuvanted with Aluminium hydroxide gel.

Cattle, buffaloes and calves : 2 ml s/c

Primary vaccination at 6 months of age and above. Revaccinate the animals annually.

(v)   H.S. Vaccine Broth (Biological Products Section, Vety. College Kanapara, Guwahati (Assam).

(vi)   H.S. Vaccine: Alum ppt; adjuvant (Institute of Veterinary Biologicals Products, Pune).

(vii)   H.S. Vaccine: Oil adjuvant (Institute of Veterinary Preventive Medicine, Ranipet, Chennai).

(viii) H.S. Vaccine Broth /adjuvant (Livestock Research Station, Patna).

(ix)   H.S. Vaccine Broth (M.P. Vaccine and Research Institute, Mhow).

(x)   H.S. Vaccine: Adjuvant/alum ppt (Punjab Veterinary Vaccine Institute, P.A.U., Ludhiana.

(xi)   H.S. Vaccine Broth/adjuvant (Regional Veterinary and Biological Unit, Vety. Hospital, Jaipur).

(xi)   H.S. Vaccine: Oil adjuvant (Veterinary Biological and Research Institute, Hyderabad).

(xiii) H.S. Vaccine Adjuvanted (Bio-Med).

RINDERPEST VACCINES

Rinderpest Tissue Culture Vaccine (I.V.R.I.): It is a live, attenuated lyophilysed vaccine, prepared from modified strain of rinderpest, propagated in cell culture.

Dose is 1 ml s/c per animal irrespective of age and species. Contents of vaccine to be reconstituted in sterile chilled normal saline as per the number of dosage (50 dosage) indicated at the time of supply.

Vaccine has life long immunity i.e. upto 11 years, however, it may be advisable to repeat vaccination every 5 year.

Rinderpest vaccine live, freeze dried, tissue cutlure (BAIF) :- One ml s/c irrespective of age and size of animals, long lasting immunity develops but annual vaccination is advised. Contents of vaccine to be reconstituted with diluent supplied as per the number of dosage (100/50/25 dosage).

Raksha Rinderpest live tissue culture vaccine (Indian Immunologicals):– One ml s/c per animal. Primary vaccination can be done at the age of 4 months. Avoid vaccination during advanced pregnancy. (25/50/100 dosage along with diluents).

Rinderpest vaccine live F.D.G.T.V. : (Haryana Veterinary Vaccine Institute, Hissar). One ml s/c. Primary vaccination at the age of 4-6 months of age. Life long immunity (100 dosage).

- Rinderpest G.T.V. –(Freeze dried) Vaccine:– Bengal Veterinary College, Mohanpur, Calcutta.
- Rinderpest G.T.V. –(Freeze dried) Vaccine: B.P. Section, Lucknow.
- Rinderpest G.T.V. –Institute of Veterinary Preventive Medicine, Ranipet, Chennai.
- Rinderpest G.T.V. –(Freeze dried) Livestock Research Station, Patna.
- Rinderpest G.T.V. –M.P. Vaccine and Research Institute, Mhow.
- Rinderpest G.T.V. –Regional Veterinary and Biological Unit, Jaipur.
- Rinderpest G.T.V. –Veterinary Biological and Research Institute, Hyderabad.
- Rinderpest T.C. adapted - Bio -Med.

THEILERIOSIS VACCINE

Rakshavac -T (Indian Immunologicals): contains attenuated shizonts.

Remove the vaccine vial from liquid nitrogen and thaw in luke-warm water. Transfer the thawed vaccine concentrate (1 ml for 2 dose or 2.5 ml for 5 dose) to the corresponding vaccine diluent vial (5 ml for 2 dose or 12.5 ml for 5 dose) and mix gently. Inject 3 ml s/c per animal (adult or calves of 2 months of age or above). Vaccination of animals in advanced stage of pregnancy should be avoided. Immunity develops in 6 weeks and remains for one year. Annual vaccination is recommended. Vaccine should be transported and stored in liquid nitrogen.

ENTEROTOXAEMIA VACCINES

Enterotoxaemia vaccine (I.V.R.I): Containing highly toxigenic strain of *Cl. welchii* type-D, grow in anaerobic medium and atoxic by formaldehyde solution. Used for prophylaxis against pulpy kidney disease (Enterotoxaemia in sheep and lambs). 2.5 ml s/c for sheep and lamb (above 3 months of age), repeat after 14 days. Immunity remains for one year. Annual vaccination is recommended. Pregnant ewes can also be vaccinated safely. The second injection should be given in about 3 weeks before lambing.

Enterotoxaemia Vaccine (Haryana Veterinary Vaccine Institute, Hissar): 2.5 ml s/c, repeat after 14 days with same dose. Immunity remains for one year.

Enterotoxaemia Vaccine (BAIF): Contains strain of *Cl. welchii* type-D and adjuvanted with Aluminox. Dose 2.5 ml s/c.

Enterotoxaemia Vaccine (BAIF): Cantains strain of *Cl. Welchii* type C and D adjuvanted with Aluminox. Dose 5 ml s/c.

Multicomponent Vaccine (BAIF): Contains *Cl. welchii* type B.C. and D., *Cl. septicum* and *Cl. oedematiens*, adjuvanted with Aluminox. Dose 5 ml s/c.

Other Sources of Enterotoxaemia Vaccines:

- Institute of Vety. Biological Products, Pune.
- Institute of Vety. Preventive Medicine, Ranipet, Chennai.
- Bio-Med.

- Karnataka Serum Institute, Hebbal, Bangalore.
- Punjab Vety. Vaccine Institute, P.A.U., Ludhiana.
- Veterinary Biological and Research Institute, Hyderabad.

SHEEP POX VACCINES

Tissue Culture Sheep Pox Vaccine (I.V.R.I.): Live freeze dried vaccine. One ml of freshly reconstituted vaccine should be injected s/c in the posterior axillary region for all age group. Vaccine provides lasting immunity for about 22 months, can be used in the face of an outbreak as well as in the healthy sheep.

Sheep Pox Formal Gel Vaccine (B.P. Section, Lucknow)

> Sheep : 5 ml s/c
>
> Lambs : 3 ml s/c

Can be used at the time of outbreak, also in healthy sheep. Pregnant ewes can be vaccinated. Immunity develops in 7-10 days and lasts for 7-8 months in lambs and 8-12 months in adult sheep.

Other sources of Sheep Pox Vaccines:

- Haryana Veterinary Vaccine Institute, Hissar.
- Bio-Med.
- Institute of Vety. Preventive Medicine, Ranipet, Chennai.
- Regional Vety. and Biological Unit, Jaipur.
- Veterinary Biological and Research Institute, Hyderabad.

SWINE FEVER VACCINES

Lapinised Swine Fever Vaccine (I.V.R.I.): It is a live vaccine used for active immunization of swine from unweaned stage to adult stage against swine fever. Dose is 1 ml IM of reconstituted vaccine per animal, irrespective of age, breed and sex. Immunity remains for about one year. Vaccine can be stored in freezing chamber of refrigerator for a period of 3 months and for 6 months in deep freeze unit at-15 to -20°C.

Lapinised Swine Fever Vaccine Live (B.P. Section, Lucknow). One ml of reconstituted vaccines s/c in all categories of animals and immunity lasts for about one year.

Lapinised Swine Fever Vaccine (Haryana Veterinary Vaccine Institute, Hissar). One ml s/c per animal. Immunity remains for one year.

ANTI-RABIC VACCINES (Post Bite)

Anti-rabic Vaccine 5% inactivated (I.V.R.I.): The vaccine consists of 5% suspension of sheep brain infected with rabies fixed virus and inactivated with beta-propiolactone to a final concentration of 5%. It is intended for immunization and treatment of all species of animals exposed to rabies infection, vaccine may be injected by s/c route.

Species	If animal has never been immunized against rabies with anti-rabic vaccine.	If animal has previously been immunised with anti-rabic vaccine.
Animal wt. under 15 kg (Dog, pup, cat, monkey)	2 C.C. daily x 14 days	2 C.C. daily x 7 days
Animal wt. between 15-100 kg (Dog, deer, sheep, goat)	5 C.C. daily x 14 days	5 C.C. daily x 7 days.
Animal wt. between 100-800 kg (Buffaloes, bullock, cow, horse)	15 C.C. daily x 14 days	15 C.C. daily x 7 days
Camel, elephant	30 C.C. daily x 14 days	30 C.C. daily x 7 days

Pups under two months of age do not respond satisfactorily to anti-rabic treatment.

For pre-exposure immunization follow schedule as in column 3.

If the wounds are severe, the dosage even if the animals have been immunized previously should be the same as given in column 2.

Anti-rabic Vaccine 5% inactivated (Haryana Vety. Vaccine Institute, Hissar).

Dosage:

- Animals wt. under 30 lbs : 2 ml s/c x 14 days.
- Animals wt. between 30 to 100 lbs: 5ml s/c x 14 days.
- Animal wt. above 100 ibs.
  (Calf, heifer, donkey, pig) :- 10 ml s/c x 14 days.
- Animals like buffalo, cow, horse, etc. : 30 ml s/c x 14 days.
- Camel, elephants : 60 ml s/c x 14 days.

Within one month after the completion of first vaccination if the animal is exposed to the rabid dog bite, one injection will be sufficient.

If exposed within 6 months, 7 injections are needed. The vaccination should be done as early as possible within 4 days after the bite by a rabid dog or other animals.

Anti-rabic vaccine 5% inactivated (Punjab Veterinary Vaccine Institute, P.A.U., Ludhiana).

Dosage and schedule same as for I.V.R.I. Vaccine.

Rabipur (Hoechst): Contains inactivated rabies antigen, used for pre- and post-exposure prophylaxis against rabies. Pre-exposure prophylaxis. : 1 ml on day 0, 7 and 21:

Post-exposure prophylaxis: 1 ml on day 0, 3, 7, 14, 30, 90

Rabisin (Serum Institute of India) used for pre- and post-exposure prophylaxis same as for Rabipur (post-exposure).

Raksharab (Indian Immunologicals) same as for Rabipur (Post-exposure).

POULTRY VACCINES

AVIAN ENCEPHALOMYELITIS VACCINES

AEM Live, freeze dried Vaccine (Bio-Med) : The vaccine must be given at 13-14 weeks of age in cold drinking water. Keep 4 waterers per 100 birds, add 8 ml of dissolved vaccine to 4 litres of cold water. The vaccine virus may cause some drop in egg production of non-immune hens, therefore, this vaccine should not be used on farms which has not been vaccinated previously with avian encephalomyelitis (inactivated) vaccine.

A.E.M inactivated, liquid Vaccine (Bio-Med): It must be given at 10 weeks of age either I/M or S/C route at the dose rate of 0.2 ml into thigh region. For the reconstitution of vaccine use 20 ml diluent for 100 birds and 100 ml diluent for 500 doses.

AVIAN INFECTIOUS BRONCHITIS VACCINES

I.B. Vaccine (BAIF): (Live, attenuated, Massachusetts strain) Primary Vaccination: at the age of 4 days, 2 drops intranasal. Booster: at 6 and 16 weeks, 2 drops intranasal or in drinking water.

I.B.Vaccine (Bio-Med): (Live, attenuated, freeze dried, Massachusetts strain):

At 3-4 weeks age.
At 16-18 weeks age.

2 drops in the nostrils or with clean, cold drinking water (1 litre water for 100 chicks). For reconstitution use 8 ml diluent for 100 doses and 40 ml diluent for 500 doses.

I.B. Vaccine should be given 10-15 days prior to or after R.D. vacccination to avoid undue stress. In layers, vaccination can result in slight drop in egg production for 10-12 days.

I.B. Vaccine (Srini Biological Laboratories, Pune): Reconstitute the vaccine in chilled diluent or drinking water (1.5 litre per 100 dose). Fresh skimmed milk at the rate of 6 gm/litre water is mixed as stabilizer.

At 2-3 weeks age – one drop intraocular.

At 4-5 weeks age – intraocular or oral, withhold water for atleast 2 hours before the supply of vaccinated water.

At 15-16 weeks age – as above.

EGG DROP SYNDROME '76'

Killed (Bio-Med): At 14-16 weeks of age I/M. Immunity for one year.

FOWL CHOLERA VACCINES

- B.P. Section, Lucknow.
- IVRI, Izatnagar.
- Institute of Veterinary Biological Products, Pune.
- M.P. Vaccine and Research Institute, Mhow.
- Vety. Biological and Research Institute, Hyderabad.
  At 6-8 weeks of age 1ml s/c
  Repeat after 21 days in breeding flock.

FOWL POX VACCINES

F.P. live, attenuated Vaccine (BAIF): Primary Vaccination – at 8 weeks of age, 2 pricks on inner surface of wing web.

Booster: At 48 weeks, 2 pricks on inner surface of wing web.

F.P. Live, attenuated, B.M. Strain (Bio-Med) 0.2 ml reconstituted vaccine (20 ml diluent for 100 doses) I/M, s/c at the age of 3-6 weeks and booster at 16-18 weeks of age.

F.P. Vaccine (Hissar): Birds above 8 weeks of age by web puncture method.

F.P. Vaccine (Vety. Biological Institute, Trivandrum, Kerala): Supplied as 0.3 gm of vaccine with 30 ml of 50% glycerine saline, administered by feather follicle method.

Other Sources of F.P. Vaccines:

- IVRI, Izatnagar.
- Institute of Veterinary Biological Products, Pune.
- Institute of Vety. Preventive Medicine, Ranipet, Chennai.
- Karnataka Serum Institute, Hebbal, Bangalore.
- Livestock Research Station, Patna.
- Punjab Vety. Vaccine Institute, P.A.U., Ludhiana.
- Regional Vety. and Biological Unit, Jaipur.
- Veterinary Biological and Research Institute, Hyderabad.

INFECTIOUS BURSAL (GUMBORO) DISEASE VACCINES

I.B.D. attenuated, freeze dried Vaccine (BAIF): Safe for use in chicks above 2 weeks of age.

Primary Vaccination : 14 to 21 days of age, 2 drops intraocular.

Booster : 7 to 8 weeks of age, in drinking water.

I.B.D. Inactivated (Killed) Vaccine (Ventri Biologicals, Pune): 0.5 ml s/c or I/M (in the breast muscle) at 16 to 24 weeks of age.

Gumboro Disease Vaccine (Indovax Pvt. Ltd.): In endemic areas, intermediate strains.

I.B.D. Georgia 11-13 days 1 drop intraocular.

I.B.D. Georgia: 28–30 days 1 drop intraocular

INFECTIOUS CORYZA VACCINE

Infectious Coryza Inactivated (Killed) Vaccine (Ventri Biologicals, Pune).

Ist dose : at 8 weeks and above, 0.5 ml s/c (midway skin of head and base of neck).

Booster dose : 3-4 weeks later.

LARYNGOTRACHEITIS VACCINE

Live, attenuated, freeze dried Vaccine (Bio-Med): Reconstitute the vaccine by using 8 ml of diluent for 100 doses.

Ist Vaccination at 8 weeks of age, put 2 drops of reconstituted vaccine in the vent, hold the bird until the vaccine is drawn inside the vent. Examine the birds for 'takes' after 4 days of vaccination. A positive 'take' is indicated by swelling and reddening of mucous membranes of vent. If 'takes' are in less than 70% bird's immediate revaccination should be undertaken.

Revaccination (eye drop method): At the age of 18 weeks, instill one drop of reconstituted vaccine in each eye.

MAREK'S DISEASE VACCINES

M.D. Vaccine, Living (BAIF): Contains FC strain of Herpes Virus of Turkey, to be given immediately on hatching.

Primary Vaccination – 1 day, 0.2 ml intramuscular. Repeat after one year, the immunity develops within 5-10 days.

M.D. Vaccine (Bio-Med) (HVT Strain–live, attenuated, freeze dried). 0.2 ml s/c, I/P or I/M in day old chicks and repeat at 3 weeks age.

M.D. Vaccine (Ventri Biologicals, Pune): 0.2 ml s/c in day old chicks.

NEW CASTLE (RANIKHET) DISEASE VACCINES

NDV living, F/Lasota Strain (BAIF): Primary -– 4-day old chick, 2 drops intranasal. Booster 4-5 weeks of age intraocular, intranasal or in drinking water.

NDV living, Mukteshwar R_2B Strain (BAIF): Highly immunogenic strain, safe for adult birds above six weeks of age 0.5 ml s/c at 8 weeks of age.

R.D.F-1 Strain live, attenuated Vaccine (Bio-Med): Administer 2 drops into the nostrils or to the eyes of 1-7 days old chicks. It gives protection for a period of 4-6 weeks. In broiler vaccination should be performed twice at 1-7 days age and at 4-5 weeks age.

R.D.Lasota Strain Vaccine (Bio-Med): For day old chicks.

R.D. R_2B Strain Vaccine (Bio-Med): A live, attenuated freeze dried vaccine intended for booster vaccination against Ranikhet disease, 0.2 ml I/M in thigh muscle at 5-8 weeks age and repeat at 16-20 weeks of age.

R.D.F. Strain Vaccine (HVVI, Hissar): For day old chicks, 2 drops intranasal.

R.D. Vaccine (HVVI, Hissar): 1 ml s/c in adult poultry.

R.D.F_1Strain Vaccine (VBI, Trivandrum): For day old chicks, one drop to nostrils or eye.

R.D. Vaccine (VBI, Trivandrum): For adult birds at the age of 6-8 weeks, 0.5 ml s/c

N.D.V., living (Lasota strain) (Srini Biologicals, Pune) : One drop intranasal or intraocular at the age of 4-10 days.

N.D.V. inactivated (killed) (Srini Biologicals, Pune): 0.5 ml S/C or 1/M at the age of 16-20 weeks.

Other sources of R.D. Vaccines:

R.D. Vaccine – B.P. Section, Lucknow.

R.D. Vaccine – Bengal Vety. College, Mohanpur, Calcutta.

RD Vaccine – B.P. Sections, Vety. College Khanapara, Guwahati.

R_2B Vaccine and R.D.F, Strain Vaccine – IVRI, Izatnagar

R.D. Vaccine and R.D. (Lasota strain) Vaccine Institute of Veterinary Biological Products, Pune.

R.D. Vaccine and R.D. (F_1 strain) Vaccine - Karnataka Serum. Institute, Hebbal, Bangalore.

R.D.(F_1 strain) and R.D. R_2 B Vaccine – Livestock Research Station, Patna.

R.D. (F strain) and R.D. (R_2B strain) Vaccine – Punjab Veterinary Vaccine Institute, P.A.U., Ludhiana.

R.D.(F strain) and R.D. (Mukteshwar strain) – Regional Vety. and Biological Unit, Jaipur.

R.D.Vaccine – Veterinary Biological and Research Institute, Hyderabad.

SERA

ANTI-ANTHRAX SERUM

Horse : - 100 ml s/c

Cattle : - 50 ml s/c

    Sheep and goat : - 20 ml s/c

Source :   . B.P. Section, Lucknow.

    . Karnataka Serum Institute, Hebbal, Bangalore.

    . M.P. Vaccine and Research Institute, Mhow.

ANTI-B. Q. SERUM

Cattle :- 15 ml s/c

Sheep and goat :- 10 ml s/c

Immunity lasts for 15 days only. The serum is not curative.

Source: . B.P. Section, Lucknow.

    . I.V.R.I., Izatnagar.

    . Karnataka Serum Institute, Hebbal, Bangalore.

    . M.P. Vaccine and Research Institute, Mhow.

H.S. ANTI-SERUM

Cattle : 4-20 ml s/c

Buffaloes: 20 ml s/c

Immunity lasts for 2 weeks. It has no curative value.

Source: B.P. Section, Lucknow.

I.V.R.I., Izatnagar.

M.P. Vaccine and Research Institute, Mhow.

ANTI-R.P. SERUM

Cattle and buffaloes : 10 ml /100 lbs b. wt. s/c

Others : 20 ml s/c

Immunity lasts for 10 days.

Source: . B.P. Section, Lucknow.

. I.V.R.I., Izatnagar.

. M.P. Vaccine and Research Institute, Mhow.

Institute of Vety. Preventive Medicine, Ranipet, Madras.

ANTI -SNAKE VENUM SERUM (Polyvalent Lyophilysed)

Used in the case of snake bite in humans and animals. Each ml of the reconstituted anti-snake venum serum neutralizes not less than the following quantities of standard venums:

Dried *Cobra* venum 0.6 mg,

dried common *Krait venum* 0.45 mg, dried *Russel's viper*

venum 0.6 mg and dried *Saw scale viper* 0.45 mg.

For all species of animals reconstitute the contents of one ampoule in 10 ml diluent (pyrogen free water). Allow to stand for one minute, use clear part only by IM, s/c or IV (very slow, dilute 5 to 10 times with glucose saline solution). Repeat after 2 hours, then 6 hourly, local infusion is advised in viper bite.

Source: Haffkine Bio-Pharmaceuticals Corporation Ltd., Parel, Mumbai.
Central Research Institute, Kasauli.

Serum Institue of India, Pune.

TETANUS ANTI-TOXIN

For the treatment and prophylaxis of tetanus in horses and other animals after exposure to infection through operation or injuries.

As prophylaxis : Subcutaneously

Horse and cattle : 1500-3000 i.u.

Calf, sheep, goat and pig : 500-1500 i.u.

Dogs, cats, lambs : 250-500 i.u.

As Therapeutic: 100 times of the prophylactic dose of anti-toxin should be given as soon as possible after the appearance of symptoms.

The initial therapeutic dose should be given IV but thereafter daily dose may be given s/c until definite improvement.

Source:

- Burroughs Wellcome India Pvt. Ltd., Mumbai.
    - (i)   Ampoule of One ml - 1500 i.u.
    - (ii)   Ampoules of Two ml - 10, 000 i.u.
    - (iii)   Ampoules of Ten ml - 50,000 i.u.
- Serum Institute of India, Pune.

Ampoules of 750 i.u., 1500 i.u., vials of 10, 000 i.u. and 50,000 i.u.

- Glaxo Laboratories, Mumbai.

TETANUS TOXOID

For prophylaxis against tetanus

Tet-vac - Glaxo Laboratories, Mumbai, 0.5 ml ampoule.

Dosage: Horse, cattle, calf, foal: 2-6 ml s/c or I.M. A second dose 4 weeks later and a booster dose a year later. Immunity develops in about 9-14 days after vaccination.

Tetanus toxoid: Haffkine Bio-Pharmaceuticals Co. Ltd., Mumbai. 0.5 ml, 1 ml, 5 ml and 10 ml ampoules, 5 ml and 10 ml vials.

Absorbed tetanus toxoid:

Serum Institute of India, Pune.

0.5 ml, 1 ml ampoules and 10 ml vials.

PHARMACEUTICS

VETERINARY PREPARATIONS
Index—Therapeutics/Brand Names

ANTHELMINTICS AND OTHERS

Babesiosis : Berenil (Hoechst), Pronil-H (Merind), Trypan blue (Ethicare).

Cestodes : Albendazole (HAL), Alben (Jeps). Albidol (Concept), Albomar Glaxo), Albonil (Alved), Analgon (Wockhardt), Cestonil (Alved), Cestophene (PCI), Cosylan (USV), Decarin (Rajshree), Eraworm (Marc), Tetzan (Jeps), Fitwom (BBB), Helmigard (Unichem), Kalbend (Karnataka), Kalmben 50% Powder (Karnataka), Kitworm-50 (IPCI), Krimos (BBB), Mebendal (VF), Minthal (Alembic), Niltape (Ethicare), Nilzan (Imkemex), Nohelm (Vetcorp), Overcid (B.C.), Panacur (Hocchst), Panfugal (Merind), Piperazine hexahydrate (Merind), Piperazine hexahydrate (Ventri), Piperazine liquid (HAL), Piperazine liquid (Morvel), Praziplus (Vet Care), Salminth (Salus), Sonex (ARC), Taenil (IH), Wormin (C.P.), Worminil (Charak), Zanil (Imkemex), Zodex (Concept), Zomar (C.P.)

Coccidiostat : Amdon (Merind), Amprol plus (Glaxo), Amprol sol 20% (Glaxo), Amprolium soluble powder (Merind; USV), Clopimix 25% premix (Piya), Coban-100 (Ventri), Codrinal (Hoechst), Coxidol (Ventri), Coxistac (Pfizer), Cycostat (Cyanamid), Dimdim liquid (Arex), Dot (Aries), Ducoxin (Glaxo), Kadiprol (CHC), Paquin (Ranbaxy), Regecoccin Premix (Themis), Stenorol (Hoechst), Sulfagon (Balloun), Sulphon (Balloun), Superdot (Vetcare), T-Cox (USV), Unistat (Unichem), Veldot (Ventri), Vets furan (VF), Zonamix (Piya), Zycox (IH),

Ectoparasites: Butox (Hoechst), Canifur-AZ (CP), Flea and Tick Collars (BC), Flurry (CHC), Herbal dog shampoo (Badri), Herbal tick powder (Badri), Ivomac (Glaxo), Larvadex (Ciba-Geigy), Lourell (Indian Herbs), Maggocite liquid (CR), Pestoban (IH), Pestovil (Herb Product), Tetmosol (IEL).

Fascioliasis: Albendole (BAIF), Albendazole (HAL), Albomar (Glaxo), Albonil (Alved), Amfanide (Merind), Analgon (Wockhardt), Carbon tetrachloride (Ethicare), Decarin (Rajshree), Deverm (Ethicare), Dewormin (CR), Distodin (Pfizer), Endex (Ciba-Geigy), Fasinex (Ciba-Geigy), Flukaphene (Ethicare), Flukin (Arex), Helmigard (Unichem), Hexachlorophene (ICC), Kalbend (Karnataka), Kitworm-50 (IPCI), Krimos (BBB), Minthal (Alembic), Nilzan (Imkemex), Okazan (Wockhardt), Oxyclozanide (USV), Rafoxanide (USV), Rafoxin (Concept), Rainil (Piya), Ranide (Glaxo), Sonex (ARC), Tolzan-F (Hoechst), Valbazen (Pfizer), Wormal (Microlabs), Zanil (Imkemex), Zodex bolus (Concept), Hexanide (Sarabhai), Alben (Jeps), Clozan (Jeps), Zomar (CP), Tetzan (Jeps), Actuss (USV), Nohelm (Vet Corp).

Lungworm: Actuss (USV), Alben (Jeps), Albendazole (HAL), Albidol (Concept), Baifomisole (BAIF), Dewormin (CR), Eraworm (Marc), Helmosol (PCI), Levamisole (Ciba-Geigy), Ivomec (Glaxo), Kalbend (Karnataka), Kalmisole powder, Bolus (Karnataka), Kitworm powder-50 (IPCI), Mebendal (VF), Mebendazole (Karnataka), Mebvet (Jeps), Nilamisol (Piya), Nilverm (IEL), Nilzan (Imkemex), Nohelm (Vetcorp), Panacur (Hoechst), Panfugal (Merind), Piperazine hexahydrate (Merind), Piperazine liquid 45% (HAL), Salworm (Salus), Tetramisole HCL (Piya), Valbazen (Pfizer), Zodex (Concept), Zomar (C.P.).

Nematodes: Albendazole (HAL), Actuss (USV), Alben (Jeps), Albidol (Concept), Albomar (Glaxo), Albonil (Alved), Almizol (Alembic), Analgon (Wockhardt), Anthelmet (Balloun), Baifomisole (BAIF), Banminth (Pfizer), Curaminth (Sarabhai), Decarin (Rajshree), Deverm (Ethicare), Dewormin (CR), Eraworm (Marc), Fenbezol powder (Ranbaxy), Fenzole (Jeps), Fetzan (Jeps), Helmex powder (Balloun), Helmigard (Unichem), Helmonil (Alved), Helmosol (PCI), Ivomec (Glaxo), Kalbend (Karnataka), Kalmeben 50% (Karnataka), Kalmisole (Karnataka), Kitworm (IPCI), Krimos (BBB), Lemasol-P (Ranbaxy), Levamisole (Ciba-Geigy), Levasol (VF), Mebendal (VF), Mebendazole 10% (Karnataka), Mebvet (Jeps), Minthal (Alembic), Nilamisol (Piya), Nilverm (IEL), Nilzan (Imkemex), Nohelm (Vetcorp), Panacur (Hoechst), Panfugal (Merind), Piperazine (Ethicare), Piperazine adipate oral (Karnataka), Piperazine hexahydrate (Merind), Piperazine hexahydrate 56.3% (Cyanamid), Piperazine liq (Glaxo), Piperazine liquid (Morvel), Piperazine liquid 45% (HAL), Praziplus (Vetcare), Salworm (Salus), Tetramisole HCL (ICCL), Tetramisole HCL (Piya), Thiabendazole (Arex), Valbazen (Pfizer), Vermitan (Themis), Vibex (CHC), Wopell (IH), Wormal (Microlab), Wormin bolus (C.P.), Wormiza (Charak), Worminga (Pharmanza), Zodex bolus (Concept). Zomar(C.P.),

Theileriosis: Berenil (Hoechst), Butalex (CHC) (C.P.), Pronil-H (Merind),

Trypanocidals : Pronil-H (Merind), Tartar emetic (Ethicare), Tribexin Prosalt (IDPL), Triquin (Workhardt), Trypnil (Merind).

TOPICAL ANTI-INFECTIVE PREPARATIONS-

Charmala (ARC), Charmil (Dabur), Dermocept Oint (Concept), Ektodex (Petcare), Flematic oil (TTKP), Hamycin-AVS (HAL), Herbal scab lotion (Badri), Herbex (BBB), Herbittol (Herb Product), Ivomec (Glaxo), Jeplon (Jeps), Neocidal 20 EC (Ciba-Geigy), Notix (Petcare), Notix Scrub (Petcare), Notix Talc (Petcare), Ostaderm Oint (VF), Povidin (Jeps, USV), Ropak (Rajshree), Scabitex (Balloun), Tetmosol (IEL).

ALLERGIC DISORDERS

Antihistamines: Alergipar (Biomedica), Alert (Morvel), Avil (Hoechst), Baifovil (BAIF), Cadistin (CHC), Chloril vet (TTKP), Cural (Merind), Histal (Vetcare), Parichlor (Biomedica), Promethazine HCL (Biomedica), Vetalog (Sarabhai), Zeet (Alembic).

ANTIBIOTICS

Ampicillin: Albercilin (Hoechst), Ampicillin (Sarabhai), Ampicillin (USV), Ampilin (Lyka), Bacipen (Alembic), Campicillin (C.P.), Conampi (Concept), Dynacil (HAL), Kampibiotic inj. (Karnataka), Marcocilin (Marc), Roscillin (Ranbaxy), Synthovet inj. (PCI), Ventricillin powder (Ventri), Vetampin (Wockhardt).

Ampicillin and Cloxacillin: Baxivet (Lyka), Binocin (Concept), Combipen (Vetcorp), Floclox (Ranbaxy), Kloxamp inj. (Karnataka), Penicure-D (Marc), Rosciclox (Ranbaxy), Vetclox-plus (Sarabhai).

Amoxicillin: Amoxysol (Pfizer), Comoxyl (Concept).

Bacitracin: Bacitrin (Microlab),

Chloramphenicol: Chloramphenicol Sod-Succinate (Lyka), Neochlor forte (Vetcare), Phenivet inj. (PCI), Piya-mycetine (Piya), Simercetin (Biomedica).

Cephlexin: Lixen (Glaxo)

Chlortetracycline: Chlortetracycline soluble powder (Cyanamid).

Cloxacillin: Cloxacillin inj. (Karnataka), Moxel inj. (Alembic), Vet clox plus, (Sarabhai) Hipenox (CHC).

Doxycycline: Doxyn (USV), Doxyterin (Sarabhai), Tetradox (Ranbaxy).

Enrofloxacin : Enrocin (Ranbaxy), Meriquin (Merind).

Erythromycin : Albac (Ranbaxy), BMD-100 (Ranbaxy), Erystrim (Themis).

Framycetin: Sofrakay sus. (Roussel).

Gentamicin: Cicin (Themis), Gentabio (Vetcare), Gentabiotic inj. (Karnataka), Gentamicin (Alved), Gentamicin (USV), Gentamicin Cream (Lyka), Gentamor (Morvel), Gentim (Merind), Gentavet inj. (PCI), Marcogenta (Marc), Primicin (HAL)

Kanamycin: Kancin (Alembic).

Neomycin: Doxyn (USV), Gass cutter tab. (Piya), Neocare forte (Vetcare), Neomix-325 (Unichem), Neomycin (Unichem), Unimycin (Unichem), Retinamycin (Biomedica), Vetbacin (Glaxo).

Nitrofurans: Altasol (Vet Farma), Avicox (Microlab), Entrodone (Salus), Fetin 5 and 20% (ICCI), Furanitro (Piya) Fue-Furan tab. (ICCI), Furalay-200 (Microlab), Furacillin cream (IPCI), Furakal Bolus (Karnataka), Furan-100 (Ethicare). Furanitro (Microlab), Furazolidone 5% and 20% (Salus), Furazolidone-200 (Karnataka), Furazolidone-224 (Vetcare), Furazolidone Premix (Ethicare), Furea bolus (Pfizer), Furex-20 (BAIF), Furavet (IPCI), Metrozal-u (Salus), Microsol (Microlab), Marcogyl bolus (Marc), Neftin-200 (Pfizer), Neful (Themis), Nefur-HC (Themis), Paquin (Ranbaxy), Scorid (VF), Vetsfuran (VF), Zolodine-200, 50 (IPCI) Bifuran (Pfizer), Furasol (Pfizer), Profidone -200 (Sarabhai).

Oxytetracyline: Oxytetracycline (USV) Inj. Oxytetracycline (Ind. Imm.), Microvet inj. (P.C.I.), Otcim (IDPL), Oxycycline tab. (Piya), Oxymor (Morvel), Oxysteclin (Sarabhai), Oxytetracycline (Alved), Oxytetracycline (Merind). Oxytra (HAL), Oxytetracycline-LA (Sarabhai), Radoxy (Radix), Telon-LA (Merind), Terramycin (Pfizer), Wolicyclin (Wockhardt).

Penicillin: Benzapen benzathine (Karnataka), Fortified Procaine Benzyl penicillin (IDPL), Fortified Procaine Penicillin (Alembic), Kalpen forte PPF 20 inj. (Karnataka), Longacillin (HAL), Penicillin intramammary (Boots), Procillin (HAL), Vetopen 2.5 (HAL), F.P.P. 20 & F.P.P. -40 (Sarabhai).

Penicillin with Streptomycin: Bistrepen (Alembic), Dicrysticin-S (Sarabhai), Munomycin forte (Glaxo), Pendistrin-SH (Sarabhai), Vetopen inj. (HAL).

Sulpha drugs: Baifidine (BAIF), Chemozine (P.C.I.) Diadin Tab, (Pfizer), Dimdim liq. (Arex), Furazol (IPCL), Hamidin (HAL), Inj. Sulphadimidine sodium (Ind. Imm), Phthalylsulphathiazole (ICCI), Saldin (Salus), Sulphadimidine (Arex), Sulphadimidine sod Inj. (IDPL), Sulphadimidine tab. (IDPL), Sulphadin bolus (VF), Sulphaguanidine tab. (IDPL), Sulphagut bolus (Karnataka), Sulphanilamide (Rhone Poulenc), Supercox (Wockhardt), Sulcoprim (Concept), Hatrix (HAL), Cosumix (Ciba-Geigy) Sulphadimidine (Sarabhai) Sugaprim (Sarabhai), Kot (Vet Corp), Micotrim (Pharmanza), Micotrim-D (Pharmanza), Pesulin (C.P.).

Tetracyclines: Alcyclin (Alembic), Hostacycline powder (Hoechst), Tetracycline bolus (Sarabhai), Tetracycline powder (IDPL), Tetrakal forte (Karnataka). Vetcycline (Salus).

Trimethoprim + Sulpha drugs: Antrima bolus (Rhone-Poulenc), Bactridox (Alved), Bactrisol (Alved), Biotrim. (Ranbaxy), Duocidal bolus (Karnataka), Eviprim vet (Hoechst), Marcoprim (Marc), Metaprim (VF), Micotrim -U (Pharmanza), Morprim (Morvel), Mortin-vet (Microlab), Oriprim (CHC), Radiprim (Radix), Salprim (Salus), Sulcoprim bolus (Concept), Sulprim-24 (Unichem), Sultrimax (BAIF), Sumetrol Inj. (Themis), Synastat (Roussel), Trepin (C.P.), Trimo-vet (Piya), Venprim SD (Ventri), Vetran (IPCI), Vetran-LA (VF), Woktrin (Wockhardt).

Miscellaneous antibacterial: Aldazin (Alved), Alincomycin (Alved), Anarobin (Unichem), Bidox (Merind), Check-o-Tox (Ranbaxy), Colistin (Vetcare), Dynamutilin (Ciba-Geigy), Fluquin (C.P.), Gass-cutter tab. (Piya), Imequyl (Rhone-Poulenc), Khorsolin-TH (Glaxo), Linco-Spectin SPO (Unichem), Linco-Spectin SS. Inj. (Unichem), Mycomulin (Concept), Pelwin (Wockhardt), Septilin (Himalaya), Sodium sulphadimethylphyrimidine (Cyanamid), Thiacetazone and Isoniazid tab. (IDPL), Unimix (Unichem), Zydaquin (CHC).

CENTRAL NERVOUS SYSTEM

Anaesthetics : Ketmin - 50 (Themis), Novocain (Hoechst).

Analgesics, Antipyretic, Anti-Inflammatory Drugs : Alfenac (Alved), Algesin vet (Alembic), Analgin (ICCI), Analgin (Karnataka), Ansed (Morvel), Atrizone (Alved), Bangshil (Alarsin), Betnesol (Glaxo), Bioril (Charak), Bolin (Merind), Butagesic (Concept), Canapar (USV), CP Vet (Rajshree), Curadex (Concept), DCF-Vet (Vetcorp), Dexamethasone (USV), Dexamethasone sod. (Alved), Dexasone (C.P.), Dexavet (Merind), Dexona (CHC), Diclovet (Alembic), Dipravet (PCI), Esgipyrin - N (SGPL Sarabhai), Feverdon (VF), Hostacortin-H (Hoechst), Iodine and Methyl salicylate ointment (Ethicare), Iodoball ointment (Balloun), Marcodex (Marc), Meparin (Morvel), Methydex (IPCI), Mordex (Morvel), Morpin (Morvel), Multifur (Vesper), Novalgin (Hoechst), Opigin (Salus), Oxalgin (CHC), Paracetol (CHC), Petofen (Marc), Polygesic (Unichem), Prednisolone (Wockhardt), Promethazine HCl (Rhone-Poulenc), Proxyvet (Wockhardt), Pyroson powder (Balloun), Pyroxin bolus (Marc), R. Compound (Alarsin), Ravnita (Biomedica), Ridalpin (Karnataka), Rnalgin (Radix), Rumalaya cream (Himalaya), Thermo-care (Vesper), Vetcort (Alembic), Zobid (Sarabhai).

Anticonvulsants: Mysoline (IEL)

Antiemetic: Atropine (BAIF), Atropine sulphate (Morvel).

Local anaesthetics: Gesicaine Vet (SGPL), Lignocaine (BAIF), Lignocaine (Radix), Morcain (Morvel).

Sedative: Sicvel (Morvel), Siquil (Sarabhai), Spasmodin (Biomedica), Sugil (Biomedica), Triflupromazine (ICCI), Xylaxin (Indian Immunologicals), Xylocad (C.P.).

CIRCULATORY SYSTEM

Hematinics: Cofecu (IH), Hematic (Ethicare), Iron copper cobalt capsule (ARC).

Hemostat: Acitron (SGPL), Adrenaline (BAIF), Stadren-V (Medinex), Styplon (Himalaya).

DIGESTIVE SYSTEM

Antibloat: Afanil (Dabur), Afron (BBB), Antiblot (IPCI), Antiflat (Charak), Bloatonil (Balloun), Bloatosil (Wockhardt), Blot (Morvel), Blotex (Rajshree), Blotinox (CR), Debloat (Ethicare), Digeplan (Rajshree), Digesto (Pee), Gasex (Himalaya), Gritona

(Anuja), Herbal-bloat liq. (Badri), Iccontor. (ICCI), Impacdon (VF), Neutex (ARC), Pashu Pachan (ARC), Rumax (Vesper), Rumicare (Intercare), Timpol (I.H.), Tympan (ARC). Tymplax (Balloun).

Antidiarrhoeal: Aspul (ARC), Bonnisan (Himalaya), Catorrhoea tab. (CR), Diadisco (BBB), Diardon (VF), Diarex (Himalaya), Diarin (Balloun), Diaroak (Dabur), Diovet (Charak) Dirol (Rajshree), Dysekal powder (Balloun), Dysentron (Herb. Prod.), Enterofur (Vesper), Herbal-Diarina (Badri), Intokam (Anuja), Pectoline powder (IPCI), Pectrol (Radix), Pesulin (C.P.), Scorid (VF), Sofrakay (Roussel), Sulfagon (Balloun), Sulphon (Balloun), Thaloxone (Ethicare).

Appetizer: Anorexon forte bolus (Pfizer), Apetone (Salus), Biovet (Wockhardt), Bonnisan (Himalaya), Digeplan (Rajshree), Digestone (Anuja), Dog Sou (Vestas), Gritona (Anuja), Herbotone (Badri), Herminsa (BBB), Himalayan Batisa (I.H), Impacdon (VF), Impactone (Salus), Kamdhenu Batisa (Herb. Prod.), Minal forte (Alembic), Movirom (Arex), Pachoplus (Dabur), Ruchamax (Dabur), Rumax (Vesper), Rumbion (I.H.), Rumenton tab. (Pfizer).

Colic: Morgan (Morvel), Valginate vet (TTK).

Deodorant: Deodorase (Vetcare).

Liver tonics/extracts: Acti-Liv forte (Anuja), Ashilive forte (Biomedica), Beekom-L (Wockhardt), Belamyl (Sarabhai), Bio Boost bolus (Lyka Labs), Bivinal forte (Alembic), Brotone (Glaxo), Crystafol parenteral vet (Medinex), Cyanoplex (BAIF), Hematol (BBB), Hepacin (BBB), Hepagest (Alembic), Inj. Vit B Complex with liver extract (Ind. Imm.), Liv-52 (Himalaya), Livogen inj. (Glaxo), Liverjet (C.P.), Livfit (Dabur). Livobex (TTKP). Livol (I.H.), Livoma (Rakesh), Livomex (Rajshree), Livomin (Herb. Prod.), Livtone (Anichem) Livertone (Ranbaxy), Livirubra (CHC), Livotonic (A.R.C.), Livovet (Charak), Livron (VF), Meriton (Merind), Nutriliv forte (Vetcare), Pepsid inj. (Concept), Ripason (TTKP), Stronic inj. (Ranbaxy), Tefroli (TTKP), Vestom Powder (Balloun), Yakrifit (Dabur), Zigup (Indian Herbs).

Rumenotorics and digestive stimulants: Anfro-plus (Jeps), Appevet (Rakesh), Biovet -YC (Wockhardt), Bovirex (Marc), Bovirum bolus (Sarabhai), Cadfeed (CHC), Catone Powder (CR), Digeplan (Rajshree), Digestovet (VF), Floratone bolus (Concept), HB strong (I.H), Herbotone (Badri), Kamdhenu batisa (Herb. Prod), Ketonex (Alved), Lacto-sacc (Vretcare), Livol PF (IH), Movirom (Arex), Norexia (Ethicare), Onfeed (C.P.), Pachoplus (Dabur), Pashupachan (ARC), Promin (Rajshree), Ruchamax (Dabur), Rumbion, Himalayan Batisa (IH), Rumen bolus (Alembic), Rumenton (Pfizer), Rumentonic (Rakesh), Ruminol - C (Pharmanza), Rumobin (Balloun), Runinol (Pharmanza), Toxol (Vesper).

EXPECTORANTS

Ballex Powder (Balloun), Bronto (Anuja), Caflon (I.H.), Cafon (ARC), Cofgon (BBB), Cof Kontrol (Biomedica), Cofodex (Rajshree), Catcough (CR), Coughdon (VF), Fluherex (BBB), Herbal Kof (Badri), Kafact (Charak), Sporin (Rajshree).

GENITO-URINARY SYSTEM

Ecbolics: Clinosol (BBB) Endoklin (Salus), Exapar (Dabur), Harboleen (Rajshree), Harira (GHPL), Herbogyne liq. (Badri), Myron (Alarsin), Replanta (IH), Uterovet (Rakesh).

Genital system drugs: Aq. Iodine sol. (Ethicare), Becline (Balloun), Entrodone (Salus), Epidosin-vet (TTKP), Fazole bolus (Unichem), Furan-U (Pharmanza), Furea bolus (Pfizer), Metrijet (Intercare), Metro-herb (Salus), Metronidazole (Rhone-Poulenc), Metrozol-U (Salus), Micotrim-U (Pharmanza), Povidone Iodine (Ethicare; USV), Sultrim (Balloun), Talsur (Kamataka), Urenit bolus (Balloun), Utrex (Vesper), Utronza (Pharnanza).

Sex tonics: Aloes compound (Alarsin), Banjhna (BBB), Cobaphos (Glaxo) Cadfeed (C.H.C.), Cyclo-herb (Salus), Estrona (Rakesh), Fortege (Alarsin), Fertivet (Arex), Prazola (Pharmanza), Gyanolactin (Jeps), Gyna-forte (Rajshree), Govardhen (GHPL), Heat-X (Herb. Prod.), Herbogyne cap. (Badri), Hormotone liq. (Charak), Onfeed Bolus (C.P.), Janova (Dabur), Prazola (Pharmanza), Rajana (ARC), Ratraj (BBB), Speman (Himalaya), Tentex forte (Himalaya), Uterotone cap. (C.R.), Utop (ARC).

Urinary system: Cystone (Himalaya drugs), L-Tona (Anuja), Remot (Morvel), Ridema (Merind).

Uterine tonic: Cad feed (C.H.C.), Fazole bolus (Unichem), Gynaecare (Vesper), Janova (Dabur), Onfeed bolus (C.D.), Prajana (IH), Proctive (Rakesh), Prolapse-cure (Rajshree), Prolapse-In (CR), Uterotone liq. (CR).

HORMONES

Corticosteroids: Betenisol (Glaxo), Curadex (Cencept), Dexamethasone (USV), Dexamethasone sod. (Alved), Dexasone (CP), Dexona (C.H.C.), Hostacortin-H (Hoechst), Marcodex (Marc), Prednisolone (Wockhardt), Vetalog (Sarabhai).

Gonadal hormones: Chorulon (Intercare), Dinolytic (BC), Duraprogen (Unichem), Folligon (Intercare), Prid (BC), Promone-E (BC), Pulp depot (Morvel), Stilbestrol inj (ICCI), Syncro-Mate-B(BC), Synchro-Part PMSG (BC).

Gonadotrophic hormones: Coriogan (BC), Cystorelin (BC), Ovaset (BC), Receptal (Hoechst), Trophovet (Ind. Imm.), Fertagyl (Intercare).

Oxytocin: Oxytocin inj. (ICCI).

PGF$_2\alpha$: Hormo P$_2$ Alpha (BC), Lutalyse (Unichem), Prosolvin (Intercare).

Miscellaneous: Adrenaline (BAIF).

INFUSIONS

Dexalt (Ethicare). Dexgyl (Radix), Dextrose 5% and sod. chloride 0.9% (Radix), Dextrose inj. 20% (BAIF), Dextrose inj. (Radix), Rintose (Wockhardt). Strong Dextrose inj. (Ethicare), Dextrose (Wockhardt).

MAMMARY SYSTEM

Galactogogue: Ascal (Alembic), Boon-o-Milk (Aries), Dugdh-dan (CR), Galog (I.H.), Gynolaclin (Jeps), Hi-milk (VF), Lactoboost (Themis), Lactivet (Alved), Lactolet-M (Rajshree), Lactotone (Rajshree), Lectocure (Herb. Product), Leptamilk Forte (Concept), Leptaden (Alarsin), Mastimin (Vesper), Milchey (Charak), Milconza (Pharmanza), Milkmax (Ethicare), Milko-herb (Salus), Milkoplex (Rakesh), Milkotone (Anuja), Milkvet (Rakesh), Payapro (Dabur), Profat (GHPL), Prolact M (GHPL), Rasol (BBB), Trace mix (Pee), Hyalactin (Jeps).

Mastitis: Cloxacillin (BAIF), Cloxampicillin (BAIF), Floclox (Ranbaxy), Masti-Care (Vesper), Mastimin (Vesper), Pendistrin-SH (Sarabhai), Penicillin (Boots), Penicure-D (Marc), Povidone Iodine Solution (Ethicare, USV), Rifijet (Intercare), Tilox (Wockhardt), Vetclox-plus (Sarabhai), Vetimast (Ciba-Geigy),

METABOLIC DISEASES

Ketosis: Dexamethasone (USV, Alved, CP). Dexona (C.H.C.), Lactosacc (Vetcare), Mordex (Morvel), Vetalog inj (Sarabhai), Vetcort inj. (Alembic).

Parturient Paresis: Baifocal (BAIF), Cabcodex (BAIF), Cal-D-plus (C.P.), Cal. borogluconate (Indian Immunologicals), Cal. borogluconate (Wockhardt), Calbomax (BAIF), Calborogluconate (Ethicare), Calcipar 25% (Biomedica), Caldee-12 (Wockhardt), Caldivet (Ranbaxy), Calife-C inj (Merind), Calmex-M (Ranbaxy). Catone Powder (CR), Glacal (Glaxo), Glamag (Glaxo), Kaldex-M (Radix), Lactaid (Hoechst), Lactaid Plus (Hoechst), Mifecal (C.P.), Mifex (Rhone-Poulenc), Thiacal (Wockhardt).

NEOPLASTIC DRUGS

Anthiomaline (Rhone-Poulenc). Inj. Lithium antimony thiomalate (Indian Immunologicals).

NUTRITION

Growth Stimulators: BMD-1000 (Ranbaxy), Caldevel (Ranbaxy), Livtone (Anichem), Stres Vin (Anichem) . 3-Care (Vetcare), 3-Nitro Hoechst (Hoechst), Acetylarsan (Rhone-Poulenc), Albac (Ventri), Aries poultry concentrate (Aries), Aureomycin (Cyanamid), Aurofac (Cyanamid), BeeKom-Forte (Wockhardt), Bio Spur (Rhone-Poulenc), Biomindif (Boots), Bivinal forte (Alembic), Cadisol plus (CHC), Cal-D-plus (C.P.), Calvit (Marc), Choline-500 (Vetcare), Cholymbi (Lyka Labs), Colistin (Vetcare), Crunch Ezz (Vestas), Digesto (Pee), Dimbpro (Dabur), Dog sou (Vestas), Egup (IH), Fura-20 (Pee), Flavomycin-40 (Hoechst), G- Probiotic (Vetcare), Geriforte (Himalaya), L-mezole plus (Vetcare), Lacto-Sacc (Vetcare), Lactomin (Vesper), Lactovet (Rakesh), Livoferol (Unichem), Lyncho (Themis), Lysocare (Vetcare), Lysomix (Aries), Merinitro (Merind), Methiocare-86 (Vetcare), Methiomin (Aris), Milkmin (Sarabhai), Minalforte (Alembic), Minarex (Rakesh), Mindif Minerals (Boots), Nutribix Economy Treats (Petcare), Nutribix rolls (Petcare), Nutricoat (Petcare), Nutripet Food Booster (Petcare), Nutripet Pet-Meal (Petcare), Nutripro (Vetcare), Polmix-B (Arex), Polmix-L (Arex), Prot-o-Liv (Aies), Protexin

(Ciba-Geigy), Provimin Forte (Rhone-Poulenc), Pup-Lick (Vestas), Retisol (VF), Riz puffs (Vestas), Roxarsone (Merind), Roxolin (Ciba-Geigy). Sharkoferrol vet (Alembic), Stafac-20 (Pfizer), Stresroak (Dabur), Super dot (Vetcare), Trimix (Vestas), Tylosin tartrate (Ventri), V-Fur-200 (Ventri), Vetkal-B$_{12}$ (Sarabhai), Vitator CLMB (Themis), Whee puffs (Vestas), Yeasacc (Vetcare), Zeetress (IH),

Minerals: Agrimin (Glaxo), Animin (Vets Farma), Aries M.M. (Aries), Ayucal (Dabur), Biomindif (Boots), Calborol (Rhone-Poulenc) Calcimin (Salus), Calcipar 25% (Biomedica), Caldhan (Dabur), Calvet (Radix), Kalzole (Glaxo), Cattlemin (Aries), Cofecu (IH), Cyclomin (Alved), Egg max (Ethicare), Electroblend WHO-Formula (IPCI) Glamag (Glaxo), Minal Forte (Alembic), Mindif Minerals (Boots), Navnid (ARC), Ossopan Vet (TTKP), Pashumin (Pee), Phosphamin (Salus), Poultrymin (Aries), Replamin (Merind) Supermindif (Boots), Tonoball Tonic Powder (Balloun), Tonophosphan (Hoechst), Tonoricin (Wockhardt), Tracemin (Aries), Venlyle (Ventri), Vetcopp (VF), Vetlick (VF), Vets Cu-Co (VF), Vets Mineral Mixture (VF), Vets Trace Minerals (VF).

Mineral and Vitamin Preparations: Anemin (BBB), Apthocare (Vesper), Ascal (Alembic), Balltone (Balloun), Bonyvet (Arex), Brolay (Anichem), Onfeed (C.P.). Cadfeed (CHC). Cadiplex-L (CHC), Calci vet (Morvel), Calci-royal (Concept), Caldivet (Ranbaxy), Calfos AD$_3$ plus (VF), Canovite-C (Ranbaxy), Cobaphos (Glaxo). Concimin (Concept), E care-Se (Vetcare), E care-Se-forte (Vetcare), Groblend (Glaxo), Gwala (Sarabhai), Gynae-forte (Vesper), Herbal kal-C (Badri), Hivit (Ranbaxy), Hylactin (Jeps). Kalayan multimin forte (Piya), Kalrol-D3 (Pharmanza), Lactivet (Alved), Merical (Merind), Merimilk (Merind), Nutri-sacc (Vetcare), Nutrical (Pfizer), Nutrilay (Pfizer), Nutrimilk (Pfizer), Nutripet (Vetcare), Olpro (Lyka Labs), Omocal B-$_{12}$ (Morvel), Oracal AD$_3$ Syrup (Rajshree), Osteocalcium (Glaxo), Pupvit (Inovetys), Robust (Anichem), Strexia (Wockhardt), Supplevite-M (Sarabhai), Vetkal-B$_{12}$ (Sarabhai), Vetmix Forte (VF), Vetril (Vestas), Visyneral Calcium with B$_{12}$ (USV), Vitavit-7 (Inovetys), Vitmix-Con (Pee), Vitrical (Pee).

Vitamins: Activit special (Vetcare), Advet-AD (IPCI), Alviton (Alembic), Ascal (Alembic), Ascoplex (BAIF), Amnovit Baifoplex (BAIF), Ballmix (Balloun), Balloun-B-complex (Balloun), B-care plus (Vetcare), B-care sol (Vetcare), Beekom-forte (Wockhardt), Beepex (Morvel), Belive (Morvel), Bicoral (BAIF), Bicoral forte (BAIF), Billipon (Biomedica), Biocare (Vetcare), Bion-12-vet (Morvel), Bovivita (CHC), C-care-100 (Vetcare), Cholidox (Vetcare), Concitone (Concept), Dicirol (Glaxo), Famitone (Ranbaxy), Formula-100 (Aries), Gromax (Themis), Groviplex (Glaxo), Hyblend AB$_2$D$_3$ (Glaxo), Hyblend AB$_2$D$_3$K (Glaxo), Kalayan B-complex Syrup (Piya), Kaysol forte (Vetcare), Livertone (Ranbaxy), Lychoplex (USV), Lyrim (C.P.), Lysovet (IPCI), Livovet (Marc), Merivit-100 (Merind), Multimin AB$_2$D$_3$ (PCI), Multisol Bovine (PCI), Neuroxin (CHC), Nurovet (Alved), Nutrliv (Vetcare), Pamibion (Biomedica), Piyamix A+B$_2$+D$_3$+K (Piya), Piya- Mycetine (Piya), Piyoplex WM Forte (Piya), Piyasol-P (Piya), Plexa-BC (Concept), Prepalin Forte (Glaxo), Polymix Multivit Plus (Ranbaxy), Retablend A (WM) (IPCI), Raprovit (Radix), Rovimix A+B$_2$+D$_3$ (Roche), Rovimix A+B$_2$D$_3$+K (Roche), Rovimix AD$_3$ Type 50/5 (Roche), Rovisol A-Oral type 100 (Roche), Rovisol AD$_3$ EC (Roche), Solvit ABDEC (Vetcare), Themineuron (Themis), Stresvel AB$_2$D$_3$+K (Ventri), Vetapine (Piya), Rovibe (Roche), Vetral (VF), Vets-AD$_3$ 50/5 (VF), Vets Bee (VF), Vets AB$_2$D$_3$+K (VF), Vetsol-B (VF), Ventrimix AB$_2$D$_3$ (Ventri), Ventrimix AB$_2$D$_3$+K (Ventri), Ventriplex-M (Ventri), Visyneral AD$_3$EC (USV), Vetstress liquid (IPCI), Vetyplex (IPCI), Veemix (Pee), Vibelan (Glaxo), Vitacept (Concept), Vitatone liq M(CHC), Vitamix AD$_3$ powder (Morvel), Vitamin AD$_3$E (Sarabhai), Vimeral (Glaxo), Vitablend AD$_3$ (Glaxo), Vitablend WM forte (Glaxo), Vitaplex AB$_2$D$_3$ (Piya), Vitator (Themis), Vitadec (BAIF), Vimicon (BAIF) Pro-Winstress (C.P.), Winner Liquid (Morvel).

SKIN

Antifungal: Charmil (Dabur), Ropak (Rajshree), Teeburb (I.H.), UTPP-5 (Vetcare), Vetcopp (VF).

Antiseptic preparation: Ball dressing (Balloun), Cream of Gamma Benzene Hexachloride and Proflavin (Ethicare), Dermatis Cream (Balloun), Dresol liquid (CR), Furazone powder (Balloun), Gabex (IPCI), Herexide (BBB), Pivipol sol. (Arex), Savlon (IEL), Povidone iodine (Ethicare, USV).

Instillations: Nanco (BBB), Paristola (Biomedica), Retinamycin (Biomedica), Simercetin (Biomedica),

Topical preparations: Ayana (ARC), Blaze (IH), Charmil (Dabur), Canifur (C.P.), Canfur-AZ (C.P.), Catgall Ointment (CR), Dermocept ointment (Concept), Flurry (CHC), Healovet (Charak), Herbal tik powder (Badri), Herbittol (Herb Product), Himax (IH), Jeplon (Jeps), Lorexane (IEL), Melicon -v (C.P.), M-Lorax (Marc), Povidin (Jeps), Ropak (Rajshree), Savlon (IEL), Vitapet (Dynamic).

Disinfectants: Disfect-S (Pfizer), Khorsolin - TH (Glaxo), Nuvan (Ciba-Geigy), Tek-trol (Ranbaxy).

Index—Pharmaceutical Companies

Index — Generic / Brand Names

195.	Clinosol	BBB	64	245.	Dexasone	C.P	72
196.	Clopimix 25% Premix	Piya	154	246.	Dexavet	Merind	135
197.	Cloxacillin	BAIF	57	247.	Dexgyl	Radix	157
198.	Cloxacillin inj	KAPL	127	248.	Dexona inj	CHC	69
199.	Cloxampicillin	BAIF	57	249.	Dextrose	Radix	157
200.	Cobaphos	Glaxo	91	250.	Dextrose and Sod. Chloride	Radix	157
201.	Coban-100	Ventri	190	251.	Dextrose inj 20%	BAIF	57
202.	Codrinal	Hoechst	103	252.	Diadin tab	Pfizer	151
203.	Cofecu	Indian Herbs	110	253.	Diadisco	BBB	64
204.	Cofgo	BBB	64	254.	Diardon	Vets Farma	207
205.	Caflon	Indian Herbs	110	255.	Diarex	Himalaya	96
206.	Cofodex	Rajshree	160	256.	Diarin	Balloun	60
207.	Colidox	Vet Care	197	257.	Diaroak	Dabur	84
208.	Colistin	Vet Care	201	258.	Dicirol granules	CP	72
209.	Combipen	Vetcorp	203	259.	Diclovet	Alembic	39
210.	Comoxil	Concept	79	260.	Dicrysticin-S	Sarabhai	174
211.	Conampi	Concept	79	261.	Digeplan	Rajshree	160
212.	Concimin	Concept	79	262.	Digesto	Pee Farma	144
213.	Conciplex	Concept	79	263.	Digestone	Anuja	47
214.	Concitone	Concept	80	264.	Digestovet	Vets Farma	208
215.	Coriogan	B.C.A.H.P.	62	265.	Dimdim	Arex	50
216.	Cosumix	Ciba-Geigy	101	266.	Dimbpro	Dabur	84
217.	Cosylan	USV	188	267.	Dinolytic	B.C.A.H.P.	62
218.	Coughdon	Vets Farma	207	268.	Diovet	Charak	77
219.	Coxidol	Ventri	190	269.	Dipravet	PCIP	142
220.	Coxistac	Pfizer	150	270.	Dirol	Rajshree	160
221.	CP-Vet	Rajshree	160	271.	Disfect-S	Pfizer	151
222.	Crunch Eez	Vestas	196	272.	Distodin	Pfizer	151
223.	Crystafol Parenteral	Medinex	134	273.	Dog Sou	Vestas	196
224.	Curadex	Concept	80	274.	Dot	Aries	51
225.	Cural	Merind	135	275.	Doxiterin	Sarabhai	174
226.	Curaminth	Sarabhai	174	276.	Doxyn	USV	188
227.	Cyanoplex	BAIF	57	277.	Dressol	Cattle Remedies	75
228.	Cycloherb	Salus Pharma	173	278.	Dugdh-dan	Cattle Remedies	75
229.	Cyclomin-7	Alved	43	279.	Dugdha Powder	Salus Pharma	173
230.	Cycostat	Cyanamid	82	280.	Duocidal bolus	KAPL	127
231.	Cystone	Himalaya	96	281.	Duocidal powder	KAPL	127
232.	Cystorelin	B.C.A.H.P.	62	282.	Duocoxin	Glaxo	91
233.	DCF Vet	Vetcorp	203	283.	Duraprogen	Unichem	185
234.	De-odorase	Vet Care	197	284.	Dynacil	HAL	98
235.	Debloat	Ethicare	86	285.	Dynamutilin	Ciba-Geigy	101
236.	Decarin	Rajshree	160	286.	Dysekal	Balloun	60
237.	Dermatis cream	Balloun	60	287.	Dysentron	HPI	95
238.	Dermocept	Concept	80	288.	E-Care-Se	Vet Care	198
239.	Deverm	Ethicare	86	289.	Eggmax	Ethicare	86
240.	Dewormin	Cattle Remedies	75	290.	Egup	Indian Herbs	110
241.	Dexalt	Ethicare	86	291.	Ektodex	Petcare	146
242.	Dexamethasone	USV	188	292.	Ektodex	Vet Care	201
243.	Dexamethasone sod phosphate	Indian Immunologicals	113	293.	Electro Care Plus	Vet Care	198
244.	Dexamethasone sod. phos	Alved	43	294.	Electroblend	IPCI	115
				295.	Emdoklin bolus	Salus Pharma	173

No.	Name	Company	Page	No.	Name	Company	Page
396.	Herbal kal-C	Badri	53	446.	Kalpen	KAPL	128
397.	Herbal kof	Badri	53	447.	Kalrod-D3	Pharmanza	148
398.	Herbal Scab lotion	Badri	54	448.	Kalyan B Complex	Piya	154
399.	Herbal-bloat liq.	Badri	53	449.	Kalzole	Glaxo	92
400.	Herbal-diarina	Badri	53	450.	Kamdhenu Batisa	HPI	95
401.	Herbal-dog Shampoo	Badri	53	451.	Kampibiotic inj	KAPL	129
402.	Herbaltik-cattle	Badri	53	452.	Kancin	Alembic	39
403.	Herbaltik-dog	Badri	53	453.	Kaysol forte	Vet Care	199
404.	Herwex	BBB	64	454.	Ketmin-50	Themis	180
405.	Herbittol	HPI	95	455.	Ketonex	Alved	43
406	Herbogyne capsule	Badri	53	456.	Khorsolin-TH	Glaxo	92
407.	Herbogyne liq.	Badri	53	457.	Kitworm powder-50	IPCI	116
408.	Herboleen liq.	Rajshree	160	458.	Kloxamp inj	KAPL	129
409.	Herbotone	Badri	54	459.	Kot	Vet Corp	203
410.	Herexide	BBB	64	460.	Krimos	BBB	64
411.	Herminsa	BBB	64	461.	L-mezole	Vet Care	201
412.	Hexachlorphene tab.	ICCI	123	462.	L-Mezole Plus	Vet Care	199
413.	Hexonide	Sarabhai	175	463.	L-Tona	Anuja	47
414.	Hi-milk	Vets Farma	208	464.	Lactaid	Hoechst	104
415.	Himalayan Batisa	Indian Herbs	110	465.	Lactivet	Alved	43
416.	Himax	Indian Herbs	110	466.	Lacto-sacc	Vet Care	199
417.	Hipenox	CHC	70	467.	Lactoboost	Themis	181
418.	Histal	Vet Care	201	468.	Lactolet-M	Rajshree	160
419.	Hivit Inj. (Vet)	Ranbaxy	165	469.	Lactomin	Vesper	193
420.	Hormo P2 alpha	BCAHP	63	470.	Lactotone	Rajshree	161
421.	Hormotone	Charak	77	471.	Lactovet Powder	Rakesh	162
422.	Hostacortin	Hoechst	104	472.	Laracare	Inter Care	201
423.	Hostacycline	Hoechst	104	473.	Larvadex	Ciba-Geigy	101
424.	Hyblend AB2D3	Glaxo	91	474.	Lectocure	HPI	95
425.	Hyblend AB2D3K	Glaxo	91	475.	Lemasol	Ranbaxy	165
426.	Hylactin	Jeps	125	476.	Leptaden	Alarsin	35
427.	Icconton	ICC	123	477.	Leptamilk Forte	Concept	80
428.	Imequyl	Rhone-Poulenc	168	478.	Levamisole	Ciba-Geigy	101
429.	Impacdon	Vets Farma	208	479.	Levasol	Vets Farma	204
430.	Impactone bolus	Salus Pharma	172	480.	Lignocaine	BAIF	57
431.	Intokam	Anuja	47	481.	Lignocaine	Radix	157
432.	Iodine and Methyl Salicylate Oint.	Ethicare	87	482.	Linco-spectin	Unichem	185, 187
433.	Iodine Sol.	Ethicare	86	483.	Lithium Antimony Thiomalate	Indian Immunologicals	113
434.	Iodoball	Balloun	60	484.	Liv-52	Himalaya	96
435.	Iron Copper Cobalt Capsule	A.R.C.	45	485.	Liv-tone	Anichem	44
436.	Ivomec	Glaxo	92	486.	Liver-tone	Ranbaxy	166
437.	Janova	Dabur	85	487.	Liverjet	CP	73
438.	Jeplon	Jeps	125	488.	Liverubra	CHC	70
439.	Kadiprol	CHC	70	489.	Livfit	Dabur	85
440.	Kafact	Charak	77	490.	Livobex	T.T.K. Pharma	183
441.	Kalayan Multimin Forte	Piya	154	491.	Livoferol	Unichem	185
442.	Kalbend (vet)	KAPL	128	492.	Livogen Inj	Glaxo	92
443.	Kaldex-M	Radix	157	493.	Livol	Indian Herbs	110, 111
444.	Kalmeben	KAPL	128	494.	Livoma Tab	Rakesh	162
445.	Kalmisole	KAPL	128	495.	Livomex	Rajshree	161

598.	Notix scrub/talc	Petcare	146	
599.	Novacain	Hoechst	105	
600.	Novalgin	Hoechst	105	
601.	Nurovet	Alved	43	
602.	Nutri Sacc	Vet Care	200	
603.	Nutribix	Petcare	146	
604.	Nutrical	Pfizer	151	
605.	Nutricoat	Petcare	147	
606.	Nutricoat	Vet Care	199	
607.	Nutrilay	Pfizer	151	
608.	Nutriliv forte	Vet Care	199	
609.	Nutriliv inj	Vet Care	201	
610.	Nutrimilk	Pfizer	152	
611.	Nutripet	Petcare	147	
612.	Nutripet	Vet Care	199	
613.	Nutripro	Vet Care	199	
614.	Nuvan	Ciba-Geigy	102	
615.	Okazan	Wockhardt	211	
616.	Olpro	Lyka	131	
617.	Omocal B-12	Morvel	141	
618.	Onfeed bolus	CP	73	
619.	Opigin bolus	Salus Pharma	172	
620.	Oracal AD$_3$ Syrup	Rajshree	161	
621.	Oriprim	CHC	70, 71	
622.	Ossopan Vet Gr.	T.T.K. Pharma	183	
623.	Ostaderm	Vets Farma	208	
624.	Ostocalcium	Glaxo	92	
625.	Otcim	IDPL	107	
626.	Ovaset	BCAHP	63	
627.	Overcid	BCAHP	63	
628.	Oxalgin	CHC	71	
629.	Oxyclozanide	USV	189	
630.	Oxycycline	Piya	154	
631.	Oxymor	Morvel	141	
632.	Oxysteclin inj	Sarabhai	176	
633.	Oxytetracycline	Alved	42	
634.	Oxytetracycline	Concept	80	
635.	Oxytetracycline	Indian Immunologicals	113	
636.	Oxytetracycline	Merind	136	
637.	Oxytetracycline	USV	189	
638.	Oxytetracycline-LA	Sarabhai	176	
639.	Oxytocin	Radix	158	
640.	Oxytocin inj	ICCI	123	
641.	Oxytra	HAL	99	
642.	Oxyzon	Piya	154	
643.	Pachoplus	Dabur	85	
644.	Pamibion	Biomedica	66	
645.	Panacur	Hoechst	105	
646.	Panfugal	Merind	136	
647.	Paquin	Ranbaxy	166	
648.	Paracetol inj	CHC	71	
649.	Parichlor inj	Biomedica	67	
650.	Paristola eye and ear drops	Biomedica	67	
651.	Pashu Pachan	A.R.C.	45	
652.	Pashumin	Pee Farma	144	
653.	Payapro	Dabur	85	
654.	Pectoline (Powder)	IPCI	116	
655.	Pectzol	Radix	158	
656.	Pelwin	Wockhardt	211	
657.	Penicillin (Intra-mammary inj.)	Boots	68	
658.	Pendistrin-SH	Sarabhai	176	
659.	Penicure-D	Marc	133	
660.	Pepsid inj	Concept	81	
661.	Pestoban	Indian Herbs	111	
662.	Pestokil	HPI	95	
663.	Pesulin	CP	73	
664.	Petofen	Marc	133	
665.	Phenivet	PCIP	142	
666.	Phosphamin tab	Salus Pharma	172	
667.	Piperazine	HAL	99	
668.	Piperazine	Morvel	141	
669.	Piperazine adipate	KAPL	129	
670.	Piperazine Hexahydrate	Cyanamid	82	
671.	Piperazine Hexahydrate	Merind	137	
672.	Piperazine Hexahydrate	Ventri	190	
673.	Piperazine liq (45%)	Glaxo	92	
674.	Piperazine liq and soluble powder	Ethicare	88	
675.	Pipirocid	Arex	49	
676.	Pivipol	Arex	50	
677.	Piyabee	Piya	155	
678.	Piyablend AD$_3$ Type 50/5	Piya	155	
679.	Piyadial (ORS)	Piya	155	
680.	Piyafin	Piya	155	
681.	Piyamenton	Piya	155	
682.	Piyamix A+B$_2$+D$_3$+K	Piya	155	
683.	Piya Mycetine	Piya	155	
684.	Piyanitro	Piya	155	
685.	Piyaphene	Piya	155	
686.	Piyaplex WH Forte	Piya	156	
687.	Piyasol-P	Piya	156	
688.	Plexa-BC	Concept	81	
689.	Polmix	Arex	50	
690.	Polygesic	Unichem	186	
691.	Polymix Multivit plus	Ranbaxy	166	
692.	Poultrymin	Aries	52	
693.	Povidin	Jeps	126	
694.	Povidone Iodine sol.	Ethicare	88	
695.	Povidone-Iodine	USV	189	
696.	Prajana	Indian Herbs	111	
697.	Prazi plus	Vet Care	202	
698.	Prazola	Pharmanza	148	

No.	Name	Company	Page		No.	Name	Company	Page
800.	Stadren-V (inj)	Medinex	134		850.	Tek-trol	Ranbaxy	167
801.	Stafac-20	Pfizer	152		851.	Telon-L.A.	Merind	137
802.	Stat	Ethicare	88		852.	Tentex forte	Himalaya	97
803.	Stenorol	Hoechst	105		853.	Terifix-M	Merind	137
804.	Stilbesterol inj	ICCI	123		854.	Terramycin	Pfizer	152, 153
805.	Streptomycin inj	IDPL	107		855.	Tetmosol soap	IEL	109
806.	Stres-vin	Anichem	44		856.	Tetracycline bolus	Sarabhai	176
807.	Stresroak	Dabur	85		857.	Tetracycline Powder	IDPL	107
808.	Stresvel AD3EC oral	Ventri	190		858.	Tetradox	Ranbaxy	167
809.	Strexia	Wockhardt	211		859.	Tetrakal	KAPL	130
810.	Stronic inj	Ranbaxy	167		860.	Tetramisole HCl	ICCI	124
811.	Styplon	Himalaya	97		861.	Tetramisole HCl	Piya	156
812.	Sugaprim	Sarabhai	176		862.	Tetzan	Jeps	126
813.	Sugil	Biomedica	67		863.	Thaloxone	Ethicare	88
814.	Sulcoprim	Concept	81		864.	Themineuron (inj)	Themis	182
815.	Sulfadimidine	Sarabhai	177		865.	Thermo Care	Vesper	195
816.	Sulfadimidine	Arex	50		866.	Thiabendazole	Arex	50
817.	Sulfagon	Balloun	61		867.	Thiacal	Wockhardt	212
818.	Sulfagut bolus	KAPL	129		868.	Thiacetazone and Isoniazid tablet	IDPL	108
819.	Sulfasys bolus	KAPL	129		869.	Tilox	Wockhardt	212
820.	Sulphadimidine	Pearl Chemical	143		870.	Timpol	Indian Herbs	111
821.	Sulphadimidine sod	IDPL	107		871.	Tolzan-F	Hoechst	105
822.	Sulphadimidine sod	Rhone-Poulenc	169		872.	Tonoball	Balloun	61
823.	Sulphadimidine sodium	Indian Immunologicals	113		873.	Tonophosphan	Hoechst	105
					874.	Tonoricin	Wockhardt	212
824.	Sulphadin	Vets Farma	205		875.	Toxol	Vesper	195
825.	Sulphaguanidine	IDPL	107		876.	Trace mix	Pee Farma	144
826.	Sulphanilamide Powd.	IDPL	107		877.	Tracemin	Aries	52
827.	Sulphon	Balloun	61		878.	Trepin	C.P	73
828.	Sulprim-24	Unichem	186		879.	Tribexin pro-salt	IDPL	108
829.	Sultrim	Balloun	61		880.	Trimix	Vestas	196
830.	Sultrimax	BAIF	58		881.	Trimo-vet	Piya	156
831.	Sultrimax-S inj	BAIF	58		882.	Triquin	Wockhardt	212
832.	Sumetrol	Themis	182		883.	Trophovet	Indian Immunologicals	113
833.	Super mindif	Boots	68					
834.	Supercox	Wockhardt	212		884.	Trypan blue	Ethicare	88
835.	Superdot	Vet Care	200		885.	Trypnil	Merind	137
836.	Supplevite-M	Sarabhai	177		886.	Tylosin tartrate	Ventri	191
837.	Supplimin	Sarabhai	177		887.	Tympan	A.R.C.	46
838.	Synastat tab	Roussel	170		888.	Tymplax	Bolloun	61
839.	Syncro-mate-B	BCAHP	63		889.	Unimix	Unichem	187
840.	Syncro-part PMSG	BCAHP	63		890.	Unimycin	Unichem	187
841.	Synthovet	PCIP	142		891.	Unistat	Unichem	187
842.	T-Cox	USV	189		892.	Urenit	Balloun	61
843.	Taenil	Indian Herbs	111		893.	Urul	BBB	65
844.	Talsur inj	KAPL	130		894.	Uterotone	Cattle Remedies	76
845.	Tapherex	BBB	65		895.	Uterovet	Rakesh	162
846.	Tartametic (2% & 4%)	Ethicare	88		896.	Utop	A.R.C.	46
847.	Teeburb	Indian Herbs	111		897.	UTPP-5	Vet Care	200
848.	Tefroli	T.T.K. Pharma	184		898.	Utrex	Vesper	195
849.	Tegeron Cream	Rhone-Poulenc	169		899.	Utronza	Pharmanza	149

Products Information

ALARSIN

Alarsin House, A/32,
Road No. 3, MIDC, Andheri (E),
MUMBAI - 400 093

Preparation	Indication	Dosage/Route	Presentation
ALOES COMPOUND (Vet) (Ovarian activator in anoestrus animals)	Infertility (non–pathogenic). Anoestrus, suboestrus, silent heat. Repeat breeding, delayed maturity in heifers. Prolonged post-partum an-oestrus conditions.	L.A: 5-10 tabs bid for 3-6 weeks, Heifer : 5-10 tab bid for 2 months max. S.A.: 2-3 tab bid for one month orally.	Pack of 100 tabs.
BANGSHIL (Vet)	G.U.T. Infection. Painful micturition, bladder disturbances. Urethritis, prostatitis. Infertility (Pathogenic) Resistant infection of urinary tract. Post-partum & post-surgical infection.	L.A: 10 tab bid x 2 weeks then 5 tab bid as long as necessary S.A: 3 tab bid x 2 week, then 2 tab bid as long as necessary. Orally.	100 tablets.
FORTEGE (Vet)	Fatigue, stress condition. Male infertility, subfertility, deficient spermatogenesis. Sluggish sex performance.	In Fatigue:- L.A: 10 tab bid x 15 days then 10 tab daily x 15 days S.A: 2 tab bid x 3 weeks. In disturbed spermatogenesis L.A: 10 tab bid x 1-2 month orally.	100 tablets and 1000 tablets.
	Note: In dogs for *enlarged prostate* fortege + bangshil 2 tab of each bid till improvement.		
LEPTADEN (Vet)	Repeat breeding habitual abortion. Prophylexis against early embryonic death.	L.A: repeat breeding 10 tab bid x 2 weeks from day of A.I. Habitual abortion 10 tab bid x 2 months after A.I. As prophylexis against early embryonic death. 5 tab bid x 2 weeks after A.I. S.A: 2 tab bid x 1 month.	100 tablets and 1000 tablets.
	Disturbed lactation due to stress condition, hypogalactia, In retention of placenta.	L.A: 10 tab bid x 1 month S.A: 2-3 tab bid x 2 weeks L.A: 15 tab bid x 3 days. S.A: 3 tab bid x 3 days, orally	
LEPTADEN(Vet) (In poultry)	For proper growth & better weight gain. Improve feed utilization. Improve egg quality. Increase egg laying capacity.	3-5 tabs in 1 kg of feed.	100 & 1000 tabs.

Preparation	Indication	Dosage/Route	Presentation
MYRON (Vet)	Genital diseases : Cervicitis, endometritis, metritis, parametritis, vaginitis, atonic reproductive tract and associated infertility. For inducing rapid involution of uterus after parturition.	L.A: 10 tab bid x 2-3 weeks. S.A. 2-3 tab bid x 2-3 weeks, orally.	100 & 1000 tablets.
R. COMPOUND (Vet)	In all skeleto-muscular and neuro-muscular inflammatory and painful condition with limitation of joint movement. *Lameness :*due to trauma, injury, arthritis. After surgery in patellar luxation, poll evil and fistulous withers in horse and dog. In management of paraplegia and post-paraplegia. For quicker healing in post-surgical trauma and wound. Supplementary treatments in mastitis.	L.A: 10 tab bid x 2-3 weeks S.A: 2-3 tab bid x 2-3 weeks, orally.	100 tablets.

ALEMBIC CHEMICAL WORKS CO. LTD.
Veterinary Div.
Alembic Road, BARODA - 390 003

Preparation	Indication	Dosage/Route	Presentation
ALCYCLIN BOLUS Each bolus contains 500 mg Tetracycline HCl	* To initiate treatment * For follow up therapy * For bacterial diarrhoea, enteritis, pneumonia etc. * For treatment of metritis, pyometra and cervicitis. * Ideal in gynaecological disorders like dystocia, abortion, retention of placenta.	Oral Cattle, sheep, horses, goats and pig; Prevention: 1 to 2 boluses/day Treatment : 4-6 boluses/day Lambs, kids, dogs and cats Treatment : 1/2 - 1 bolus/day I/U : Cow, buffaloes and mares : 1-2 Boluses inserted deep into the uterus. Ewes and Sows: 1/2 - 1 Bolus inserted into the uterus. Bitches 1/4 -1/2 bolus inserted into the uterus	Strip of 4 boluses.
ALGESIN VET Each ml Algesin Veterinary contains : Phenylbutazone Sod. 200 mg Lidocain 10 mg	* Non-specific fever * Pain and swelling * Joint diseases such as arthritis tendosynovitis, fibrositis, osteoarthritis, myositis, neuritis, neuralgia etc.	I/M route only L.A. : 3-12 ml S.A. : 1-4 ml	Ampoules of 3 ml.
ALMIZOL Water soluble powder Levamisol Hydro- chloride 300 mg/gm	*In case of livestock* Can be safely used in pregnant and lactating animal * Active against Benzimidazole Resistant spp. * Highly effective against Lungworm * Effective against heart worm * Active against sexually mature and immature worms. * Act better and longer by virtue of its immunopotentiating effect. *In case of poultry* * Broad spectrum activity * Reduces more no. of worms * Deworming free period can be extended * Least stress.	Cattle, sheep, pig and goat : Dissolve 5 gm Almizol in 200 ml water. One ml of the solution to be given orally per kg body weight Poultry 5 gm Almizol for 80-100 birds dissolved in 4 lits drinking water and 100 gm for 1500-2000 birds dissolved in 80 lits drinking water.	Pouch of 100 and 5 gm.

Preparation	Indication	Dosage/Route	Presentation
ALVITON Each 5 ml contains : Vit A 2,50,000 IU Vit D3 25,000 IU Vit E 150 IU Vit C 500 mg	Ideal for alleviating stress, improve resistances against disease Ideal supportive therapy against infertility. Helps in faster growth and proper bone formation.	Cattle and buffaloes :- 10 ml daily for 7 days Calves : 5 ml daily for 7 days Dogs : 3-5 ml daily for 7 days Poultry : 5-10 ml/100 birds.	Bottle of 20 ml, 110 ml 500 ml and 1 lit plastic container.
ASCAL Each 5 ml contains : Calcium Phosphate 0.24 gm Vit D3 500 IU Vit B 12 7.5 mcg	Ascal ensures more milk and better health as it provides calcium and phosphorus in right proportions and higher concentrations of vit D3 and B12.	Cattle and horses: 50 ml bid daily Calves : 20 ml twice daily Dog : 5 ml twice daily Poultry : 20-60 ml/100 birds.	Bottle of 110 ml and 450 ml.
BACIPEN Injection of Ampicillin Sodium	Calf scours, enteritis, pneumonia, metritis, H.S., retained placenta, mastitis, B.Q., salmonellosis, brucellosis, wound, infection etc.	2-7 mg/kg b.w. daily by i/m or i/v route.	Vial of 1 gm, 2 gm and 2.5 gm.
BISTREPEN Procain penicillin G 15,00,000 units, Penicillin G.Sodium 5,00,000 units, streptomycin sulphate 2.5 gm **BISTREPEN** Contains : Procain Penicillin G 3,00,000 units Pen. G Sodium 1,00,000 units Streptomycin Sulphate 1 gram	For treating mixed infections caused by G +ve and G -ve organism. For treating unidentified organism.	L.A: 2 ml/50 kg body weight i/m S.A: 1 ml/5 kg body weight Preparation : To each large dose vial add 7.5 ml sterile distilled water to make 10 ml suspension and 2 ml sterile distilled water to each small dose vial to make 3 ml suspension.	Vial of 1 gm and 2.5 gm.
BIVINAL FORTE Each ml of Bivinal Forte Vet. contains : Vit B1 50 mg, Riboflavin 5 mg, Vit B6 5 mg, Niacinamide 100 mg. DL. Panthenol 10 mg Inositol 2 mg Methionine 5 mg, Liver extract derived from 2 gm of fresh liver having vit B12 activity equivalent to 0.2 mcg of cyanocobalamine	* Non-specific anorexia and off feed conditon * Liver disorders * Debility and general weakness. * Eczemas * Growth and development of young animals * Vitamin B complex deficiency * Neurological disorders * Blood protozoan diseases.	*Large animals:* 5 ml twice weekly. *Small animals:* 0.5 ml - 1 ml twice weekly By I/M route only.	10 ml vials.

Preparation	Indication	Dosage/Route	Presentation
DICLOVET (Inj. Vet). Each ml contains Diclofence sod. 25 mg.	Various conditions associated with joints such as arthritis, tenosynovitis, osteoarthritis, Myositis, neuritis, neuralgia, swelling, etc.	1 mg-1.2 mg/kg b.w. I/M route only.	30 ml vial.
FORTIFIED PROCAIN PENICILLIN 20,00,000 units. Each vial contains Procain Pen. G 15,00,000 units, Pen. G Sod. 5 Lacs units. FORTIFIED PROCAIN PEN 40 Lac Units Each vial contains Procain Pen. G 30 Lac units Pen. G Sod. 10 lac units	Treatment of infections caused by Srtreptococci, Straphylococci Clostridia, Corynebacteria, Bacillus anthracis, Actinomyces bovis, etc.	*Preparation:* Add 4 ml distilled water to F.P.P. Veterinary 20 lacs vial and 8 ml to 40 lacs vial. Large and medium sized animals (cattle, horses, calves, foals, sheep, goats and swine) 4,000 unit/kg b.w. at 24 hrs interval Small Animals (Poultry, dogs and cats) 2,00,00 to 4,00,000 units at 24 hrs interval.	Vials of 20 lac and 40 lac
HEPAGEST Liquid Herbal liver tonic	Nutritional deficiencies due to liver disorders, cirrhosis of liver, aflatoxicosis, hepatitis, anorexia dyspepsia, stress.	L.A. : 15-20 ml twice daily S.A. : 2-5 ml twice daily	Bottle of 250 ml and 1 litre; Jar of 5 litre.
KANCIN Kanamycin acid sulphate equivalent to 1 gm of kanamycin base	*Large Animals:* * To achieve higher rate of conception in repeat breeding cases. * To achieve predictable results in the treatment of coli-mastitis and staphylococcal mastitis. *Other indications:* * Respiratory tract infection * Calf scours, enteritis and umbilical infection due to *E. coli* and Salmonella. *Small Animals:* * Infection of repiratory and urogenital tracts * Secondary bacterial infection associated with viral diseases viz. Distemper, Parvo virus etc. Post-surgical sepsis. *Poultry:* * Infection due to *E. coli* and Salmonella CRD and Bronchitis complicated by E. coli organisms. To prevent early chick mortality	*Preparation:* Dissolve the contents of the vial with 10 ml water for injection. 5-10 ml/100 kg b.w. by I/M. Repeat breeders : 5-10 ml deep i/u, 24 hrs post insemination Endometritis : 5-10 ml i/u Repeat after 24-48 hrs interval. Small animals : 0.1-0.2 ml/kg body weight. To prevent early chick mortality 1 gm to be dissolved in 300 ml of water to treat 600 chicks.	1 gm vial

Preparation	Indication	Dosage/Route	Presentation
MINAL FORTE Mineral mixture	Improves productivity, milk production, prevents infertility, protects from deprived appetite, helps digestion and prevents anorexia, ensures faster recovery.	Mixing rate : 1 kg Minal forte/100 kg of feed Daily dose : Adult animals : 28 gm Young animals : 5-15 gm	1 kg polybag.
MINTHAL (i) Minthal bolus 200 mg Albendazole 200 mg (ii) Minthal bolus 600 mg Albendazole 600 mg (iii) Minthal powder Albendazole 5% W/W (iv) Minthal Suspension Albendazole 2.5%W/V	Broad spectrum anthelmintic.	Worm dose : Sheep and goat : 5 mg/kg b.w. Cattle 7.5 mg/kg b.w. Fluke dose : Sheep and goat : 7.5 mg/kg b.w. Cattle : 15 mg/kg b.w.	Boluses : 200 mg & 600 mg Powder : 30 mg pouch and 300 gm container suspension : Bottle of 30 ml.
MOXEL Inj. Each 2.0 gm vial contains Amoxycillin Sodium 1 gm Cloxacillin Sodium 1 gm	Moxel inj. is indicated in severe infections.	5-10 mg/kg b.w. by i/m or i/v route.	Vial of 2 gm
RUMEN BOLUS Each bolus contains : Ferrous sulphate 1 gm Cobalt chloride 200 mg Copper Sulphate 50 mg Vit B_{12} 20 mcg Vit B_1 25 mg Yeast 300 mg	Restores rumino-reticular motality, ideal rumenotoric and restores appetite.	2 bolus twice daily orally for 3-5 days.	Strips of 5x4 boluses.
SHARKOFERROL Vet Each 15 ml contains Malt extract 4.52 gms, Saccharated iron oxide 1.8 gms, calcium gluconate 0.18 gm, Vit A 7,500 i.u., Vit D_3 600 i.u., Niacinamide 45 mg, Vit B_1 5 mg, Vit B_2 5 mg	*In Livestock :* * General debility * Under developed growth * Iron deficiency anaemia * Vitamin A deficiency * Rickets, osteomalacia, anorexia * Convalescence, pregnancy, milk fever, lactation, prolapse etc. *Poultry :* Stress conditions, proper feed utilization, growth & egg production, rickets, thin shelled eggs, vitamin deficiency, calcium deficiency etc.	By oral route: Calves, cattle and horses : 10 to 50 ml daily. Poultry : 20-60 ml/100 birds in water. Either alone or after mixing with jaggery or water. Similarly for dogs, Sharkoferrol Veterinary can be mixed with milk.	Bottle of 1 kg.

Preparation	Indication	Dosage/Route	Presentation
VETCORT Inj (Vet) Each ml contains : Dexamethasone Sodium phosphate equivalent to 4 mg of Dexamethasone Phosphate	Bovine ketosis, arthritis and related disorders. Allergic and dermtological conditions, anaphylactic shock, septic shock. Pregnancy toxaemia, inflammation of respiratory tract and urinogenital tract, local inflammatory condition etc.	By l/M or I/V Cattle and horses : 4 to 20 mg daily i.e. 1 to 5 ml daily. Calves, pig, sheep & goats : 2 to 4 mg daily. Dog and cat : 0.5-2 mg daily.	5 ml vial.
ZEET Inj. Each ml contains : Chlorpheniramine maleate 10 mg	Eczema, dermatitis, urticaria, insect bite, allergy, itching of unknown origin, rhinitis, anaphylactic shock, bloat, mastitis, pregnancy toxaemia, retained placenta etc.	L.A: 3-5 ml S.A. : 0.5-2 ml By I/M route:	Vial of 10 ml and 30 ml.

ALVED PHARMA & FOOD PVT. LTD.
No. 2, 21st Avenue, Ashok Nagar
CHENNAI - 600 083

Preparation	Indication	Dosage/Route	Presentation
Antibiotic/Antibacterials			
ALDAZIN Inj. Sulphamethoxypyridazine 250 mg/ml	To treat any bacterial infection.	I.M., S.C. or IV Livestock : 1 ml/10 kg body weight.	30 ml vial.
ALINCOMYCIN Inj Lincomycin as HCl. 20 mg/ml	Intrauterine or intramammary infusion against bacterial/mycoplasmal infection.	As infusion L.A.: 10-20 ml S.A.: 5-10 ml daily for 5 days.	30 ml vial.
ALINCOMYCIN - Vet. Inj. Lincomycin (as HCl.) 300 mg/ml	Against gram (+) bacteria and mycoplasma, useful in treating deep seated infection of bones, ears, skin etc.	By I.M. or I.V. L.A: 1 ml/30 kg b.w. S.A: 1 ml/15 kg b.w.	5 ml vial.
BACTRIDOX Inj. Sulphadoxine 200 mg Trimethoprim 40 mg in 1 ml	To treat a wide spectrum of bacterial infections.	By I.M., I.V. use in all animals 1 ml/10-15 kg b.w. Repeat only in chronic and obstinate cases.	30 ml vial.
BACTRISOL Inj. Sulphadiazine 400 mg Trimethoprim 80 mg in 1 ml	Against a wide range of systemic and local bacterial infections.	Deep I.M. Livestock: 3ml/100 kg body weight.	10 ml & 30 ml vial.
BACTRISOL BOLUS Sulphadiazine 1.0 gm Trimethoprim 0.2 gm in each bolus	Broad spectrum antibacterial useful in G.I. tract infections.	Oral 1 bolus for 40 kg body weight.	10 x 10's.
BACTRISOL Powder Trimethoprim 2% w/w Sulphadiazine 10% w/w	Broad spectrum antibacterial against primary and secondary bacterial infections.	Oral 1 gm/4 kg b.w.	100 gm, 250 gm and 1 kg.
BACTRISOL SUSPENSION Trimethoprim 80 mg, Sulphadiazine 400 mg in 1 ml.	Broad spectrum antibacterial against specific and non-specific bacterial infections.	Calf, sheep, goat 1 ml for 16 kg body weight.	100 ml, 1 litre.
GENTAMYCIN Inj. Gentamycin 40 mg/ml.	Broad spectrum antibiotic.	1 ml/ 25 to 50 kg b.w. IV or I.M.	30 ml vial.
OXYTETRACYCLINE Inj. Oxytetracycline Hydrochloride 50 mg/ml.	Broad spectrum antibiotic.	1-2 ml/ 25 kg b.w. by, IV, I.M., S.C. Route	30 ml vial.
Anthelmintics			
ALBONIL Powder Albendazole 5% w/w	Wide spectrum dewormer against nematode, cestode and flukes.	Round/tape worm : 1 gm/10 kg body weight. Flukes : 1 gm/5 kg b.w.	100 gm.
ALBONIL 150 Tab Albendazole 150 mg/tab.	Wide spectrum dewormer against nematode, cestode and flukes.	Round/tape worm : 1tab/30 kg body weight. Sheep and goat: 1 tab/20 kg body weight. Fluke - Double dosage.	10 x 10's.
CESTONIL Tab Praziquantel 50 mg/tab	Tapeworm infestation	1 tab/10 kg body weight at 6 weeks interval.	10 x 10's.

Preparation	Indication	Dosage/Route	Presentation
HELMONIL Soluble Powder Levamisole HCl. 30% w/w	Dewormer against all types and stages of nematodes.	Livestock: 1 gm/40 kg b.w.	250 gm & 100 gm.
HELMONIL-150 Tab. Levamisole - HCl 150 mg/tab	Broad spectrum dewormer against all types and stages of nematodes.	Livestock : 1 tab/20 kg b.w.	10 x 10's.
HELMONIL Inj. Each ml contains: Levamisole HCl 182 mg/ml.	Immunostimulant in viral infections, as an adjunct in chemotherapy. To prevent mastitis, metritis and calf mortality.	I.M. Inj. cattle : 1 ml/70 kg b.w. for 2-3 days; for pregnant cattle same dosage weekly once for 3 weeks before delivery.	10 ml & 30 ml.

Analgesics/Antipyretics/Corticosteroids

Preparation	Indication	Dosage/Route	Presentation
ALFENAC Inj. Diclofenac sod 25 mg/ml	Analgesic, anti-inflammatory and painful syndromes.	I.M. Inj. L.A: 6-12 ml. S.A: 1-3 ml.	100 x 3 ml amps.
ARTIZONE - S Inj. Each ml contains : Phenylbutazone 200 mg - Sodium salicylate 20 mg	Antipyretic, anti-inflammatory, Ephemeral fever, pyrexia, lameness, arthritis etc.	By slow I.V. or I.M. L.A: 10-20 ml/day for 3-5 days.	30 ml vial.
DEXAMETHASONE Sod. Phos. Inj. Each ml contains : Dexamethasone phosphate 4 mg/ml.	Corticosteroid therapy in ketosis, stress, as an anti-inflammatory agent.	Parenteral : L.A: 2.5 ml - 10 ml S.A: 0.5 to 1 ml. Intra-articular : L.A: 0.5 - 2 ml Periarticular : S.A. 0.25 - 1 ml.	10 ml vial.

Others

Preparation	Indication	Dosage/Route	Presentation
CYCLOMIN - 7 Bolus Slow release preparation containing Co, I, Zn, Mn, Cu, Fe & Se.	Trace mineral supplement for improving breeding efficiency.	1 bolus once a week.	10 x 10's.
KETONEX Bolus Each bolus contains : Nicotinic Acid 1.5 gm, Dried yeast 1.5 gm, Sodium Hyd, Phos. 0.375 gm.	Rumen tonic to correct metabolic disorders and anorexia.	Livestock : 1-2 bolus bid Sheep and goat : 1/2 bolus bid Ketosis (Prevention) - 1/2 Bolus bid x 10 days	10 x 10's.
KETONEX Powder Nicotinic acid 24% w/w Dried Yeast 24% w/w Sodium Acid Phosphate 6% w/w	- do -	L.A: 20-25 gm daily, S.A: 5-10 gm. To prevent and control ketosis 30 gm/day for 10 days before and after parturition.	50 gm & 250 gm.
LACTIVET Powder	Phosphorus enriched vitamin mineral supplement to boost lactation.	20-30 gm/day	2.5 kg, 500 gm.
NUROVET Inj. Each ml contains : Vit B_1 33 mg, Vit B_6 33 mg, Vit B_{12} 333 mcg.	Anorexia, vomiting, diarrhoea, fatigue and general debility, anaemia, neurological disorders.	Deep I.M. Cattle/Horse/Camel/ Pig : 5 ml- 10 ml Calves/Sheep/goat : 2- 5 ml.	10 ml.

ANICHEM INDIA LTD.
16/A, Dutt Vihar Society, Race Course
BARODA - 390 007

Preparation	Indication	Dosage/Route	Presentation
BROLAY GRAND (Poultry Feed Supplement) Contains Vitamins & Minirals	Increases body weight, thin shell egg production is checked. Improves growth.	Mix 2.5 kg brolay grand per tonn of poultry feed.	10 kg.
LIVTONE (Herbal Poultry feed supplement)	Liver booster, better growth and production, provide dietary safe guards to liver against afla toxins, restore normalcy in the reduced feed intake.	Poultry : 2.5 Kg Livtone per tonn of feed with complete mixing.	2 kg
ROBUST (Poultry feed supplement) each 5 ml contains- Calcium 100 mg Phosphorus 50 mg Vit D_3 400 Iu Vit B_{12} 5 mcg Vit B_6 0.62 mg Biotin 4 mcg Lysine 3 mg Methionine 3 mg.	For complete bone growth and weight gain in broilers.	Chicks: 20 ml per 100 birds. Growers : 50 ml per 100 birds. Layers : 100 ml per 100 birds.	5 litre jar.
STRESVIN (Herbal Poultry feed supplement)	Recommended in stressful conditions like vaccination, debeaking, transportation, cage fatique, over crowding, abrupt change in climate or feed, to overcome peak production.	Chicks : 5 gm/1000 birds per day. Growers, layers and broilers : 10 gm/1000 birds per day.	10 gm & 100 gm packs.

ANIMAL RESEARCH CENTRE (A.R.C)
44, New Colony
JAIPUR - 302 001

Preparation	Indication	Dosage/Route	Presentation
ASPUL (astringent powder)	Diarrhoea, dysentery.	*Oral* Cattle & horses : 25-40 gms. Calves, colts, sheep, goat: 10-15 gms. Camel: 60-100 gms.	100 gm and 1 kg pack.
AYANA (dressing oil for pains etc.)	Yoke gall, horn cancer, swelling of udder, primary stage of mastitis, all sorts of pain and sprain.	Topical application	100 ml and 500 ml bottle.
CAFON (Cough & Cold powder)	Respiratory problems : pneumonia, bronchitis, pharyngitis, anti-inflammatory, expectorant.	*Oral as electuary* Cattle : 25-40 gms - Calves & colts : 10- 15 gms - Sheep and Goat : 15-20 gms. Camel: 80-100 gms.	100 gm and 1 kg pack.
CHARMALA (Skin ointment)	Eczema, scabies, tail gangrene, dagnala and other skin diseases.	*Topically* Rub for 10 days on alternate days. For tail gangrene rub after every two or three days for a month.	100 gms pack.
IRON COPPER COBALT Capsule: Each capsule contains : Copper Sulphate 0.5 gm, Cobalt chloride 0.5 gm Ferrous Sulphate 0.5 gm	Indigestion, irregular heat, late maturity, blood deficiency, diarrhoea, loss of appetite.	*Oral* L.A: 2 Cap daily for 10 days. S.A: 1Cap daily for 10 days	20 Capsules and 100 Capsules pack.
LIVOTONIC (Liver Tonic)	Damaged liver, hepatitis, jaundice, chronic fever, oedema, ascites.	*Oral* Cow, buffalo, horse: 10-15 gms. Calves, heifer, pig : 5-7 gms. Sheep and Goat: 3-5 gms Poultry: 1% mixed with feed.	1 kg and 100 gms pack.
NAVNID (Mineral mixture)	Loss of normal health, anorexia, decreased productivity, deficiency of trace elements.	*Oral* L.A: 50 gms in feed, daily S.A: 20 gms in feed, daily.	1 kg and 25 kg pack.
NAVNID HERBAL Salt bricks (with mineral, urea and molasses)	Deficiency of trace elements, pica.	Put the brick in the manger or hang with the help of a rod or stick so that it can lick easily.	2 kg pack.
NEUTEX (anti-tympany)	Gaseous, frothy tympanitis.	*Oral or intra-ruminal* Large animals: 100 ml. Small animals: 50 ml. Goats/Pig: 25 ml.	100 ml botttle.
PASHU PACHAN (Stomachic and tonic powder)	Anorexia, listlessness, off feed, indigestion, loss of milk yield, atony of rumen, sore mouth, constipation, distension of stomach, gas formation.	Oral with gur or concentrate Cow & buffalo : 50 gms. Horses & mules : 40 gms - Camel and Elephant : 100 gms. Colt, sheep, goat: 10 gms.	100 gms , 200 gms , 400 gms and 1 kg pack.

Preparation	Indication	Dosage/Route	Presentation
RAJANA (Oestrus inducer)	Anoestrus, irregular oestrus, non-functional ovary, delayed maturity.	*Orally with gur in bolus form* Cow, buffalo, mare, heifer : 3 cap Sheep & Goats: 2 cap, for 3 days.	6 capsules and 2 capsules pack.
SONEX (broad spectrum anthelmintic)	Roundworms, hookworms, tape worms, threadworms, whip-worms etc. Copper deficiency, improve wool texture, irregular heat.	*Drench in water* Poultry : 0.5-1 gm. Sheep, goat, pig, calf: 2-5 gms. Cow, buffalo, horse : 10-20 gms. Camel : 30-50 gms.	20 gms, 100 gms 500 gms pack.
TYMPAN (Anti-bloat powder)	Bloat	Cow, buffalo, horse : 50 gms. Calves, colts, heifers : 25 gms. Sheep and goat : 10-15 gms.	100 gm, 1 kg.
UTOP (Uterotonic powder)	Retained placenta.	Sheep and goat : 40 gms. Large animals : 100-200 gms.	100 gms, 1 kg.

ANUJA PHARMACEUTICALS
5, Rajmahal Shopping Centre, Mathura Das Vasanji Road
Andheri (East), MUMBAI-400 069

Perparation	Indication	Dosage/Route	Presentation
ACTI-LIV FORTE Each gm has : Kadu 90 mg, Kalmegh 220 mg, Bhrungraj 170 mg, Bandal 5 mg, Punaranava 180 mg, Arjun 165 mg, Bhumiamalki 170 mg	Effective in cirrhosis of liver, inappetance, loss of vigour, vitality, weight and RBC and corrects constipation.	Cow, buffalo, horse and adult Pig : 10-14 gm orally Sheep/goat : 5 gm orally Dog/cat/piglet : 2-3 gm orally Poultry : 1-2 gm orally.	100 gm.
BRONTO Each gm has: Bhiringni 200 mg, Calamus Indicus 100 mg, Tyestimadha 200 mg, Vasa 300 mg, Pure Yavashar 100 mg, Somalata 100 mg	Coryza, nasal catarrh, colds, moist cough, whooping cough, bronchitis, pneumonia, influenza and chronic eosinophilia, contraindicated in dry cough.	Cattle/buffalo/horse/adult pig : 10-14 gm orally. Sheep/goat : 3-5 gm. dog/cat/piglets : 2-3 gm Poultry : 1-2 gm.	100 gm.
DIGESTONE Each gm has : Harda 300 mg, Chitrak 150 mg, Sunth 75 mg, Shank Bhasma 75 mg Triphala 150 mg, Kali Mirch 50 mg, Vidanga 100 mg, Gulvel 100 mg	Indigestion, inappetance and other digestive disorders in livestock and poultry.	Cow/buffalo/horse/adult pig : 10-14 gm. Sheep/goat : 5 gm Dog/cat/piglet : 2-3 gm Poultry : 1-2 gm orally daily.	100 gm.
GRITONA Each gm has : Dil 200 mg, Ajovan 200 mg, Nutmeg 50 mg, Kakchai 200 mg, Harda 200 mg, Ashwagandha 150 mg	Carminative and digestive powder, useful in bloat, dyspepsia, other digestive disorders, tympany, emphysema and impaction, contraindicated in diarrhoea and bleeding.	Cattle/buffalo/horse/adult Pig : 10-14 gm orally. Sheep/goat : 5 gm Dog/cat and piglets : 2-3 gm Poultry : 1-2 gm.	100 gm.
INTOKAM Each gm has : Indrajav 300 mg, Belfal 300 mg Kadachhal 300 mg, Nagarmotha 100 mg	Diarrhoea and dysentery in livestock.	Cattle/buffalo/horse/adult Pig : 10-14 gm. orally. Sheep/goat: 5 gm Dog/cat/piglets: 2-3 gm. Poultry: 1-2 gm	100 gm.
L-TONA Each gm has : Ashoka 330 mg, Lodhra 330 mg, Dhakti flowers 200 mg, Nagkesar 70 mg, Ulatkambal 70 mg	Leukorrhoea, acts as uterine sedative and nervine tonic in livestock. Effective in urinary calculi.	Cattle/buffalo/horse/adult pig : 10-14 gm orally. Sheep/goat: 5 gm, Dog/cat/piglet: 2-3 gm.	100 gm.

Preparation	Indication	Dosage/Route	Presentation
MILKOTONE Each gm has : Shatavari 350 mg, Jeavanti 200 mg, Ashwagandha 100 mg, Kavach 150 mg, Vidari 20	Gives vitality, increases milk yield, used as general tonic in debility for the regain of health and vigour.	Cow/buffalo/horse : 10-14 gm orally daily. Sheep/goat/pigs : 5 gm. Dog/cat/piglet : 2-3 gm Poultry : 1-2 gm.	100 gm.
WORMAHAL Each gm has : Vidanga seeds 400 mg, Kalijeeri 200 mg, Palasa seeds 400 mg	Effective against roundworms, whipworms, hookworms and tapeworms and their allied symptoms like colic, anorexia weakness, oedema etc.	Cattle/buffalo/horse/adult pig: 10-14 gm orally. Sheep/goat : 5 gm Dog/cat/piglets : 2-3 gm Poultry : 1-2 gm.	100 gm.

AREX LABORATORIES PVT. LTD.
Botawala Building, 21 Sitla Devi Temple Road
Mahim, MUMBAI-400 016

Preparation	Indication	Dosage/Route	Presentation
BONY VET Contains : Calcium along with Vit A, D and B$_{12}$	For normal growth in pups, to improve appetite and to remove calcium deficiency.	Pups : 1 tsf bid orally Dog : 2-3 tsf bid orally.	100 ml and 450 ml bottle.
DIMDIM LIQUID Contains : 16% sulfadimidine sodium	Caecal and intestinal coccidiosis in poultry.	Add water upto mark and add 8-10 ml per litre of drinking water or 100 ml/8 kg feed for 3 days. Repeat 2 days later for 3 days.	100 ml and 450 ml.
FERTIVET Each tab has : Cis-clomiphene citrate 180 mg. Trans-Clomiphene citrate 120 mg	Corrects delayed puberty in heifer, anestrus, repeat breeding, inactive gonads, oestrus synchronisation in cows, ovulation in mares and super ovulation in sows.	Anoestrus : 1 mg/kg b wt. for 5 days orally. Non-ovulatory oestrus/Repeat breeding : 1.5 mg/kg b.wt. for 3 days by dissolving in water, orally. Precaution — Before fertivet administration, close rumino- reticular groove by drenching 1% copper sulphate solution.	5 tabs.
FLUKIN Contains : 100 mg Hexachlorophene per tab	Liverfluke infestation in sheep and goats.	Adult sheep and goat : 1-2 tabs orally or 10-15 mg/kg b.w. Lambs : 1/2 tab orally. Repeat 1 day later if needed. Give at weekly interval in divided doses in debilitated animals.	50 tabs.
FLUKIN FORTE Contains : 1 g Hexachlorophene per tab	Paramphistomiasis and liverfluke infestation in cattle and buffaloes.	Cattle and Buffalo : 1-2 tab preferably at 4 months interval. Calves : 1/2 tab. Debilitated animals should be given in two divided doses at one week interval.	50 tabs.
MOVIROM Each tab has : Antimony Potassium tartrate 2 g, Ferrous sulphate 2 g	Ruminal atony, indigestion due to impaction and loss of appetite.	Cattle/buffalo: 2-3 tabs daily for 2-3 days. Sheep/Goats: 1/2 tab for 2 days. Provide sufficient water during treatment.	50 tabs.
PIPIROCID LIQUID Piperazine hexahydrate equivalent to 0.82 g piperazine per 5 ml	Roundworms of livestock and poultry, nodular worms of swine and pinworms and strongylosis in horses.	Cattle/buffalo: 15-30 ml/50 kg b. wt. Horses : 15 ml/30 kg b.wt. Swine : 15 ml/25 kg b. wt. Calves : 5 ml /10 kg b.wt. Dog/cat : 2.5 ml/10 kg b. wt. Poultry : 4-6 weeks age: 30 ml/100 birds in 3-4 litres of water. Over 6 weeks :- 60 ml/100 birds in drinking water.	100 ml 450 ml 4.5 litres.

Preparation	Indication	Dosage/Route	Presentation
PIVIPOL (Sol.) Pivipol wash solutions has : 1% W/V Povidone iodine. Pivipol Forte Solution has 10% W/V Povidone iodine.	General antiseptic, mastitis, metritis, vaginitis, trichomoniasis, as a bath to pets for skin affections, as a substitute for Lugol's iodine.	Apply twice or thrice daily after cleaning the area. Pivipol forte should be diluted 10 times for mucosa but can be used directly on the skin.	Pivipol wash solution 10 ml Pivipol Forte 50 ml.
POLMIX-B Powder Contains : Clomiphene citrate along with calcium and phosphorus	For hypothalamo-pituitary stimulation and additional weight gain for broiler.	2 g/10 kg broiler mash at 5th and 6th week age.	10 g, 100g.
POLMIX-L Contains: Clomiphene citrate	For hypothalamo-pituitary axis stimulation and increased egg production in layers.	2 g/10 kg of layers feed at 30th to 31st week of age.	10 g, 100g.
SULFADIMIDINE Each tab has : 5 g sulfadimidine	Broad spectrum chemotherapeutic agents effective against gram positive and gram negative bacteria, and protozoa.	L.A. : 2 tab/50 kg b. wt. Ist day and then 1 tab/50 kg b.wt. daily for 3-4 days SA : 1 g/5 kg b.wt. Ist day followed by 1/2 g/5 kg b.wt. daily for 3-4 days.	10 tabs 50 tabs.
THIABENDAZOLE Solution Each 10 ml has : 1.33 g Thiabendazole	Effective on both mature and immature roundworms, stomachworm and intestinal worms of livestock.	Cattle/buffalo : 66-110 mg Thiabendazole/kg b.wt. Sheep/goat : 44-66 mg Thiabendazole/kg b.wt. Pig : 50 mg Thiabendazole/kg b.wt. Repeat the treatment 14-21 days later.	450 ml bottle.
THIABENDAZOLE (Bolus/Tab) Bolus has 2 g Thiabendazole; Tablet has 500 mg Thiabendazole	Useful in roundworm, stomach worm and intestinal worms and lungworms of calves, sheep and goats.	Calves : 60-100 mg/kg b.wt. Sheep/goat : 40-60 mg/kg b.wt. Lungworm : 88 & mg/kg b.wt. Lambs/kids : 1/2-1 bolus Ewes (over 25 kg): 1-1/2 bolus Rams/bucks (over 50 kg): 1-1 1/2 bolus Repeat the treatment 14-21 days later.	50 bolus 100 tab.
THIABENDAZOLE PRE-MIX Each 100 g provides : 33.33 g of Thiabendazole	Gastrointestinal roundworms infestation in livestock.	All animals 50-100 mg Premix/kg b.wt. Repeat 21 days later.	250 g, 1 kg.

ARIES AGRO-VET INDUSTRIES PVT. LTD.
Aries House, Plot No. 24
Deonar Govandi (East), MUMBAI-400 043

Preparation	Indication	Dosage/Route	Presentation
ARIES M.M. (Mineral feed supplement for cattle with salt or without salt) Contains : Ca, P, NaCl, Fe, I$_2$, Cu, Mn, Co.	A complete mineral mixture for cattle and buffaloes for regular use.	With feed. Mix @ 1 kg (with salt)/100 kg feed and 0.7 kg (without salt)/100 kg feed. Adult cattle and buffaloes: 28 g daily.	1 kg 50 kg pack.
ARIES M.M. (Mineral feed supplement for poultry with salt or without salt). Contains: Ca, P, Cu, Co, Mn, I$_2$, Zn, Fe, Mg, NaCl.	A complete mineral mixture for poultry.	*With feed* Mix. @ 2.5 kg (with salt)/100 kg and 2 kg (without salt)/100 kg poultry feed and use daily or 28 g/100 birds daily.	50 kg pack.
ARIES POULTRY CON-CENTRATE Contains : essential amino acids, such as L-Lysine and DL-methionine, animal proteins, Vitamin A, Vitamin B$_2$, Vitamin D$_3$, Vitamin K, Vitamin B$_{12}$, anti-oxidants, anti-aflatoxins, flavouring agent, coccidiostat, anti-bacterials.	Feed supplement for poultry.	Mix @ 50 kg/500 kg of poultry feed and give daily.	50 kg bag.
BOON-O-MILK Contains : non-hormonal galactagogues.	Improves milk yield, better fat and breeding efficiency. Controls milk fever.	*Orally or with feed :* Cattle and buffaloes : 15 g daily for 15 days or 500 g/100 kg feed.	450 g/1 kg. jar.
CATTLEMIN (with salt or without salt) Contains _ Ca, P, NaCl, Fe, I$_2$, Cu, Mn, Co, F$_2$, Zn, Acid Soluble Ash.	Complete mineral mixture for dairy animals for optimum production.	*Orally or with feed* Cattle and buffaloes : 30 g with salt or 20 g. without salt, daily. *with feed:-* 1% (with salt) and 0.7% (without salt).	1 kg, 50 kg.
DOT Dinitro-ortho-toluamide (Vet) 25%	The best coccidiostat with very pronounced activity against *E. tenella* and *E. nicatrix.* Also protects other micro-nutrients of the finished ration.	500 g/ton poultry feed for regular use.	Pack of 500 gm and 1 kg jars.

Preparation	Indication	Dosage/Route	Presentation
FORMULA - 100 Each kg contains : Vitamin B_{12}-100 mcg	Improves weight gains and feed efficiency in poultry, pigs, and calves. Increases egg production in poultry.	*With feed* For broilers : 220 g/ton feed *Layers*: 100 g/ton of feed *Breeders*: 150 g/ton of feed *Turkeys*: 220 g/ton of feed *Baby pigs*: 450 g/ton of feed, *Suckling pigs*: 370 g/ton of feed *calves*: 150 g per ton of feed.	1 kg, 5 kg.
LYOMIX Contains : L-Lysine HCl	For balanced lysine level in feed, makes ingredients suitable for poultry consumption which are unfit for human.	*With feed*: *Layers*: 0.5% lysine requirement. *Broilers*: 0.3% lysine requirement. Add 100 g/ton of poultry feed.	100 g.
METHIOMIX DL- Methionine	Improves growth rate and egg production in poultry and pigs.	*With feed* Normally starter feed should contain 0.4%, Grower feed -0.35%, Layer feed -0.3% of DL- Methionine. Add 100 g/ton feed.	100 g.
POULTRYMIN Contains : Ca, P, Mn, I_2, Zn, F, Cu, Fe.	Mineral and trace element supplement for poultry.	1 kg/50 kg poultry mash.	1 kg, 50 kg.
PROT-O-LIV. Contains : per kg Protein - 58% Fibre - 1.32% Metabolizable energy - 3000 kcal	Provides high quality animal proteins containing essential amino acids, improves growth as well as production in poultry.	With feed.	
TRACEMIN Contrains: Ca, Cu, Co, Mn, I_2, Fe, Zn (in poultry ration)	Trace mineral supplement for cattle and poultry for optimum health and production.	*Mixing rate - For cattle and Buffaloes:*- 1 kg Tracemin + 9 kg bone meal or dicalcium phosphate/ton cattle feed. *Poultry :*- 1 kg Tracemin + 10 kg bone meal + 5 kg common salt + 9 kg limestone powder/ton poultry feed.	1 kg.

BADRI BIOLOGICALS PVT. LTD.
C-261/3, Rajendra Nagar
BAREILLY

Preparation	Indication	Dosage/Route	Presentation
HERBAL-BLOAT Liq. (Antizymotic and surfactant)	Gaseous and frothy tympany, impaction and colic.	Cattle & buffalo : 100 ml orally. Horse & dunkey : 50 ml orally. Calves, sheep and goat : 25 ml orally. To be administered with lukewarm water.	100 ml 450 ml.
HERBAL-DIARINA (Antidiarrhoeals)	Gastroenteritis, dysentery and diarrhoea.	Cattle & buffalo: 30-50 gm bid orally. Calves, sheep & goat : 10-15 gm bid orally. Administered with rice gruel.	1 kg.
HERBAL DOG SHAMPOO (Skin & hair tonic)	Skin and hair tonic, protects against ectoparasites.	Wet the hair coat, rub with sufficient quantity of shampoo, leave for 10-15 minutes & then wash with clean water.	100 ml.
HERBOGYNE Capsule (Heat inducer)	Anestrus condition, silent and irregular heat and anovulatory heat.	Cattle & buffalo : Ist day-5 caps, IInd day-4 caps. IIIrd day- 3 caps. To be given with gur.	Packs of 500 & 100 capsules.
HERBOGYNE Liquid (Ecbolic and cleansing draught)	Retained placenta, uterine inertia, perpural uterine infection, pyometra, anestrus, weak and irregular heat, as cleansing draught after calving, also in case of incomplete let down of milk.	Cattle & buffalo: Retained placenta: 100 ml bid for 4 days. Cleansing draught : 100 ml bid x 4 days. Anestrus and uterine infection : 50 ml daily for 4 days. Mares : half of the dose of cattle. to be administered with enough lukewarm water.	4.5 Litres.
HERBALKAL-C Syrup (Vitaminised calcium syrup)	Hypocalcemia, rickets, osteoporosis, maintenance of normal calcium levels during lactation & as a general tonic.	Cattle & buffalo : 100 ml bid x 2-3 days ; 450 ml as single dose in acute deficiency. Calves, sheep & goat : 25 ml bid for 3-6 days. Dogs: 10 ml bid.	450 ml, 4.5 Litres
HERBALKOF Powder	Cough due to pneumonia and other pulmonary diseases, lungworm infestation, common exposure due to cold etc.	Cattle & buffalo : 30-40 gm Horses & mules : 20-30 gm Sheep & goats: 10-15 gm To be given as electuary, twice daily.	1 kg.
HERBALTIK-CATTLE Powder (Ectoparasiticidal)	Infestation of ticks, mites, lice & fleas.	Apply the dry powder on the body with the help of clean cloth and rub it. Bath the animal after 7 days.	100 gm, 500 gm.
HERBALTIK-DOG Powder (Ectoparasiticidal)	Infestation of ticks, mites, lice & fleas.	Apply the dry powder on the body with the help of clean cloth	

Preparation	Indication	Dosage/Route	Presentation
		and rub it. Bath the animal after 7 days.	100 gm.
HERBAL-SCAB Lotion. (Multipurpose skin disease lotion)	Mange, ringworm, specific & nonspecific dermatitis.	Clean the lesion and apply lotion with a piece of cloth/cotton. The application may be repeated after 2-3 days, if required.	100 ml, 450 ml.
HERBOTONE (Stomachic and general tonic)	Depraved appetite, indigestion, atony of rumen and constipation.	Cattle & buffalo : 40-50 gm. Calves, sheep, goat: 15-30 gm. Horse : 30-50 gm. To be administered in warm water or in molasses twice a day.	400 gm, 1 kg.

BAIF LABORATORIES

Briahnagar, Off Nagar Road, WAGHOLI - 412 207, Dist. PUNE

Preparation	Indication	Dosage/Route	Presentation
ADRENALINE Each ml. contains: Adrenaline Acid Tartarate 1.8 mg	Effective sympathomimetic therapy.	Horse/cattle: 8-16 µg/kg b.wt. Dog : 10-30 µg/kg. body weight Route S.C. or I.M.	10 ml vial.
ALBENZOLE Contains: Powder 15% : 150 mg albendazole per gram Suspension 2.5%: 25 mg albendazole per ml, Bolus: 600 mg albendazole	Effective dewormer against several species of parasites in animals.	Cattle/buffaloes: 50 mg/10kg b.wt. Sheep, goat, pig: 50 mg/10 kg b.wt. Dogs: 50 mg/3.5 kg b.wt. Poultry (Powder): 255-375 mg/100 birds. Liver Fluke : Cattle, buffaloes : 50 mg/5kg b.wt. Sheep, goat: 50 mg/6.6 kg b.wt.	Powder: 50 gm, 250 gm Suspension: 30 ml, 500 ml Bolus : 600 mg.
AMNOVIT Contains : vit A, D_3, E, B_2, B_6, B_{12}, K, Niacinamide, calcium pantothenate, folic acid, choline chloride, L Lysine, L-Methionine, L-Tryptophane.	Stimulates milk production, enhances fat content in milk, increases disease resistance, prevents chick mortality, improves growth rate, checks abnormal oestrous period in cattle resulting in better fertility.	10 gm. per 25 litre of drinking water.	200 gm and 1 kg.
ASCOPLEX Each ml contains: Thiamine hydrochloride 35 mg Riboflavine 0.5 mg Pyridoxine hydrochloride 7 mg, Niacinamide 23 mg. Ascorbic acid 70 mg	Concentrated vitamins (B+C) Inj. Adjunctive therapy with antibiotics and post-operative condition. Cerebro-cortical necrosis. Bacterial toxaemia, ketosis, fodder poisoning, liver damage, restores the animal to normal after prolonged exertion.	Cattle/horses: 20-30 ml. Calves, foals, sheep: 5-10 ml. Dogs over 15 kg: 5-10 ml. Dogs below 15 kg and cats: 5 ml (IM route).	10 ml vial.
ATROPINE Each ml contains: Atropine sulphate 1.0 mg	Partial antidote in organo-phosphorus poisoning.	Horse/cattle: 30-60 µg/kg b.wt. Pig: 20-40 µg/kg b.wt. Dog/cat: 30-100 µg/kg b.wt. Route - S.C.	10 ml vial.
BAIFIDINE Bolus Each bolus contains: Sulphadimidine 5 gm.	In treatment of H.S., Foot-rot, Mastitis, Metritis, Pneumonia, calf-scour, calf-diptheria, secondary bacterial complications associated with RP, and wound infections.	200 mg/kg body weight for all species i.e. 2 bolus/50 kg b.w. followed by half the dose daily oral or intrauterine.	5 gm. bolus available in containers of 10 and 50 bolus.
BAIFIDINE Inj. Each 100 ml contains: Sulphadimidine sodium 33.3 gm.	Treatment of calf pneumonia, calf-scours, intestinal infections, foot-rot and septicaemia.	For all species initial dose 0.2 gm. per Kg b.wt. Maintenance dose 0.1 gm per kg. body weight. Route I.V./S.C./I.P.	100 ml vials.

Preparation	Indication	Dosage/Route	Presentation
BAIFOCAL Each 100 ml contains : Cal. gluconate 20.8 g Boric Acid 4.2 g	To overcome milk fever syndrome. Quickly recovers from hypocalcaemia. Efficiently restores normal calcium levels.	Cattle & buffaloes: 200-350 ml. Sheep, goats & pigs: 50-75 ml Dogs: 2-3 ml I/V or SC route.	450 ml bottle.
BAIFOLPLEX Each ml contains: Thiamine hydrochloride (B$_1$) 50 mg, Cyanocobalamin 350 mcg, Pyridoxine hydrochloride 35 mg	Treats vit. B. complex deficiency syndromes. Nervous disorders. Cerebro-cortical necrosis. Anaemia. Acute Ketosis. Sress conditions.	Horses/cattle: 10-15 ml Sheep/goat: 3-5 ml. Dogs: 1-2 ml (IM/SC route).	10 ml vials.
BAIFOMISOLE Each 100 ml contains: Levamisole 15.0 gm.	Broad spectrum anthelmintic injection. Active against adult and larval gastrointestinal nematodes, lungworms. Acts as immunostimulant in poultry and livestock.	Cattle/sheep/goat/Pig: 7.5 mg per kg body weight. As immunostimulator: Poultry 0.75 mg/kg body weight by IM or SC route 1.5 mg/kg body weight by drinking water.	10 ml, 30 ml and 100 ml packings.
BAIFOVIL Each ml contains: Chlorpheniramine maleate 22.75 mg.	Allergic reactions & anaphylactic shocks, congestion of lungs and brain, pulmonary oedema, urticaria, eczema and dermatitis.	Large animals: 10 ml. Small Animals: 5 ml. Route - I.M.	10 ml vials.
BICORAL Each 25 ml contains: Vit B$_2$, B$_6$, B$_{12}$, Biotin, Pantothenyl alcohol, Niacinamide, L-Lysine, L-Methionine	Used as feed supplement for livestock and poultry to increase growth rate, weight gain, optimises feed conversion, to improve disease resistance, to overcome stress conditions, in poultry to improve egg-production, growth rate, weight gain, to prevent curled toe paralysis, perosis, fatty liver and kidney syndrome, enhances hatchability.	Cattle/buffalo/horse: 100 ml/animal. Calf/sheep/goat: 50 ml/animal Poultry: 25 ml/100 birds Dog: 10-25 ml/animal.	500 ml and 5 litre.
BICORAL Forte	Same as above.	Cattle/buffalo/horse : 20ml/animal. Calf/sheep/goat: 10ml/animal Poultry: 5 ml/100 birds. Dog: 2-5 ml/animal.	1 litre and 2.5 litre.
CABCODEX Each 100 ml contains: Cal. gluconate 20.0g Boric acid 3.6 g, Magnesium hypophosphite 3.25 g Dextrose anhydrous 20.0 g	Milk fever syndrome complicated by low levels of magnesium and phosphorus. Helps recovery from concurrent acetonaemia Meets increased sugar needs	Cattle & buffaloes: 200-350 ml Sheep: 25-75 ml IV/SC route.	450 ml bottles.

Preparation	Indication	Dosage/Route	Presentation
CALBOMAX Each 100 contains: Cal. gluconate 20.0 g, Boric acid 3.6 g, Magnesium hypophosphite 3.25 g	Treats milk fever syndrome Hypocalcaemia Hypomagnesaemia Hypophosphataemia.	Cattle & buffalo: 200-350 ml Sheep, goat & pigs : 25-75 ml IV/SC route.	450 ml bottles.
CLOXACILLIN Each tube contains : Cloxacillin 200 mg Quick release base Q.S.	Effective control of bovine mastitis during lactation.	Infuse one tube into each infected quarter by gently emptying contents of the tube into the teat canal. Repeat the treatment for two more days.	3 g collapsible tubes.
CLOXAMPICILLIN Each tube contains: Cloxacillin sod. 200 mg, Ampicilin sod. 75 mg, Quick release base Q.S.	Therapy for bovine mastitis. Broad spectrum bactericidal against major causative organisms.	Infuse one tube into each affected quarter after complete milking once every 24 hrs till the affected quarter and milk appear normal.	3 g collapsible tubes.
CYANOPLEX Thiamine hydrochloride, Riboflavin, Pyridoxine hydrochloride, Niacinamide, B_{12}, Liver extract.	Prevents & treats B complex deficiency, anaemia, anorexia, impaired metabolism, stunted growth, debility; supportive therapy in parasitic infestations, bacterial and viral infections.	LA: 10 ml/day for 3 or more days IM or deep S.C. route SA: 1-2 ml/day I/M.	10 ml vials.
DEXTROSE Inj. 20% 100 ml contains: Dextrose anhydrous 20 g	An important nutritional supportive therapy. In case of hypoglycaemia, ketosis, acetonemia & pregnancy toxaemia.	Cattle : 400-450 ml Calves : 50 ml Piglet : 4 ml Dogs : 10-50 ml (I.V. route).	500 ml bottles.
FUREX - 20 100 gm. contains: Furazolidone 20 gm	Improves egg production in layers, increases weight gain in broilers, enhances disease resistance, reduces chicks mortality, encourages hatchability.	Mix 25 g furex - 20 per 100 kg of feed.	1 kg.
LIGNOCAINE Each ml contains: Lignocaine HCl 21.3 mg Sodium chloride 6 mg	Fast acting local anaesthetic, blocks paravertebral and regional nerves.	Horse/bovine: upto 200 ml Sheep/goat/pig: 60 ml. Dog: 25-50 ml. Cat: 5ml Route S.C. Paravertebral anaesthesia in bovines: 7 ml in each nerve route, caesarean & abdominal surgery: 40-50 ml S.C.; nerve block in canine 1-2 ml.	30ml and 100 ml vials.

Preparation	Indication	Dosage/Route	Presentation
SULTRIMAX Bolus Each bolus contains : Sulphadiazine 1.00 gm Trimethoprim 0.20 gm	In treatment of enteritis, neonatal septicaemia, diarrhoea, acute undifferentiated diarrhoea of calves, peritonitis, acute mastitis, metritis, pyometra, systemic nephritis, pyrexia, undifferentiated pneumonia of calves & pigs.	Large animals : 2-4 bolus daily Small animals : 1-2 bolus daily oral or intrauterine.	1.2 gm bolus in containers of 4 and 10 bolus.
SULTRIMAX Inj. (I/M) Each ml contains: Sulphadiazine sod. 400 mg. Trimethoprim 80 mg	Therapy for infections of respiratory tract, urinary tract, alimentary tract, genital tract, skin, joints and wounds.	For all species Sulphadiazine 12.5 mg Trimethoprim 2.5 mg per kg body weight daily for five days I/M.	10 ml, 30 ml and 100 ml vials.
SULTRIMAX-S Inj. (I/V) Each ml contains: Sulphadiazine 200 mg Trimethoprim 40 mg	Same as above.	Same as above, I/V.	30 ml, 100 ml vials.
VIMICON Contains: Vit A, D_3, E, B_2, B_{12}, Vit K, Niacinamide, choline chloride, calcium pantothenate, calcium, phosphorus, manganese, iodine, iron, zinc, copper, cobalt.	Helps in overcoming stress condition. Improves feed conversion, egg production, egg shell quality with reduced convalescent period after illness.	Mixing rate per 100 kg feed Poultry: starter, finisher and breeder: 500 gm, Growers/layer: 250 gm Cattle/horse/sheep/goat/pigs: 250 gm. Pig starter: 500 gm.	250 gm. and 2.5 kg.
VITADEC Contains: Vit A, D_3, E and Vit C	Water miscible formulation for overcoming stress condition, increasing disease resistance. Promoting growth & fertility, improves egg shell quality.	Cattle/buffalo: 10-15 ml/animal Calf/sheep/goat:5-10 ml/animal Poultry: 2-5ml/100 birds. Treat for a week. Administer daily in drinking water.	500 ml and 1 litre.

BALLOUN PHARMACEUTICALS
Bharath Illam, Tirunagar,
MADURI-625 006

Preparation	Indication	Dosage/Route	Presentation
ANTHELMET Powder Contains: Tetramisole HCl 30% w/w	For nematodal infection of gastrointestinal as well as respiratory tract.	Cattle/buffalo : 150 mg/100 kg b.wt. as drench. Sheep: 15 mg/kg b. wt as drench.	100 g bottle.
BALL DRESSING Contains : Boric acid, Zinc oxide, Acriflavin, Copper sulfate, Oleum Margosa, Yellow soft Paraffin.	Antiseptic wound dressing after castration and dehorning, prevents ulcers and maggot infestation.	Local application.	450 g bottle.
BALLEX Powder Contains: Extractum Belladona Sicum 6% w/w, Camphor 1.8% w/w, Pot. iodide 0.9% w/w, Ammon. Chloride 31%w/w Glycerrhiza 36% w/w.	Acute or chronic bronchitis, spasmodic cough and other respiratory disorders.	Cattle/buffalo/horse: 30-45 g tid orally. Calves/sheep/goat : 10- 15 g tid orally.	200 g, 1 kg.
BALLMiX Each gm has : Vit A 50,000 I.U., Vit D$_3$ 5,000 I.U.	Feed supplement.	250 g/ton feed.	2 kg, 5 kg and 10 kg.
BALLOUN-B-COMPLEX Each ml contains: Vit B$_{12}$ 6.25 mcg, Riboflavin 1.25 mg, Niacinamide 37.5 mg, Vit B$_6$ 0.62 mg, Cal. Pantothenate 1.25 mg.	Deficiency of Vitamin B Complex.	Cattle/buffalo/horse: 15-20 ml/day. pig/calves/dogs: 5 ml/day orally.	100 ml bottle.
BALLTONE Tablets Each tablet contains: Ferrous sulfate 17.5 mg, Thiamine HCl 25 mg, Vit B$_{12}$ 20 mcg, Choline chloride 9.5 mg, Copper sulfate 2.5 mg, Cobalt sulfate 50 mg, Manganese sulfate 2.5 mg.	Primary and secondary inappetance.	Adult cattle and buffalo : 2 tabs daily for 2-3 days orally.	20 tabs 450 tabs.
BECLINE Tablets Each tablet contains: Oxytetracycline HCl 500 mg.	For prevention and treatment of metritis, pyometra and cervicitis caused by gram positive and gram negative bacteria.	Cows/buffalo/mare: 1-2 tab i/u. Ewe/sow : 1/2 tab i/u.	25 tab.
BLOATONIL Contains: Silica in Dimethicone suspension 1% W/V, Arachis oil 10% W/V	Chronic as well as acute tympany in ruminants.	Cattle/buffalo: 100 ml orally, dose can be doubled in acute cases.	100 ml bottle.

Preparation	Indication	Dosage/Route	Presentation
DERMATIS Cream Contains: Cetrostearyl alcohol 50 g, Liquid paraffin 500 ml.	Antiseptic and bactericidal for both gram positive and gram negative organisms. Lubricants and protective cream prior to rectal and uterine examination.	Local application.	100 g, 500 g bottle.
DIARIN Powder Contains: Chalk 30% w/w, Kaolin 30% w/w, Black Catechu 20% w/w, Ginger Powder 20% w/w.	Useful in non-specific diarrhoea in livestock.	Cattle/buffalo/horse : 25-35 g orally. Sheep/goat : 10-15 g.	200 g, 1 kg.
DYSEKAL Powder Contains: Kaolin 66% w/w, Mag. carbonate 16.5% w/w, Sod. bi carb 16.5% w/w.	All forms of non-specific diarrhoea in livestock.	Cattle/buffalo/horse 30-45 g tid orally. Sheep/goat : 10-15 g bid orally.	200 g, 1 kg.
FURAZONE Powder Contains : Nitrofurazone 0.2% w/w.	Superficial wounds, burns, ulcers and skin infections.	Local application.	10 g.
HELMEX Powder Contains : Levamisole HCl 30% w/w in a soluble powder base	Gastrointestinal and respiratory tract nematodal infection in livestock.	Cattle/buffalo/sheep/ Calves/pigs : 7.5 mg/kg, b.wt.	100 g bottle.
IODOBALL Ointment Contains : Iodine 55 w/w and Methyl salicylate 5% w/w.	Rheumatism, sprains, arthritis, swellings and contusions.	Rub well on to the affected area liberally. Precaution - Do not apply on broken skin.	20 g tube.
PYROSON Powder Contains : Sod. salicylate 40% w/w, Ginger powder 20% w/w.	For all types of non-specific fever in livestock.	Cattle/buffalo/horse : 70 g daily orally. Sheep/goat 15-20 gm. daily	200 g, 1 kg.
RUMOBIN Tablet Each tab contains: Antimony Pot. Tartrate 2 g, Dried Ferrous sulfate 2 g.	Hypomotility of rumen and simple i digestion and inappetance. Contraindication– should not be used in emaciated animals. Plenty of water should be provided to the animal under treatment.	Adult cattle and buffalo: 2-4 tab/day orally for 3-4 days.	2 tabs, 50 tabs bottle.
SCABITEX Contains: Benzyl benzoate 25% w/v	Scabies and pediculosis in livestock except cat.	Applied on to the affected area at an interval of 3-6 days.	100 ml bottle.

Preparation	Indication	Dosage/Route	Presentation
SULFAGON Tablet Each tablet has: Sulfaguanidine 5 g.	Bacterial dysentery and diarrhoea and coccidiosis.	SA: 1 g/5 kg. b. wt. followed by 0.5 g/5 kg. b.wt. subsequently every 24 hours orally for 4-5 days. LA : 2 tabs/50 kg. b.wt. followed by 1 tab/50 kg. b.wt. daily orally.	50 tabs bottle.
SULPHON Tablet Each tablet contains: Sulfadimidine 5 g	Infections caused by gram positive and gram negative bacteria, calf scour, pneumonia and bacterial or coccidial enteritis.	SA: 1 g/5 kg. b.wt. followed by 0.5 g/5 kg. b.wt. subsequently every 24 hours orally. LA: 2 tab/50 kg. b.wt. followed by 1 tab/50 kg. b.wt. daily orally. Caution–should not be continued for more than 10 days.	40 tabs box.
SULTRIM Tablets Each tablet contains: Trimethoprim 200 mg, sulfadiazine 1 g.	Bacterial infection, metritis, endometritis and retention of placenta.	Cows/buffalo: 2-4 tabs i/u.	50 tabs.
TONOBALL Tonic Powder Contains: Zinc oxide 2%, w/w, Dried Ferrous sulfate 7% w/w, Thiamine HCl 0.2% w/w, Copper sulphate 5.4% w/w, and Mag sulph 3% w/w.	Trace mineral supplement.	Cattle/buffalo/horse : 30 g daily orally. Sheep/goat/calves : 15g. Dog: 5-10 g.	200 g, 1 kg.
TYMPLAX Comprises: Formalin 3%, Arachis oil 35%.	Tympany, gaseous bloat in ruminants.	Adult cattle and buffalo: 100-140 ml orally.	100 ml bottle.
URENIT BOLUS Each bolus contains : Nitrofurazone 60 mg and urea 6 g.	Metritis, vaginitis and cervicitis in cattle	Cow/buffalo: 2-4 bolus in each uterine horn. Repeat 24 hours later.	4 boluses.
VESTOM Powder Contains: Dried Ferrous sulfate 12%, Nux-vomica powder 12%, Sod. bicarb 30% Chiretta powder 30%.	For the relief of flatulence, digestive disorders, liver dysfunctions and to improve appetite.	Cattle/buffalo/horses: 30-40 g daily orally. Calves : 15-20 g.	200 g 1 kg.

B.C. ANIMAL HEALTH PRODUCT PVT. LTD.
1 - AB, Sitabagh Colony, Dhenu Market,
INDORE -452 003 (M.P.)

Preparation	Indication	Dosage/Route	Presentation
CORIOGAN Each ml contains : Chorionic gonadotrophin - 250 i.u.	*Cow, mare and sow:* ovarian hypofunction, prolonged heat, anovulatory heat, ovarian cyst, agalactia etc. Bull, horse, ram or boar: Frigidity, impotence, cryptorchidism	Cow/mare: Prolonged heat: 1500 i.u. Anovulatory heat : 2000 i.u. Ovarian cyst : 5000-10000 i.u. inject : 1500-2000 iu every 48 hrs until the cyst disappears. Agalactia : 4000-5000 i.u. Sow : Absence of heat by a functional cyst 1000 i.u. repeat after 21 days if necessary. Agalactia: 1000 i.u. cystic follicles: Two injections of 1500-2000 i.u. at two days interval to be administered by I/M or I/V route.	Vials of 1000 i.u. and 2000 i.u.
CYSTORELIN Each ml contains: Gonadorelin (GnRH) diacetate tetrahydrate - 50 mcg.	To control ovarian cysts. To improve reproduction efficiency.	Cow/buffaloes: 100 mcg I/M or I/V.	Vial of 2 ml & 10 ml.
DINOLYTIC Natural PGF$_2$ alpha 5 mg/ml.	Cattle: * Subestrus. * Oestrus synchronization in cycling animal. * Induction of abortion. * Induced Parturition. * Pyometra. * Horse: * Estrus induction. Swine * Induced Parturition.	 25 mg (5ml) I/M. (Heat appears after 2-4 days of injection). 25 mg I/M inject twice with a period of 10-12 days between injections. 25 mg I/M between 50-120 days of pregnancy (abortion within 4 days) abortion not certain if injected between 120-270 days of pregnancy. 25 to 35 mg I/M after 270 days of pregnancy (Parturition will induce after 1-8 days of injection). 25 mg I/M, antiseptic treatment of uterus must be carried out after Dinolytic inj. 5 mg I/M between 4-13 days of cycle. 10 mg I/M, 2-3 days before end of pregnancy.	10 ml vial.
FLEA AND TICK COLLARS (impregnated with organophosphorus compound)	Fleas and ticks infestation in dogs.		

Preparation	Indication	Dosage/Route	Presentation
HORMO P$_2$ ALPHA Each ml contains: Prostaglandin F$_2$ alpha (Dinoprost) 5 mg.	Anestrus treatment due to PCL, Synchronization of estrus, abortifacent between 5 and 100 days of pregnancy, metritis, pyometra etc.	Cow/buffaloes : 5 ml I/M repeat after 11 days. Sow : 2 ml I/M.	Vial of 5 ml.
OVA SET Two separate vial of FSH & LH i) Each 9 ml vial of FSH contain FSH- 0.480 mg. ii) Each 3 ml vial of LH contains LH - 0.420 mg. iii) Each vial of solvent contains Physiological saline sol. 12 ml.	To improve quality and yield of superovulation in ovine and bovine and for embryo transfer.	Treatment consists of 8 I/M inj (2 inj/day during 4 days) Day 1 - 6 ml bid. Day 2 - 5 ml bid. Day 3 - 3 ml bid. Day 4 - 2 ml bid.	9 ml vial of FSH. 3 ml vial of LH. 12 ml of solvent.
OVERCID Tablets Each tablet contains: Praziquantel 50 mg.	Highly effective against Tapeworms infestation in dog & cat.	5 mg/kg b.wt. orally.	2, 10, 50, 100 and 1000 tablets.
PRID (Vaginal coil) Each coil contains: Progesterone (in inert Silicon elastomer) 1.55 gm estradiol benzoate (in gelatin capsule)-10 mg.	Functional anestrus, delayed puberty, post-partum anestrus, synchronization of estrus in cows and heifers.	Insert PRID into the vagina. Duration of treatment is 12 days. The coil is withdrawn by gently pulling on the string.	
PROMONE-E Each ml contains : Medroxy progesterone Acetate 50 mg.	For the prevention of estrus in anestrus bitches.	1 ml (50 mg) during anestrus, repeat at intervals of 6 months by s/c route.	5 ml vial.
SYNCRO-MATE-B Norgestomet implant and norgestomet/estradiol valerate inj.	For synchronized breeding of cycling cows and heifers.		6 x 25 dose, 16 x 10 dose, 3 x 35 dose, 3 x 10 dose.
SYNCRO-PART PMSG 400 : 400 i.u. PMSG SYNCRO-PART PMSG 500 : 500 i.u. PMSG SYNCRO-PART PMSG 600 : 600 i.u. PMSG SYNCRO-PART PMSG 700 : 700 i.u. PMSG SYNCRO-PART PMSG 6000 : 6000 i.u. PMSG Solvent vial - Normal : Saline solution	Initiation and synchronization of estrus and ovulation as it has activity similar to pituitary FSH and LH.	Ewe: Syncro-part 400 to 700 reconstitute with 2 ml solvent and inject i/m. PMSG 6000 reconstitute with 20 to 40 ml solvent to obtain 600 to 300 i.u. PMSG/ml.	Vials of Synchro-part PMSG 400, 500, 600, 700 and 6000 i.u.

BHARTIYA BOOTEE BHAWAN
21 Mangal Nagar,
SAHARANPUR-247 001

Preparation	Indication	Dosage/Route	Presentation
AFRON	Tympanitis in cattle, buffalo, sheep and goat.	Cattle/buffalo: 50 g in 1/2-1 litre lukewarm water. Sheep/goat: 15-20 g orally.	100g, 1 kg.
ANEMIN	As a general tonic & used as a mineral feed supplement.	Horse/Cattle: 25-30 gm sheep/goats/calves: 5-15 gm once in a day with feed.	1/2 kg, 1 kg.
BANJHNA	Anoestrus in livestock.	Cattle/buffalo (Large size): 3 capsules daily for 2 days. (Small size) : 2 caps daily for 2 days orally.	Pack of 6 capsules.
CLINOSOL	Used as Ecbolic & for early involution of uterus.	Horse/cattle: 50-60 gms Sheep/goat : 20-30 gms. Bitch: 10-20 gms in lukewarm water or as electuary.	100 gm, 1 kg.
COFGO	Respiratory diseases, pneumonia, bronchitis and cough.	Cattle/buffalo/horse: 30-40 g bid orally. Calves/sheep/goat: 10-15g bid orally. Dog: 2-4 g bid daily.	100 g, 1 kg.
DIADISCO	All forms of diarrhoea and dysentery in livestock.	Cattle/buffalo: 25-35 g orally. Calves : 10-15 g. Sheep/goat: 5-10 g. Dog : 2 g.	100 g, 1 kg.
FITWOM	Tapeworms infestation.	Cattle /horse : 40-60 gms sheep/goat, calves: 10-20 gm. Dog/piglet: 4-6 gm (Poultry 1-2% of feed) as Treacle for 3 days.	100 gms, 1 kg.
FLUHEREX	Cold & nasal discharge.	Horse/cattle: 20 gms. Sheep/goat : 10 gms orally in lukewarm water.	100 gms, 1 kg.
HEPACIN	Liver Stimulant & Tonic Powder, Also used in loss of appetite, constipation, anaemia.	Horse/cattle : 30-50 gms. Calves/goat/sheep: 10-30 gm orally with Gur.	100 gms, 1 kg.
HEREXIDE	Dressing powder on wounds, burns and ulcers as antiseptic powder.	Applied locally.	100 g, 1 kg.
HERMINSA	Dyspepsia, inappetance, indigestion, general debility and anaemia.	Cattle/buffalo/horse: 30-50 g bid Calves/goat/pig : 10-20 g bid Dog : 3-7 g orally bid.	100 g, 200g, 400 g, 1 kg.
HERWEX	Open wound, ringworm, dermatitis, oedematous swellings.	To be applied locally.	50 g, 1 kg.
KRIMOS	Round worms, tapeworm and liver fluke infestation in all animals and hookworms in dogs.	Cattle, buffalo/horse: 50-60g Sheep/Goat: 15-20 g. Calves : 10 g. Dog/pig : 20-30 g orally. Repeat after 1 week.	100 g, 1 kg.

Preparation	Indication	Dosage/Route	Presentation
NANCO	Conjunctivitis, watery eye, keratitis & eye injury	5 drops in eye bid.	10 ml.
RASOL	Used as galactogogue.	Cow/buffalo: 20-40 g bid Sheep/goat: 10-15 g bid orally for 10-35 days.	100 g, 200 g, 1 kg.
RATRAJ	Decreased sex libido & poor quality of semen in bulls, stallion, rams.	Bulls-25-45 gms, stallion, 25-30 gms; Boars: 8-12 gm; Dogs, buck and ram: 4-5 gm once a day orally with molasses.	100 gm, 1 kg.
TAPHEREX	Efemeral fever.	Horse/cattle: 30 gm. Sheep/goats : 15 gm orally with lukewarm water.	100 gm, 1 kg.
URUL	Urinary calculi in male animals.	Male cattle/Buffaloes : 40-60 gms; goats/sheep : 15-30 gms orally in lukewarm water bid.	100 gm 1 kg.

BIOMEDICA (P) LTD.
736 - Industrial Area B
LUDHIANA-141 003

Preparation	Indication	Dosage/Route	Presentation
ALERGIPAR Inj. Each ml contains: Pheniramine maleate 22.7 mg	Potent antihistaminic, useful in allergies, serum allergy, burns, pruritus, bloat and conditions where histamine is released.	LA : 5-10 ml Q12 h or Q24h I/M, I/V SA: 0.5-1 ml, I/M, I/v	10 ml vial.
ASHILIVE Forte Each ml contains: Vit B$_{12}$ 30 mcg, B$_1$ 25 mg, B$_6$ 5 mg, Niacinamide 100 mg, choline chloride 15 mg, DL-Panthenol 5 mg, Lignocaine 1%, Liver extract with vit. B$_{12}$ activity 2 mcg, Phenol 0.5%	Disorders of liver and B-complex deficiency, anorexia, debility and convalescence.	LA: 10 ml for 3-4 days I/M SA: 1-2 ml for 3-4 days	10 ml vial.
BILLIPON Contains: Vit B$_{12}$ 100 mcg, B$_1$ 100 mg, B$_2$ 3 mg, B$_6$ 150 mg, DL-Panthenol 5 mg, Lignocaine HCl 1%, Phenol 0.5%	B-complex vitamin deficiency, anaemia, weakness, inappetance and convalescence.	LA: 10 ml I/M for 3 days SA: 1-2 ml I/M for 3 days	10 ml vial.
BILLIPON Syrup Each 5 ml has: L-Lysin Mono HCl 50 mg, Sodium glycerophosphate 80 mg, Thiamine mononitrate 1.5 mg, Riboflavin 1 mg, Pyridoxine HCl 10 mg, Niacinamide 15 mg, DL-Panthenol 1.5 mg, Flavoured base q.s.	Debility, general weakness, stress, pregnancy and anaemia.	Cattle/buffalo/horse: 20-25 ml daily orally Calves/foals/pig/sheep/goat: 10-15 ml bid. Dog/cat: 5 ml bid	100 ml, 200 ml bottles.
CALCIPAR 25% Contains: Calcium borogluconate 25%	Hypocalcemia, milk fever, osteomalacia, and general weakness.	Cattle/buffalo/horse : 400 ml or more I/V, S/C. Calves/goat/sheep: 50-70 ml slow I/V.	400 ml.
COF KONTROL Each ml contains : Chlorpheniramine maleate 2 mg Diphenylamine HCl 12 mg Ammon. chloride 100 mg Sod. citrate 40 mg, Antimony Pot. Tartrate 0.5 mg, Chloroform 0.008 ml, Menthol 1 mg, Flavoured base q.s.	Bronchitis, cough, pneumonia.	Calves/foal/pig/sheep/goat: 10 ml bid orally Dog/cat: 5 ml bid after meals.	100 ml, 200 ml, bottles.
PAMIBION Each ml contains: Vit B$_1$ 200 mg, Vit B$_6$ 50 mg, Vit B$_{12}$ 1000 mcg	Hypothiaminosis, anaemia, neuritis and pregnancy.	Cattle/buffalo/horse: 10 ml I/M for 3-5 days Calves/foals/pig/sheep/-goat: 3 ml I/M Dog, cat: 1-2 ml daily.	2 ml ampoule, 10 ml vial.

Preparation	Indication	Dosage/Route	Presentation
PARICHLOR Inj Each ml contains: Chlorpheniramine maleate 10 mg Chlorocresol 0.1%	Antihistaminics used in various forms of allergic conditions.	Cattle/buffalo: 2.5-5 ml I/M Sheep/goat/pig: 1-2 ml I/M Dog/cat: 0.5-1 ml I/M.	10 ml vial.
PARISTOLA Eye and Ear drops Contains : Sulfacetamide sod. 10% and Prednisolone 0.3%	All types of infections of eyes and ear in domestic animals.	Cattle/buffalo/horse: 4-6 drops Q12 h in eyes 8-10 drops in ear Calves/sheep/goat/large dogs : 3-4 drops bid; Small dogs : 2-3 drops bid.	10 ml vial.
PROMETHAZINE HCl Inj Contains: 2.5% or 5% Promethazine	A potent antihistaminic, used in allergy, burn, dermatitis etc.	Cattle/buffalo/horse: 0.5-1 mg/kg b.wt I/M Pig 1-4 mg/kg b.wt I/M sheep/goat: 2.5-10 mg/kg b.wt. I/M dog/cat: 2.5-12.5 mg/kg b.wt. I/M.	10 ml vial.
RAVNITA Inj Each ml contains: Dexamethasone sod. Phosphate 4.4 mg, Methyl paraben 0.15%, Propyl paraben 0.03%, Lignocaine HCl 1%	Antiinflammatory, useful in acute mastitis, metritis, pneumonia, drug allergy and shock.	LA: 5 ml or more I/M, I/V SA: 0.5 ml I/M, I/V.	2 ml and 3 ml ampoule.
RETINAMYCIN Eye or Ear drops Contains: Dexamethasone sod Phosphate 0.1%, Neomycin sulphate 0.5% and Phenyl mercuric nitrate 0.002%	Conjunctivitis, Keratitis and eye infections, otitis and ear infection.	Instill 4-6 drops tid or Q 6 h Dog/Cat : 2-4 drops.	10 ml vial.
SIMERCETIN Ear drops Contains: Chloramphenicol 5% W/V and Benzocaine 1% W/V	Ear infections.	Instill 2-4 drops or more bid.	10 ml vial.
SIMERCETIN Inj Each ml contains: Chloramphenicol 100 mg Chlorocresol 0.1% and Lignocaine HCl 1%	Broad spectrum antibiotic, very effective against enteric infection by *S. typhimurium*, Also effective against rickettsia.	LA: 10-20 ml (2-4 mg/kg b.wt.) I/M SA: 2 ml.	10 ml vial.
SPASMODIN Each ml contains: Codein phosphate 16 mg, papaverine HCl 32 mg, atropine sulfate 0.4 mg	Colic pain in the abdomen, chronic diarrhoea.	LA: 5-10 ml x 3 days I/M Sheep/goat/calves/pigs: 2 ml daily.	10 ml vial.
SUGIL Contains: Triflupromazine HCl 20 mg/ml or 10 mg/ml	Sedative, used in vomition and to control the animals, pre-anaesthetic. Caution–The horse may show reaction.	Cattle/buffalo: 0.1-0.2 mg/kg b.wt. I/M, I/v Horse: 0.2-0.3 mg/kg b.wt. I/M, I/v. Sheep/goat: 0.1 mg/kg b.wt. I/M, I/v Dog/cat: 0.5- 1 mg b.wt. I/M, I/v.	5 ml, 10 ml vial.

BOOTS PURE DRUGS CO. (INDIA) LTD.
17, Nicol Road
MUMBAI-1

Preparation	Indication	Dosage/Route	Presentation
BIO MINDIF Provides: Calcium 28%, Phosphorus 5%, Copper 10 ppm, Cobalt 50 ppm, Iodine 10 ppm, Iron 3500 ppm, Sod. Chloride 20%, Aureomycin 0.04%.	For rapid growth, better feed utilization, increased weight gain and egg production and low mortality in poultry.	Poultry: 2.5 kg/100 kg dry or wet mash.	1 kg, 50 kg.
MINDIF MINERALS (Pigs) Provides: Calcium 25.8%, Phosphorus 4.5%, Copper 480 ppm, Cobalt 90 ppm, Manganese 800 ppm, Iodine 215 ppm, Iron 2.9%, Zinc 0.8%, Sod. Chloride 23.5%.	For improved growth, fertility, sturdy bones and to prevent piglet anaemia.	Pig : 1.5 kg/100 kg feed or 14 g/weaner daily or 21 g/fattener daily.	50 kg.
MINDIF MINERAL (Poultry) Provides: Calcium 28%) Phosphorus 5%, copper 100 ppm, Cobalt 50 ppm, Manganese 200 ppm, Iodine 10 ppm, Iron 0.35%, Sod. Chloride 23%.	Promotes growth, egg production and fertility in poultry.	Poultry : 1 kg/10 kg dry or wet mash.	1 kg, 50 kg.
MINDIF MINERAL (Sheep & Horse) Contains: Calcium 20.8%, Phosphorus 6.2%, Copper 200 ppm, Cobalt 70 ppm, Manganese 740 ppm, Iodine 250 ppm, Iron 0.4%, Sod. Chloride 35.8%.	Minerals supplement for sheep and horse for better growth and production.	Sheep: 1 kg/33 kg sheep ration. Horse: 60-120 g daily with ration. Yearling: 30-60 g daily with ration. Foals: 8-30 g daily.	50 kg.
PENICILLIN (Intramammary) Contains : 1,00,000 units of Penicillin G Potassium salt per 5 ml.	Mastitis caused by streptococcal or staphylococcal infection.	Following complete milking, one tube in each quarter is infused daily for 3-5 days. Withdraw milk for 72 hours of last treatment.	Tube of 5 ml.
SUPERMINDIF Contains : Calcium 22%, Phosphorus 9.5%, Copper 0.09%, Cobalt 0.015%, Manganese 0.1% Pot. iodide 0.25%, Sulphur 0.15%, Iron 5% and Sod chloride 30%.	Mineral supplement for cattle.	With concentrate - 500 g/50 kg feed; without concentrate - 20 g/head daily.	1kg, 50 kg.

CADILA HEALTH CARE
Aqrovet Division, Khemka House, Drive In,
AHMEDABAD-360 052

Preparation	Indication	Dosage/Route	Presentation
BOVIVITA SPECIAL (Feed Supplement) Each 5 G Contains:- Vit A 50,000 IU Vit D$_3$ 5,000 IU Vit E 5 mg fortified with Ca & P	Milk fever, muscular dystrophy, to improve fertility, to increase productivity, fat contents of milk & growth in animals.	Pregnant/milking cow and buffalo: 5 g per day Horses : 5 gm per day, calf, sheep, goats and pig: 2 g per day.	100 g, 1 kg.
BUTALEX Inj. (Buparvaquone 5%)	For treatment of theileriosis.	1 ml/20 kg body wt. 1/m only. In severe cases, a second dose to be given within 48-72 hrs.	20 ml multidose vial.
CADISTIN Inj. Each ml contains:- Chlorpheniramine maleate 10 mg.	Allergic reactions to drug, blood transfusion & allergic disorders with manifestation of respiratory signs, eczema, dermatitis, urticaria, insect bite etc.	0.5-1.0 mg/kg body wt. Large animal: 5-10 ml 1/M. Small animal: 0.5-1 ml 1/M.	10 ml & 30 ml vials.
CADISOL PLUS Liquid, each ml contains: Cal. gluconate 833 mg, vit D$_3$ 1600 IU, vit B$_{12}$ 16.7 mcg Ferric amm. citrate 167 mg, Stomach extract 3.30 mg.	Vitamins, Iron & Stomach extract to improve digestion, growth & production & to prevent calcium deficiency.	To be given orally through drinking water. Cattle, buffalo & horse:- 60 ml bid. Calf, sheep, foal, goat, pig: 25 ml bid. Dog : 10 ml bid. Poultry (100 birds) Chicks: 10 ml daily, growers & broilers: 20 ml daily, layers : 50 ml daily.	100 ml 500 ml, 1 litre & 5 litre.
CADIPLEX -L Each ml contains : Riboflavin 1.25 mg, vit B$_6$ 0.62 mg, vit B$_{12}$ 6.25 mcg Nicotinamide 25 mg D-panthenol 0.62 mg Choline chloride 10 mg Lysine mono hydro chloride 5 mg	To improve the productivity of animals and poultry and to prevent vit B-complex dificiencies.	Poultry : 10-20 ml/100 birds Pigs & calf : 3-5 ml Dog : 2.5 - 6.0 ml Horse : 10 - 20 ml to be given daily through drinking water or as wet meal.	500 ml, 1 litre & 5 litres.
CADFEED Bolus Containing vitamins, minerals, herbal, yeast & essential amino acids.	To check the nutritional deficiencies & metabolic disorders.	Calf, sheep & goat :- 1 bolus 10 daily for 3 days. Cattle & buffalo: 4 boli daily for 3 days, in case of delayed puberty or anoestrus regular supplementation of 1 bolus daily for 20 days.	Strip of 4 boli.
DEXONA Inj. Each ml contains: Dexamethasone sodium phosphate 4.4 mg	Ketosis, inflammation of respiratory tract, local inflammatory conditions, arthritis, surgical shock, anaphylactic shock, traumetic shock, severe shock of haemorrhage, surgical & septic		

Preparation	Indication	Dosage/Route	Presentation
	pregnancy toxaemia, shock, as an aid in inducing parturition & acute mastitis.	Cattle, buffalo & horse: 4-20 mg daily 1/M or slow 1/V. Calves, pig, sheep & goat : 2-4 mg daily 1/M or slow 1/V. Dog & cats: 0.5-2.0 mg daily 1/M or slow 1/V; the above dosage regimen should be divided wherever possible.	Vials of 2 ml & 5 ml.
FLURRY Liquid (herbal dog shampoo)	Antiseptic, antimicrobial, ectoparasiticidal, antidandruff, for conditioner, hair growth promotor for canines.	Wet the dog/cat with water & rub 5-8 g into depth of hair coat for 5 min. & then wash with water. Repeat, if required. In heavy infestation, apply 5-8 g directly on the affected area & then wash.	120 g bottle.
HIPENOX 1000 AND 2000 Each Vial Contains: Amoxicillin sodium 500 mg, 1 gm. Claxocillin sodium 5000 mg, 1 gm.	In haemorrhagic septicaenia, black quarter, mastitis, calf scours, brucellosis, salmonellosis, metritis & retained placenta, pyelonephritis, & post-surgical treatment.	5 mg/kg body wt. by I/V a 1/M In severe case, dose may be doubled. Dissolve the content Hipenox 1000 in 9 ml & Hipenox 2000 in 18 ml of sterile water for injection.	Hipenox 1000 & Hipenox 2000 injection.
KADIPROL Each 100 gm. contains: Amprolium hydrochloride 25 g, vit K_3 250 mg.	To prevent coccidiosis in poultry	1gm/ litre of drinking water continued for 5-7 days.	25 gm & 500 gm.
LIVERUBRA Inj. Each ml contains : (Liver extract from 8 g of liver having vit B_{12} activity equivalent to not less than 2 mcg of cyanocobalamine, lignocaine hydrochloride 1% W/V	Liver tonic.	Large animal : 5-10 ml daily 1/M Small animal : 1-2 ml daily 1/M.	30 ml.
NEUROXIN-12V Inj. Each ml contains : Thiamine HCL 30 mg Pyridoxin HCL 13.75 mg Cyanocobalamine 500 mcg	Nervine tonic.	Cattle, buffalo & horses: 5-10 ml 1/M daily for 3-5days Dog : 2-3 ml 1/M daily for 3-5 days.	10 ml.
ORIPRIM Bolus Each bolus contains: Trimethoprim 400 mg Sulphamethoxazole 2 g	Antimicrobial.	Large animal : 4 boli daily Small animal : 1/2-1 bolus daily.	Strip of 2 boli.
ORIPRIM Inj 1/M, each ml contains: Trimethoprim 40 mg Sulphamethoxazole 200 mg	Antimicrobial.	1 ml/20 kg body wt 1/M daily.	5 ml.

Preparation	Indication	Dosage/Route	Presentation
ORIPRIM Inj. 1/V, each ml contains: Trimethoprim 80 mg Sulphamethoxazole 400 mg	Antimicrobial.	Large animal : 15-30 ml daily Small animal : 2-5 ml daily.	30 ml.
ORIPRIM 'U' Bolus Each bolus contains: Trimethoprim 100 mg Sulphamethoxazole 500 mg Urea 6000 mg.	Antimicrobial/intrauterine.	Place 2-4 boli in uterus after par-turition, Repeat after 24 hrs. If cervix is not fully open, triturate & dissolve 2 boli in 30 ml sterile distilled water & infuse into the uterus with an A.I. pipette.	Strip of 4 boli.
ORIPRIM Powder Each gm contains : Trimethoprim 100 mg Sulphamethoxazole 500 mg	Antimicrobial.	Poultry : for 100 birds upto 6 wks- 2 g; upt 6-13 wks - 4g; 12-18 wks - 6 g. above 18 wks - 8 g with drinking water or 100 g / 100 kg of feed. Other species : 2g/40 kg body wt with water.	100 g.
OXALGIN DS Bolus Each bolus contains: Diclofenac sodium. 200 mg Paracetamol 1500 mg	Antiinflammatory, analgesic, an-tipyretic.	Large animal : 1-2 bolus twice daily Small animal : 1/4-1/2 bolus twice daily	Strip of 4 boli.
PARACETOL Inj. Each ml contains: Paracetamol 150 mg	Analgesic, antipyretic.	Large animal-10-30 ml prefera-bly by deep 1/M route Small animal : 1-5 ml deep 1/M.	30 ml.
VIBEX Bolus Each bolus contains: Al-bendazole 750 mg	Anthelmintic.	For roundworm, tapeworms & lung worms : Cattle, buffalo, horses, sheep, goat, pig : 5 mg / kg body wt.	Strip of 4 boli.
VIBEX Suspersion (2.5%) Each 5 ml contains : Al-bendazole : 125 mg		Dog, cat : 10-25 mg/kg body wt. for Fluke: Cattle, buffalo : 10 mg/kg body wt. sheep & goat : 7.5 mg/kg body wt.	60 ml, 500 ml & 1 litre 250 gm.
VIBEX Powder (15%) Each gm contains : Albendazole 150 mg			
VITATONE - LM Each 5 ml contains : Vit A : 2,50,000 IU vit D 3 : 25,000 IU, Vit C : 500 mg Vit E acetate : 150 mg Lysine HCL : 25 mg DL Methionine : 10 mg	For higher egg & meat produc-tion in poultry.	For Chicks : 2 ml/100 birds in drinking water, for growers : 3 ml / 100 birds in drinking water, for layers : 5 ml / 100 birds in drinking water.	100 ml, 500 ml & 1 litre.
ZYDAQUIN Each gm contains: Flumequine 100 mg	Antimicrobial.	Chicks: 2 g/ litre drinking water growers, layers & broilers 1g/litre drinking water.	100 gm.

CADILA PHARMACEUTICALS (Veterinary Division)
B.D. Patel House, Nr. Sardar Patel Colony, Naranpura
AHMEDABAD-380 014

Preparation	Indication	Dosage/Route	Presentation
CAMPICILIN Inj. Contains : Ampicillin Sod. 250 mg, 500 mg, 1 gm and 2 gm	Calf scours, pneumonia, calf enteritis, septicaemia due to salmonella infections, mastitis due to *E.Coli*, metritis & retained placenta, pyelonepritis in cattle. Enteritis, pneumonia, erysepelas, metritis in pigs. Enteritis, septicaemia, metritis respiratory infection, strangles in horses.	Oral: 4-10 mg/kg BW Parenteral:- 2-7 mg/kg BW.	250 mg, 500 mg, 1000 mg, 2000 mg, vials.
CANIFUR (Herbal dog shampoo)	Anti dandruff, ectoparasiticidal, hair growth promoter and fur conditioner.	Bath the dog to ensure complete wetting, apply 10-20 gm of canifur & rub thoroughly into the depth of hair coat to obtain foam, leave the foam on the body for 5-10 min. & then wash with water.	120 gm bottle.
CANIFUR-AZ (Herbal ingredients)	Ectoparasiticidal, kills lice, ticks, mites instantaneously.	Apply on the affected area with full strength.	120 gm bottle.
CAL-D-PLUS Contains: Cal. gluconate 833 mg Vit D$_3$ 1200 IU Vit B$_{12}$ 16.7 mcg Ferric amm. citrate 167 mg. Stomach extract 3.30 mg	To stimulate growth in puppies, calves, foals etc. To prevent milk fever. To maintain high milk yield. To correct macrocytic anaemia, rickets. To prevent connibalism, thin shelled eggs.	Cattle, horses: 50 ml bid daily Calves, foals, sheep, goats & pigs: 25 ml bid daily. Dog : 10 ml bid daily. Poultry : 10 ml/100 birds Growers/broilers : 20 ml/100 birds per day.	100 ml, 500 ml, 1000 ml, 5000 ml.
DICIROL GRANULES Each gm. contains: Cholecalciferol (vit D$_3$) 6,00,000 IU	To prevent deficiency of vit D (rickets, osteo malacia, milk fever).	2 gm / torn of feed.	5 gm sachet.
DEXASONE Inj. Each ml contains : Dexamethosone sodium phosphate 4.4 mg.	Ketosis, inflammation of respiratory tract, urogenital tract, local inflammatory conditions, arthritis, surgical shocks, pregnancy toxaenia. c/I :- John's disease, diabetes mellitus, cardiac insufficiency, advanced pregnancy.	Depends upon severity Cattle/Horse-4-20 mg/day. Calves, sheep, pigs, goats:- 2-4 mg daily. Dog & cats : 0.5-2.0 mg/day.	2 ml, 5 ml vials.
FLUQUIN Each gm contains : Flumequine 100 mg	Antimicrobial	Chicks : 0.5 gm/litre drinking water . Growers, layers, broilers : 1 gm/litre drinking water.	100 gm.

Preparation	Indication	Dosage/Route	Presentation
LIVERJET Each ml contains : liver extract (derived from 8 gm of liver) having vit B_{12} more than 2 mcg, Lignocaine HCL 1% w/v	Anorexia & protective of liver from the fatty degeneration in hepatitis & jaundice, for normal haemopoiesis & check anaemia, neurological disorders. To maintain healthy skin and pancreatic metabolism.	Large animal : 5-10 ml daily Small animal : 1-2 ml daily I/M injection.	Vials of 10 ml & 30 ml.
LYRIM Contains:- Vit A, Vit D_3, Vit E, Vit C. Lysine & methionine	To promote growth & production in poultry.	Chicks - 2 ml/100 birds in drinking water. Grower: 3 ml/100 birds in drinking water. Layers: 5 ml/100 birds in drinking water	100 ml, 500 ml & 1 litre.
MELICON-V (Herbal ingredients)	All types of skin infections. (antiimcrobial, antiinflammatory, antifungal, maggoted wound, fly & insect repellant.	Clean the affected area & apply gently (don't rub) as a thick layer twice a day.	15 gm & 60 gm tubes.
MIFECAL Calcium gluconate 20.8% Boric acid 4.2 % Mag. hypophosphite 5% Anhd. dextrose 20% Chlorocresol 0.1%	Milk fever due to hypocalcemia which may be accompanied by hypomagnesemia hypophosphatemias & ketosis.	Cows & buffalo: 250 ml to 500 ml as a single dose IV or SC; in case of relapse treatment may be repeated.	500 ml bottle.
ONFEED Bolus Herbal liver stimulant, vitamin, minerals, yeast, amino acid, digestive stimulants.	Anorexia & anestrus.	Cattle & buffalo : 4 boli daily for 3 days. Calves, sheep, goats : 1 bolus bid for 3 days. Anestrus cattle & buffalo : 1 bolus daily for 20 days.	Strips of 4 bolus.
PESULIN Bolus Each bolus contains : light kaolin 3 gm. phthalyl sulphathiazole 1 gm Pot. Chloride 15.6 mg Sod. Chloride 37.8 mg Pot. Citrate 67.9 mg Sodium acid phosphate 26.4 mg. PESULIN Suspension also	Calf scours, diarrhoea, dysentery etc.	Large animal: 4-8 boli Small animal : 2-4 boli Suspension: Cattle & horses: 100-150 ml bid. Sheep, goat, & calves: 15-60 ml bid Dogs : 15-30 ml bid.	Strips of 4 boli.
PRO-WINSTRESS (Anti Stress Liquid Feed Supplement) Contains: Vit. A, D_3. E, B_{12}, lysine & methionine.	To counteract the various types of stress.	To be given daily in drinking water. Chicks : 2-3 ml / 100 birds Growers : 5 ml / 100 birds Layers : 10 ml / 100 birds.	100 ml & 1000 ml bottles.
TREPEN Inj. Each 5 ml contains Trimethoprim 80 mg Sulphamethoxazole 400 mg	Broad spectrum antimicrobial.	Large animals : 15-30 ml daily Small animals : 2-5 ml daily by I/V route.	30 ml vials.

Preparation	Indication	Dosage/Route	Presentation
TREPEN 'U' Bolus Each bolus contains :- Trimethoprim 100 mg Sulphamethoxazole 500 mg Urea 6000 mg	Antimicrobial / intrauterine.	Place 2-4 boli in uterus after parturition, repeat after 24 hrs.	Strip of 4 boli.
TREPEN Powder Each gm contains: Trimethoprim 100 mg Sulphamethoxazole 500 mg	Antimicrobial.	Poultry : (for 100 birds) upt 6 wks : 2 gm: 6-13 wks:- 4 gm; 12-18 wks : 6 gm. above 18 wks : 8 gm with drinking water or 100 gm/100 kg feed.	100 gm.
WORMIN Bolus Each bolus contains: Mebendazole 500 mg	Broad spectrum anthelmintic, kills all the stages of round-worms, tapeworms & liver fluks.	Cattle, horse: 5-10 mg/kg Bw Sheep & goats & pigs : 5 mg/Kg Bw. Dog & Cat : 5-10 mg/kg BW.	Strip of 4 boli.
WORMIN Powder Each gm cantains : Mebendazole (50%) 500 mg	Broad spectrum anthelmintic.	Sheep : 5 gm/kg BW. Poultry : 10 gm for 500 birds OR one 50 gm pack for 2500 birds.	50 gm pack.
XYLOCAD Contains : Xylazine 2 %	Sedative, potent analgesic, muscle relaxant, anaesthetic.	Ruminents : 0.25-1.0 ml/100 kg BW. Horses : 10 ml/100 kg BW Dog : 0.5-1.5 ml / 10 kg BW Cat : 0.1 - 0.2 ml/kg BW by 1/M route.	5 ml & 30 ml.
ZOMAR Bolus Each bolus contains : Albendazole 600 mg.	Broad spectrum anthelmintic.	Roundworms /tape worms / lung worms : Cattle, buffalo, horses, sheep, goats & pigs : 5 mg/kg bwt. Dog, Cat : 10-25 mg/kg Bwt. Flukes : Cattle, buffalo : 10 mg/kg BW. Sheep, goat : 7.5 mg/kg BW	Strip of 4 sole.
ZOMAR Suspension (2.5%) Each 5 ml contains: Albendazole 125 mg	Broad spectrum anthelmintic.	-do-	60 ml, 500 ml & 1 litre.

CATTLE REMEDIES
Sirsa Ganj - 205 151 (U.P.)

Preparation	Indication	Dosage/Route	Presentation
BLOTINOX	Acute & chronic tympanitis, frothy bloat.	Cattle & buffalo : 100 ml orally Horse & donkey : 50-100 ml orally. Sheep & goat : 50 ml orally.	100 ml, 225 ml, 450 ml.
CATCOUGH (Electuary)	Bronchitis, laryngitis, Nasal catarrh & broncho pneumonia.	Cattle & buffalo : 25-30 gm orally Horse: 20-25 gm orally Sheep & goat : 10-15 gm orally Dog : 3- 5 gm orally (To be given twice or thrice daily).	100 gm, 250 gm, 1 kg.
CATGALL Oint	Myositis, muscular sprain, contusion, yolkgall etc.	Clean the affected part & apply the ointment and rub gently.	50 gm, 100 gm, 500 gm.
CATONE Powder	Malnutrition, anorexia, anaemia, indigestion, impaction, ruminal atony, flatulence, ketosis, milkfever.	Cattle & buffalo : 40-50 gm orally Horse: 30-40 gms orally Calves, colts, pigs: 20-30 gm orally Sheep & goat : 10-15 gm orally.	100 gm, 200 gm, 400 gm, 1 kg.
CATORRHOEA Powder	Indigestion, diarrhoea, non specific diarrhoea, amoebic dysentery.	Cattle & buffalo : 25-50 gm orally Horses : 20-30 gm orally Sheep & goat : 10-20 gms orally Dog : 5-10 gm orally (Twice or thrice daily with rice pith).	100 gm, 200gm, 1 kg.
CATORRHOEA Tablet	In intestinal infection, acute & chronic amoebic dysentery, bacillary dysentery, diarrhoea, enteritis, enterocolitis, giardiasis.	Cattle & buffalo : 3-5 tabs orally Sheep & goat : 2-3 tabs orally Dog : 1-2 tabs orally (Twice or thrice daily in rice pith).	Box of 8 x 6 tabs.
DEWORMIN Powder	(Dewormer) threadworm, hookworm, roundworm, tapeworm, correct the indigestion, diarrhoea, loss of appetite, constipation, colic, anaemia & irregular bowel.	Cattle & buffalo: 35-45 gm Horses: 25-30 gm Sheep & goat: 10-15 gm (Once or twice daily with matha or gur for 3 days).	100 gm, 200 gm, 1 kg.
DRESSOL Liquid	Surgical wound, abrasion bleeding, wound, delayed healing, otorrhoea.	Clean the wound aseptically dressed with gauge soaked in dressol liquid then apply bandage.	25 ml, 50 ml, 100 ml 450 ml.
DUGDH-DAN (Glactogauge)	Low milk yield due to advanced pregnancy, weekness due to malnutrition, as galatogauge after parturition.	Cattle : 3-5 tabs twice daily Goat & ewes : 1 tab twice daily for 15 days preferably with syrup.	Box 8 x 6 tabs.

Preparation	Indication	Dosage/Route	Presentation
MAGGACITE Liquid	It kills maggots, ticks and lice etc.	Swab dipped in Maggacite liquid may be packed in maggot wounds for at least a day. The wound may be cleaned with A/S and dead maggots may be removed, repeat application for better result.	25 ml, 50 ml, 100 ml 450 ml.
PROLAPSE-IN	Infection of vaginal mucous membrane, irritation in genital organs, anxiety, to check and correct prolapse of uterus and rectum.	Wash the inverted or prolapsed portion aseptically; dry up with clean soft cloth & apply powder mixed with glycerine on the inverted surface and then reduce the prolapsed organ. In post-parturient inversion administration of 100 ml uterotone liquid twice daily for 4-5 days ensures cure and reduces the chances of reinversion. 5 tabs of Prolapse-in with 100 gm of butter or ghee or lard twice daily for 2-3 subsequent days and feed the animal laxative diet.	Box 5 x 6 tabs with 20 gm powder pack.
UTEROTONE Liquid	Retention of placenta, silent heat, delayed involution, endometritis, pyometra, purpural fever, lowered milk yield associated with breeding diseases.	Cow & buffalo: 100-125 ml Mare: 50-75 ml Ewe and goat: 20-40 ml Bitch: 10-25 ml twice daily with drenching bamboo orally.	225 ml, 450 ml, 900 ml.
UTEROTONE Capsule	Silent heat and delayed ovulation.	Cow & buffalo: 2-3 caps daily for 4 days. Mare: 1-2 caps daily for 4 days. Goat & ewe: 1 cap daily for 4 days. In retention of placenta the above doses may be repeated at four hourly interval till the foetal membranes are expelled out.	Box 6 x 8 capsules.

CHARAK PHARMACEUTICALS (INDIA) LTD.
MUMBAI- 400 011

Preparation	Indication	Dosage/Route	Presentation
ANTIFLAT Powder	Tympany, impaction, indigestion, flatulence & bloat in ruminants, dyspepsia & indigestion.	Cow/buffalo: 15-25 g twice a day, orally. Sheep/goat: 8-10 g twice a day orally.	Packets of 100 g.
BIORIL Powder	Fever of varied etiology.	Large animals: 25-30 g bid Small animals: 15-20 g bid Dog & cat: 5-30 g bid	100 g, 500 gm.
DIOVET Syrup, Powder & Bolus	Diarrhoea & dysentery.	Cow, Buffalo, Horse: Syrup : 40-50 ml. Powder : 30-50 g. Bolus : 3-4 boluses. Calf, goat, sheep, pig: Syrup : 25-30 ml. Powder : 20-25 gm. Bolus : 1-2 Boluses Dog, Cat & Piglets: Syrup : 5-10 ml. Powder : 5-10 gm Bolus : 1/2 - 1 bolus. *Poultry :* Syrup 10 ml/100 birds Powder : 0.5% mixed with feed.	Syrup : 100 ml, 200 ml & 450 ml. Powder : 50 gm, 100g, & 1 kg. Bolus : strip of 4 boluses.
KAFACT Powder :	Sore throat, pharyngitis, laryngitis, common cold, bronchitis and pneumonia.	Cow, buffalo, horse: 30-50 gm bid. calf, goat, sheep, pig: 20-25 g. Dog, cat, piglet: 10-15 g bid.	100 g & 500 g.
HEALOVET Ointment	Pest infestation, repellent, wounds, sores, foot & mouth lesions, mange eruptions.	Clean the affected area and apply Healovet ointment 3-4 times/day.	Bottles of 50 gm containers of 450 gm
HORMOTONE Liquid	Hypoestrinism, anovulation, retained placenta, delayed or unsatisfactory uterine involution.	Large animals: 150 ml/day for minimum 7 days Sheep/dog: 75 ml/day.	Bottles of 200 ml 450 ml, 1 lit and 5 lit.
LIVOVET Powder, Syrup	Restoring feed intake & stimulating liver function. Counteracting damage by aflatoxin. Good supporative therapy along with oral antibiotics, sulfonamides and anthelmintics.	*Powder:* Cow/buffalo: 15-20 g twice a day with jaggery Sheep/goat/calf : 10- 15 gm twice a day. Layers: 150 gm/100 kg feed. *Syrup:* Cow/buffalo : 30 ml twice a day. Sheep/goat/calf : 15 ml twice a day.	Packets of 100 g, 1 kg & 5 kg. Bottles of 200 ml 450 ml & 5 litres.

Preparation	Indication	Dosage/Route	Presentation
		Broilers: 0-2 weeks : 4 ml/100 birds. 3-4 weeks : 8 ml/100 birds. 5th week onwards-15ml/100 birds. Layers: Chicks : 4 ml/100 birds. Growers : 8 ml/100 birds. Layers : 15 ml/100 birds.	
MILCHEY Tablet, Powder	Agalactia owing to stress, infection or metabolic disorders. Let down problems.	*Tablets:* 10 tab/twice a day (Ist day), followed by 4 tab/twice a day (for 10 days). *Powder:* 25 gm/twice a day (Ist day) followed by 15 gm/twice a day (for 10 days).	Packs of 100 & 1000 tabs. Packets of 100 g & 1 kg.
WORMINIL Powder	Anthelmintic.	Cow, Buffalo Horse & camel : 25-30 g bid. Goat, sheep & pig : 15-20 g bid. Dog & cat. 5-10 g bid.	100 gm, 500 gm.

CONCEPT PHARMACEUTICALS LIMITED
167 C.S.T. Road, Santa Cruz (East)
MUMBAI - 400 098

Preparation	Indication	Dosage/Route	Presentation
ALBIDOL Bolus Albendazole 1.5 g. Powder: Each g. contains Albendazole 150 mg, Tablet Albendazole 150 mg	Total spectrum anthelmintic & highly effective in the treatment of all types of worm infestation, eg. roundworms, lungworms, tapeworms and liverflukes in all species of animals.	For roundworms, lungworms, tapeworms; 5 mg of Albendazole/kg b.wt. For liver flukes: 10 mg/kg body weight.	Bolus 1.5 gm, Tablets 150 mg, Powder 15%- 100 gm.
BINOCIN Each vial contains (1 & 2gm vial) Ampicillin Sod. 500 mg; & 1 gm. Cloxacillin sod. 500 mg; & 1 gm	Broad spectrum antibiotic.	Large animal: 2 g. Small animal: 6 mg/kg body weight. Medium sized animal: 1g IV/IM Route.	Vial of 1 & 2 g.
BUTAGESIC Inj. Contains: Diclofenac Sodium 25 mg per ml.	Acute and chronic inflammatory and painful conditions, pyrexia due to various causes, mastitis, metritis.	Cattle/horse : 10-15 ml IM Calf/sheep/ goat : 2-5 ml IM Dog/cat : 1-2 ml IM The dosage in cattle/horse may be doubled depending on the severity of infection.	Vials of 10 ml and 30 ml.
CALCI-ROYAL Powder Calcium phosphorus with Vit C, D_3 & B_{12}, citric acid	Prevents rickets, in pica, increases milk yield, in milk fever, stimulates muscular and skeletal growth.	Cattle/horses: 40 gm daily. Calves/sheep/goat: 10 gm daily. Dogs: 2-5 gms daily orally.	100 gm sachets and 1 kg pack.
COMOXYL Vet Powder contains : Amoxycillin Trihydrate 500 mg per 5 ml	Calf scours, enteritis, pneumonia, mastitis and metritis in cattle, metritis and respiratory infections in horses, sheep and goat.	Horse/cattle : 20 gm orally for 3-5 days Calves/sheep/goat : 5 gm orally for 3-5 day Chicks : 1 gm in 4 lit drinking water Grower/broiler/layer / 1 gm in 2 lit of drinking water.	Containers of 100 gm and 500 gm.
CONCIMIN Powder contains : Vitamin + Mineral feed supplement	Corrects nutritional deficiencies, improves quality of feed and feed conversion. In poultry stimulates growth and increases egg production.	Cattle/horse : 20 gm daily Calves/sheep/goat : 5-10 gm daily Poultry: 2.5 kg/ton of feed.	Pouch of 250 gm and 2.5 kg.
CONAMPI Each vial contains: (a) Ampicillin sod 500 mg (b) Ampicillin sod. 1000 mg (c) Ampicillin sod. 2000 mg	Broad spectrum antibiotic.	Large Animal: 2 gm daily Medium sized animals: 1 gm daily Small animal : 500 mg daily.	Vials of 500 mg, 1000 mg & 2000 mg.
CONCIPLEX High potency Vit-B complex for parenteral use	Anorexia, G.I. atony, nervous disorder, muscular weakness, anaemia.	Large animal: 5 ml. Small animal: 2 ml. Deep IM.	Vials of 10 ml & 30 ml.

Preparation	Indication	Dosage/Route	Presentation
CONCITONE Multivitamin Liquid feed supplement	Used as general tonic to improve growth and production in poultry & livestock	Chicks : 5 ml/100 birds Growers/broilers : 7 ml per 100 birds Layers: 10 ml per 100 birds Cattle : 20 ml Calves/sheep/goat : 10 ml Dogs : 5 ml.	Bottle of 30 ml and 500 ml.
CURADEX Each ml contains: Dexamethasone sodium phosphate - 4 mg	In acute illness, allergy, toxaemia, shock, etc.	Large animal : 5 ml Small animal : 2 ml.	2 ml and 5 ml vial.
DERMOCEPT Ointment Antiseptic, fly repellent cream (Herbal preparation)	Mechanical & surgical wound, infected & septic wounds, maggot wounds, mange, eczema and dermatitis. Allergic skin conditions.	Wash the affected area with luke-warm water or saline water. Apply ointment gently over the area twice daily.	25 gm tube.
FLORATONE Bolus A combination of yeast, B complex, methionine with cobalt & copper in bolus form	In calves, sheep & goat for rapid recovery after diarrhoea & dysentery. Cattle & horses : Dyspepsia, rumen indigestion or dysfunction due to ketosis, toxaemia, ruminal acidosis, to improve the ruminal function after treatment with antibiotics and sulphonamide.	Calves/sheep/goat:1bolus Cattle/horses: 4 boluses bid orally.	Catch cover containing 4 boluses.
LEPTAMILK Forte Contains : Vitamins minerals and herbal feed supplements	Used as a general tonic to increase milk yield, growth promoter and appetite stimulater. Reduces incidences of placenta retention and prolapse. Increases egg production in poultry.	Cattle/horse : 30-40 ml bid orally Calves: 15-30 ml bid orally Dog : 2.5-5 ml bid orally Poultry for 100 birds Chicks/growers : 1-2 ml Broilers: 5-10 ml Layer : 10-20 ml in water.	460 ml bottle.
MYCOMULIN 45% Soluble granules	Chemotherapeutic agent for mycoplasmosis and gram positive/gram negative bacterial infections	Prevention : 5 gm / 1000 chicks for 3 days during first week of life. For subsequent medication : 27 mg/kg bwt for 2 days. Treatment : 54 mg per kg bwt daily for 3-5 days.	Container of 30 gm.
OXYTETRACYCLINE Inj. Contains : Oxytetracycline HCL 50 mg/ml .	Bacterial infections of respiratory, UTI, septicaemia, anthrax, black leg. calf diphtheria, H.S. pasteurellosis, mastitis, metritis, strangles, wounds, actinobacillosis, actinomycosis, anaplasmosis, leptospirosis.	Cattle/horse : 1-2 ml per 25 kg bwt I/M, I/V, S/C. Small animals: 1 ml per 10 kg bwt IM/IV/SC	Vials of 30 ml and 100 ml.

Preparation	Indication	Dosage/Route	Presentation
PEPSID Inj. B complex with liver extract	Anorexia, liver dysfunction, nervous weakness, anaemia, debility, after recovery from parasitic infestation, laminitis, systemic acidosis.	Cattle/horses: 3-5ml daily Calf/sheep/goat: 0.5-1ml Dog: 0.25-1 ml deep IM Inj.	Vial of 10 & 30 ml.
PLEXA BC Powder Feed supplement containing Vita. B. Complex & Vita. C for poultry and livestock.	Poor digestion and metabolism, effective feed utilization, better growth, increased egg, meat and milk production.	Cattle/horse : 10-20 gm. Calves/sheep/goat : 5-10 gm Dogs : 2-5 gm. Poultry : 5-10 gm for 100 birds or 500 gm per ton of feed.	1 kg container.
RAFOXIN Bolus Rafoxanide 2 gm Tablets : Rafoxanide 200 mg Powder: 10gm pouch contains Refoxanide 2 gm	For treatment of acute and chronic fascioliasis in sheep, goats and cattle.	7.5 mg of Rafoxanide per kg body weight.	Bolus 2 gm; Tablets 200 mg packed in 5 x 4 corton; Powder: 10 gm pouch.
SULCOPRIM Bolus Each bolus contains: Trimethoprim 400 mg, Sulphadiazine 2000 mg.	Treats all infection of GI tract, respiratory tract, reproductive tract and urinary tract.	Large animal : 2 boluses twice daily Small animal : 1 bolus twice daily	Pack of 10's.
SULCOPRIM Powder Each 5 gm contains: Trimethoprim 400 mg. Sulphamethoxazole 2 gm	Poultry: *E. Coli*, salmonellosis, bacillary white diarrhoea, fowl typhoid, coryza, infectious dermatitis.	Poultry: for 100 birds. Chicks : 2.5 gm Growers : 5 gm Layers : 10 gm Given orally in feed or water.	Packs of 100 gm and 500 gm.
VITACEPT Inj. Vitamin A 250000 I.U. Vitamin D$_3$ 25000 I.U. Vitamin E 100 mg	Infertility associated with Vit A deficiency, night blindness, xerophthalmia, karatomalacia, rickets, stunted growth, muscular dystrophy.	Cattle/horse: 2 vials/week; Calves, sheep, goats: 1 vial/week. Dogs : 1/2 to 1 ml.	5 ml vial.
ZODEX Bolus Each bolus contains: Mebendazole 1000 mg Powder : 5 gm contains : 500 mg mebendazole	Unique ovicidal & larvicidal action, removes all stages of worms: roundworms, tapeworms, hookworms, lungworms.	Cattle/horse : 2 to 4 boluses Calves/sheep/goat: 1 bolus Dogs : 1/2 bolus for 3 days.	Strips of 4's. 100 gm and 500 gm.

CYNAMID INDIA LIMITED
Animal Health Division, Nyloc House, 254-D2 Dr. Annie Besant Road
P.O.B. 9109, MUMBAI - 400 025

Preparation	Indication	Dosage/Route	Presentation
AUREOMYCIN (Nutritional Formula) Chlortetra-cycline HCl, Vit A, Vit. D3, Vit. E, Vit B6, Menadione, Niacin, Calcium pantothenate, Riboflavin, Cyanocobalamin, sodium sulfate, potassium chloride, sucrose.	Supportive therapy in all stress conditions such as transportation, change of weather, debeaking, deworming, peak egg production, change of house etc, for chicks, broilers, laying & breeding hens.	One teaspoonful dissolved in 5 lit. of drinking water, prepare fresh solution daily.	Packs of 960 g, 450 g & 200 g.
AUROFAC (Has two formulations), Aurofac-20, containing 44 g Aureomycin per kg & Aurofac-100-A, containing 100 g Aureomycin per kg.	Growth promotion & improved feed efficiency, prevention of diseases during stress, aid in prevention of early chick mortality by sensitive organisms, to maintain health and prevent chronic respiratory disease and synovitis and blue comb in laying hens and broilers.	Aurofac - 20 : 1.15 kg/tonne of feed. Aurofac-100-A: 500 g/tonne of feed.	Aurofac-20 20kg bags. Aurofac-100-A 20 kg bags.
CYCOSTAT 1 kg Cycostat contains: Robenidine - 66 gm.	For prevention of Emeria infection in broilers and cockerels.	500 gm of Cycostat per metric tonne of feed from day old to the marketing.	1 kg & 10 kg.
CHLORTETRACYCLINE Soluble Powder. 100 g CTC soluble powder contains 5.5 g of Chloretetracycline hydrochloride.	For prevention and treatment of chronic respiratory disease, synovitis, blue comb, hexamitiasis, infectious sinusitis and secondary infection.	Chickens: CTC powder in drinking water. Prevention Treatment C.Resp. Dis. 1TSF/10 lt 2-4TSF/10 lit B. Comb,. 1TSF/10 lt 2 TSF/10 lt Hexamitiasis Synovitis 2 TSF/10 lt 4TSF/10 lt Fowl cholera 4 TSF/4 lt drinking water early chick 2 TSF/10 lt for first 2 weeks mortality then 1 TSF/10 lt continuously.	100 g and 500 g pouches.
PIPERAZINE HEXA-HY-DRATE 56.3%. Contains piperazine hexahydrate 56.3% w/v equals 16.9g hexahydrate or 7.5 g base active ingredient in 30 ml product or 25% w/v solution on active ingredient basis.	Removal of large roundworms in poultry.	20 ml in 3.5 lt of water for 100 birds under 6 weeks of age. 40 ml in 5-10 lt of water/100 birds over 6 weeks of age.	450 ml bottle & 4.5 lt jar.

Preparation	Indication	Dosage/Route	Presentation
SODIUM SULFADIME-THYLPRIMIDINE PLUS CHLORTETRACYCLINE Soluble Powder. Sodium sulfadimethyl pyrimidine has a strength of 12.5%. Chlortetracycline soluble powder contains 5.5g chlortetracycline HCl/100 g	For coccidiosis, fowl cholera, fowlpox, coryza in chicks.	For 100 birds/day in drinking water SDW soln. CTC soln. For first 2 days 150 ml 5-10 TSF For next 4 days 75 ml 5-10 TSF	Bottles of 500 ml & 5 litres Jerry Can of sodium sulphadimethyl pyrimidine. 100 gm & 500 gm packs of chlortetracycline soluble powder.

DABUR AYURVET LIMITED
B-25, Sagar Apartments
6, Tilak Marg
NEW DELHI-110 001

Preparation	Indication	Dosage/Route	Presentation
AFANIL	Tympany, simple & frothy bloat, as a co-therapy for the impaction in horses.	Cows, buffaloes & horses: 50 ml Calves, heifer & colts: 25 ml Sheep & goats : 15 ml, twice daily for 2 days orally, may be administered intraruminally also.	100 ml, 250 ml glass bottle.
AYUCAL	Ca & P deficiency in birds, supplementation during high demand periods of high egg production, growth & weight gain. Better egg shell strength & improves carcass & meat quality. Prevents rickets & lameness due to mineral deficiency, prolapse, cannibalism, cage layer fatigue, osteoporosis and osteomalacia.	Broilers @ 0.1% (1kg/ton) mixed in feed. Layers (per 100 birds) Chicks : 5 gm Growers : 10 gm Layers : 15 gm mixed in feed for 7-10 days.	500 gm poly bag, 10 Kg container.
CALDHAN	Metabolic disorders due to deficiency of Ca & P. Supplementation during pregnancy & after calving. Milk fever, prolapse, retention of placenta infertility due to the P deficiency.	Cattle & horses 50 ml. calves, colts & helfers : 20 ml Sheep & goats : 10 ml Twice daily for 5-7 days.	500 ml bottle.
CHARMIL	Wound of all types, mange, Eczema, foot lesions in FMD, ringworm & dermatomycosis, broken horn, sinuses, fistulae, sores, fissures.	Clean the affected area & apply Charmil once daily.	Tube of 50 gm.
DIAROAK	Diarrhoea of different aetiology, calf scours.	Cows, buffaloes, horses & camels: 30 gm Calves, heifers, colts : 10-15 gm Sheep, goat, pig: 7.5-10 gm Adm. orally twice daily.	30 gm.
DIMBPRO	Increases egg production, restoration of egg production in various diseases. For sustained egg production & minimising broodiness in layers.	Given @ 50 gms per 100 kg feed for 10 days.	50 gm sachet.
EXAPAR	For expulsion of retained placenta, regulation of lochial discharge, delayed involution.	Cows, buffaloes & horses: 50 ml Ewes & does : 20 ml To be given after calving or in case of retained placenta double dose is given twice on Ist day and single dose for 3-5 days.	250 ml 500 ml glass bottles.

Preparation	Indication	Dosage/Route	Presentation
JANOVA	Non-specific anestrus, silent estrus, non-ovulatory estrus. For inducing timely post-partum estrus and for regulating ovarian function.	Cows, buffaloes, heifers & mares: 3 capsule per day ewes, bitches and sows: 2 caps/day orally for two consecutive days. Repeat after 10 days in case no estrus is observed	Strip of 6 capsules.
LIVFIT Vet Liquid	Restoring reduced feed intake, fighting aflatoxins, improving liver functions, better feed utilization, growth, livability and production.	Chicks : 5 ml / 100 chicks Grower: 10 ml / 100 chicks Layer/broilers 20 ml / 100 chicks In morning drinking water for 7 days. Regular usage is recommended for improving growth and livability.	Bottle of 500 ml and 5 lit Jar.
LIVFIT Vet Premix	- do -	2 kg premix/tonne of feed.	1 kg & 5 kg.
PACHOPLUS	Simple indigestion, anorexia, ruminal stasis, as co-treatment in secondary anorexia and impaction.	Cows, buffaloes, horses and camel: 2 boli Calves, heifers and colts: 1 bolus Sheep and goat: 1/2 to 1 bolus orally twice daily for 2-3 days.	Strip of 4 boluses.
PAYAPRO	Hypogalactia, agalactia, irregular or suppressed lactation; as adjuvant therapy in mastitis for restoring milk yield, for increasing milk production and higher lactation yield.	Cows and buffaloes : 4 Ewes and dogs : 1-2 orally once daily for 10-15 days.	Strip of 4 boluses.
RUCHAMAX	Inappetance, dyspepsia, impaired ruminal functions. Poor digestion, convalescence	Cows, buffaloes, horses: 15 gm Calves, heifers, colts: 5-7.5 gm Sheep, goats : 3-5 gm. oral route once or twice daily for 2-3 days.	15 gm pack.
STRESROAK Liquid	Counteracts stress due to vaccination, debeaking etc. Reduces early chick mortality, increases body resistance. For optimum feed utilization, growth and productivity.	Dosage/day/100 birds: Chicks : 5 ml Growers : 7.5 ml Layers/broilers : 10 ml in drinking water for 5-7 days.	500 ml bottle.
YAKRIFIT Liquid	For liver dysfunction & damage. Used as a tonic for liver and as a growth promoter.	Cows, buffaloes & horses : 50 ml Calves, colts & pigs : 20-25 ml Sheep & goats : 15-20 ml given twice daily for 5-7 days.	125 ml 250 ml bottles.
YAKRIFIT Bolus	Same as above.	Cows, buffaloes & horses : 2 boli Calves, colts & pigs : 1 bolus Sheep & goats : 1/2-1 bolus.	4 boli strips.

ETHICARE LTD
Fraser Raod
PATNA - 800 001

Preparation	Indication	Dosage/Route	Presentation
AQUEOUS IODINE SOLUTION Contains: Iodine 5% w/v, Pot. iodide 10% w/v	Metritis and vaginitis.	5 ml of the solution is mixed with 250 ml water and is irrigated into uterus.	100 ml, 400 ml, 500 ml.
CALCIUM BOROGLUCONATE Contains: 25% solution of calcium borogluconate	Milk fever, acute hypocalcaemia, treatment and protection of liver from chloroform and carbon tetrachloride poisoning.	Cattle/buffalo/horse: 200-350 ml I/V, S/C Sheep/goat/pig : 30-60 ml I/V, S/C Dog : 2-5 ml I/V, S/C.	450 ml bottle.
CARBON TETRACHLORIDE	Liver fluke infestation in sheep, goat and cattle, Caution - causes liver disorders.	Adult cattle 5 ml as emulsion or by probang; repeat 3-4 weeks later once or twice. Sheep/goat: 1-1.5 ml; Repeat after 3-4 weeks.	450 ml bottle.
CREAM OF GAMMA BENZENE HEXACHLORIDE AND PROFLAVINE Contains: 0.1% pure gamma isomer of BHC and 0.1% Proflavine sulfate	Blow fly larvae in wound and as dressing cream on all types of wounds.	To be applied locally.	200 g and 500 gm Jar.
DEBLOAT Contains: 1% silica in Dimethicone suspension	Frothy or gaseous bloat in ruminants.	Cattle/buffalo: 100 ml orally or intraruminal.	100 ml bottles.
DEVERM Contains: Tetramisole HCl 30% w/v	Gastrointestinal nematodes of cattle, sheep and pigs, also effective against lungworms.	Orally or mix 10 g in 300 ml water Cattle/buffalo/sheep: 15 mg/kg b.wt. or 1.5 ml/kg b.wt. Pig: 1 g/22.5 kg b.wt. orally repeat after 21 days.	10 gm sachet and 100 gm container.
DEXALT Each 27.5 g sachet contains: Sod. chloride 3.5 g, Sod. bicarb 2.5 g, Pot. chloride 1.5 g and Dextrose 20 g	Oral rehydration therapy.	Dissolve in 1 litre of water and give orally.	27.5 g sachet.
EGGMAX Contains: moisture max 3%, calcium (min) 28%, phosphorus (min) 5%, Iron 0.35%, iodine 10 ppm, copper (min) 100 ppm, manganese (min) 200 ppm, zinc 1200 ppm, fluorine (max) 0.03%, cobalt (min) 50 ppm, magnesium 800 ppm, sod. chloride (max) 15%	Feed supplement (minerals) for poultry.	1 kg/40-50 kg poultry mash orally.	1 kg, 10 kg.

Preparation	Indication	Dosage/Route	Presentation
FLUKAPHENE Contains: Hexachlorophene 20% w/w	Used in liverfluke and paramphistome infections in livestock.	Cattle/buffalo/calves/sheep/goat: 1-1.5 g/20 kg b.wt. orally. For prevention repeat at 5 months interval.	250 g, 10 g.
FURAN-100 AND, FURA-ZOLIDONE PREMIX Each kg contains: Furazolidone 100 g and 240 g respectively	Primary and secondary bacterial diseases and protozoan diseases in poultry.	Routine use - 22.5 g Furazolidone or 50 g Furan- 100/100 kg feed for 1 week. Treatment - 400 g Furan-100 for 10 days or 180 g Furazolidone Premix for 10 days Prophylaxis-100 g Furazolidone Premix for 2 weeks Antistress-45 g Furazolidone Premix/100 kg feed for 2 weeks.	50 g sachet and 500 g container.
HEMATIC Each 5 g contains: Dried ferrous sulfate 4.5 g, copper sulfate 300 mg, Mag sulph 100 mg, cobalt sulfate 100 mg.	Weakness, anaemia and neonatal ataxia, piglet anaemia.	Cattle/buffalo: 5-10 g orally Horses: 1-5 g orally Sheep/pig: 1/2-1g is given orally bid or sid.	50 g, 500 g.
IODINE AND METHYL SALICYLATE Oint. Contains: Iodine 5% w/w and methyl salicylate 5% w/w	Pain and swelling associated with bruises, abrasions, contusions and sprains.	Apply externally and rub well on to the affected area.	5 g, 200 g Jar.
MILKMAX Contains: moisture(max) 7%, calcium (min) 22% phosphorus (min) 9%, sod. chloride (min) 22%, iron 0.4-0.6%, iodine 0.02-0.1%, copper 0.06-0.1%, manganese 0.09-0.12%, cobalt 0.01-0.02%, fluorine (max) 0.03%	Trace minerals supplement.	Adult cattle and buffalo: 25-30 g/day orally or 1 kg/ 100 kg concentrate.	1 kg, 10 kg bag.
NILTAPE Contains: Lead Arsenate 20% w/w.	Tapeworm infestation in livestock.	Cattle/buffalo: 5-10 g orally Calves/sheep/goat : 2.5-5 g orally.	10 g, 500 g.
NITROFURAZONE Ointment Contains : 0.2% w/w Nitrofurazone in water soluble base.	Bacterial infection of traumatic origin, wounds etc.	Apply locally on the area for 7-10 days.	200 g, 500 gm Jar.

Preparation	Indication	Dosage/Route	Presentation
NOREXIA Each 5 g contains: Cobalt sulfate 250 mg, Dried ferrous sulfate 200 mg, Zinc sulfate 150 mg and Nux Vomica powder 4.4 g.	Rumentorics and appetizer.	Cattle/buffalo/horse: 4-5 g orally Sheep/goat 2 g orally sid or bid x 3-5 days.	25 g, 250 g.
PIPERAZINE Liquid and soluble powder Each 5 ml contains : Piperazine Hexahydrate 1.85 g equal to 0.82 g. Piperazine Powder contains: 44% Piperazine	Roundworms in livestock, nodular worms in swine, pinworms and strongyles worms in horse.	Cattle/buffalo: 15-30 ml/30 kg b.wt. or 11 g/30 kg b.wt. Horse/calves: 15 ml/30 kg b.wt. or 5.5g/30 kg b.wt. Swine : 15 ml/25 kg b.wt. Dog/cat: 2.5 ml/10 kg b.wt. orally; repeat after 2-3 weeks.	10 ml, 450 ml bottle 34 g and 225 g container.
POVIDONE IODINE Solution Contains: Povidone iodine 10% equal to 1% w/v of available iodine	Post-partum endometritis and infertility associated with mild endometritis.	Post-partum endometritis Cattle/buffalo: Dilute 1:5 in water and infuse 100 ml I/V at 1-3 weeks of calving and 50 ml 3 weeks onward.	100 ml and 500 ml bottle.
STAT Each 10 g contains: Furazolidone 400 mg, Kaolin 64 g, calcium carbonate 32 g.	Effective in bacterial enteritis, non-specific diarrhoea and food poisoning due to gram positive and gram negative bacteria.	Cattle/buffalo/sheep/goat/pig: 10 g/40 kg b.wt. bid for 3-5 days with molasses or gruel.	50g, 500g.
STRONG DEXTROSE Inj. Contains: 50% Dextrose in water	Ketosis, hypoglycaemia or intravenous glucose tolerance test (IVGTT).	Cattle/buffalo : 500 ml I/V For IVGTT - 1 ml/kg b.wt. I/V within 30 minutes.	375 ml bottle.
TARTAMETIC (2% and 4%) Contains: 2% and 4% aqueous solution of Antimony Potassium tartarate	Trypanosomiasis and schistosomiasis in cattle and horses. Caution–should not be used in gastroenteritis, cardiac, renal or hepatic insufficiency and very old and debilitated animals. S/C or I/M injection causes pain and tissue necrosis.	Schistosomiasis–Cattle: 1 ml (2%)/10 kg b.wt. on alternate day for 2 weeks I/V. Trypanosomiasis–Cattle/horse: 1ml (2%) per 10 kg b.wt. daily for four days I/V.	25 ml vial.
THALOXONE Each 10 g contains: Sulfadimidine 5 g, Phthalylsulfathiazole 4g, Furazolidone 1 g.	Useful in non-specific diarrhoea, calf scour, bacterial gastroenteritis and protozoal (coccidial) dysentery.	Orally for all species of livestock 1 sachet/50 kg b.wt.	10 g sachet.
TRYPAN BLUE Contains: Trypan blue 1 g/vial	Babesiosis or piroplasmosis in cattle, horse, sheep and dogs.	Cattle and horses : 1-4 g slow I/V Sheep : 0.5-1 g I/V.	1 g vial.

GANGETIC HERBS PVT LTD.
A-C/123A, Shalimar Bagh,
DELHI- 110 052

Preparation	Indication	Dosage/Route	Presentation
GOVARDHAN Feed I and II	Anestrus, repeat breeder, delayed maturity in heifers.	Feed I : 100 ml daily for first 5 days Feed II : 50 gm daily for next 10 days with gur.	Feed I : 500 ml Feed II : 500 gm.
HARIRA (Herbal cleansing draught)	Retention of placenta, to induce ovulatory heat, inflammatory condition of genital tract, to improve milk production.	Cow/buffaloes: 100-150 ml daily x 10 days. Mare: 75-100 ml daily x 10 days. Sheep/goat : 25-50 ml daily x 10 days.	Bottle of 500 ml & 1 litre.
PROFAT	To increase fat percentage & SNF in milk.	Cow/buffalo: 200 gm/day.	1 kg, 4kg & 10 kg.
PROLACT-M Powder	To increase milk production, to restore milk production in the animals recovered from disease, to improve let down of milk, to improve fertility in animals.	Cow/buffalo: 100 gm/day x 10 days orally. Sheep/goat: 20 gm/day x 10 days orally.	100 gm 500 gm.

GLAXO INDIA LTD (AGRIVET FARMCARE)
Dr. Annie Besant Road
MUMBAI - 400 025

Preparation	Indication	Dosage/Route	Presentation
AGRIMIN Each kg provides: Copper 312 mg, cobalt 45 mg, Magnesium 2.114 g, Iron 979 mg, Zinc 2.13 g, Iodine 156 mg, DL-Methionine 1.92g. L-Lysine Mono HCl 4.4 g, calcium 30%, Phosphorus 8.25%	Mineral mixture with essential amino acids. Ideal for better growth, fertility and production.	Large animal: 20-30 g daily orally Small animal: 5-10 g daily orally	Packs 1 kg, 10 kg.
ALBOMAR (Powder, suspension) Powder contains: 15% Albendazole; suspension contains: 2.5% Albendazole	Highly effective and safe broad spectrum anthelmintic, eliminates roundworm, tapeworm and liverflukes completely. It is ovicidal, larvicidal, cysticidal and wormicidal.	Orally @ 5 mg Albendazole/kg b.wt. Large animal Powder 0.33 g/kg b.wt. suspension 0.2 ml/kg b.wt. Poultry : (100 birds) - Powder: 4-5g in feed x 3 days in divided dose. Suspension: 20-30 ml in water x 3 days in divided doses.	Powder tins 50 g and 250 g Suspension-bottle of 30 ml, 60 ml and 500 ml.
AMPROL PLUS (Amprolium and ethopabate)	Use as a prophylactic anticoccidial agent.	500 gm/ton of feed.	10 x 1kg & 20 kg bag.
AMPROLSOL 20% 30 g Amprolsol contains: Amprolium HCl 6 g	For the treatment of coccidiosis, for prevention of coccidiosis.	Outbreaks: 30 g amprolsol in 25 litre of drinking water for 5-7 days. Prevention: Provide amprolsol 20% @0.006% amprolium (30 g in 100 litre of drinking water).	30 g & 150 g pouch.
BETENESOL Inj. Each ml contains : Betamethasone 4 mg	Ketosis, arthritis and related disorders, alergic and dermatological conditions, anaphylactic shock, local inflammatory condition etc.	Cattle and buffaloes : 4-20 mg I/M, I/V. Calves, sheep, goat : 2-4 mg I/M, I/V. Dogs, cats : 0.5-1 mg I/M, I/V	2 ml sampoule.
BROTONE Contains fresh liver extract 1.25g with Vit B$_{12}$ activity equivalent to 7.5 mcg cyanocobalamin, yeast extract 0.4 g, Thiamine 2.5 mg, Nicotinamide 24 mg and alcohol 1 ml in each 10 ml.	For toning up and boosting the function of liver. For regular use in layer and whenever there is climatic stress.	Orally through drinking water Cattle/buffalo/horse: 40 ml x 3 days, Calves/sheep/goat: 15ml x 3 days. Broiler (2-6 wks) : 5-10 ml/100 Birds daily x 10 days. Growers & layers (19 wks old) 20 ml/100 bird daily x 10 days. In layers, repeat in every 3 months.	Bottle 120 ml & 500 ml.

Preparation	Indication	Dosage/Route	Presentation
COBAPHOS Forte Each 1 ml contains : Sod. salt of phosphonic acid 125 mg, Vita B$_{12}$ 50 mcg.	Tonic in general metabolism, debility, disorders of bone formation and as a roborant, anestrus.	Large animal : 5-10 ml S/C or I/M on alternate days. Small animal : 1-2 ml S/C or I/M on alternate days.	5 ml, 30 ml.
DUOCOXIN (Amprolium 16.67%, Sulphaquinoxaline 16.67%)	To control coccidiosis outbreaks.	0.01% amprolium & 0.01% sulpha quinoxaline in drinking water for 7 days (30 gm in 50 litres of drinking water.	30 gm pouch.
GLACAL 25 Calcium borogluconate sol. 25%	Hypocalcaemia, milk fever, liver damage prevention due to drugs.	Cow, buffalo, horses: 200-350 ml S/C, I/V. Sheep, goat, pig: 2-5 ml S/C, I/V.	450 ml.
GLACAL 40 Calcium borogluconate 40%	-do-		450 ml.
GLAMAG Calcium borogluconate, magnesium, phosphorus	Milk fever due to hypocalcaemia or associated deficiencies of magnesium and/or phosphorus.	Cow/buffaloes: 200 to 250 ml S/C ot I/V.	450 ml.
GROBLEND Each 2 kg contains: Vit A 5 x 10^6 iu, Vit B$_2$ 2 g, Vit B$_6$ 400 mg, Cal. Pantothenate 4 g, Vit B$_{12}$ 5600 mcg, Vit D$_3$ 6,25,00 iu, Vit E 800 iu, Choline chloride 10 g, Copper 2 g, Manganese 27.5 g, Iron 7.5 g , Zinc 15g, Iodine 1 g, Calcium 27.25%, Phosphorus 7.45%, antiodixant qs.	Avitaminosis, mineral deficiency and for boosting the health and production in poultry and livestock.	With feed or orally Large animal: 20-25 g daily Small animal: 5-10 g daily. Poultry : 2 kg/1-1.5 ton feed.	Plastic jar 2 kg
GROVIPLEX Each 5 ml contains: Vit B$_2$ 1.25 mg, D-Panthenol 0.65 mg, Vit B$_6$ 0.62 mg, Vit B$_{12}$ 6.25 mg, Nicotinamide 37.5 mg, choline chloride 10 mg, Lysine mono HCl 10.0 mg	Provides extra power for better growth, production and resistance to liver of poultry. It rejuvenates the ruminal microflora.	With feed or water, mix 15-30 ml/100 birds in water or with feed daily. Cattle/buffalo : 50-100 ml/day.	Bottles 500 ml Jars 5 litres.
HYBLEND AB$_2$ D$_3$ Each g contains: Vit A 40,000 iu, Vit B$_2$ 25 mg, Vit D$_3$ 6000 iu	As feed supplement to promote growth, protects from infection, rickets and cures curled toe paralysis in poultry.	1 kg/5 ton of poultry feed.	1 kg.
HYBLEND AB$_2$ D$_3$ K Each g contains: Vit A 82,500 iu, Vit B$_2$ 50 mg, Vit D$_3$ 12000 iu, Vit K 10 mg	Provides strength to muscles and bones for excellent growth and production in poultry, should be used as feed supplement regularly.	Mixed in poultry feed at the rate of 1 kg/10 ton.	1 kg tin.

Preparation	Indication	Dosage/Route	Presentation
IVOMEC Oral (Ivermectin)	G.I.T. roundworms, lung-worms, nasal bots, maggoted wounds, lice, ticks etc for sheep and goat.		50 ml, 500 ml.
IVOMEC (Ivermectin w/v 1%)	GIT roundworms, lungworms, nasal bots, lice, ticks, microfilariasis, maggoted wounds.	0.5 ml/25 kg b.w. S/C.	7 ml, 20 ml vial & 1 ml ampoule.
KALZOLE Granules contains calcium, phosphorus, manganese	Thin shelled eggs, prolapse, con-nibalism, leg weakness etc in poultry.	100 gm/100 kg feed.	1 kg, 5 kg.
KHORSOLINTH Each 100 ml contains: Glutaradehyde trihydrate 7gm	Antibacterial and antifungal in action. Used to disinfect equip-ment, hospital premises, poultry house, milk sheds etc.	—	100 ml, 500 ml.
LIVOGEN Inj. Each ml contains: Vit B_1 25 mg, Panthenol 5 mg, vit B_2 1.37 mg, Nicotinamide 100 mg, Vit B_{12} 30 mcg, choline chloride 15 mg, liver injec-tion crude derived from 8 g fresh liver with 2 mcg of cya-nocobalamin	Anorexia, liver degeneration, fatty liver and liverfluke infesta-tions.	Large animal: 10 ml x 3 days deep I/M. Dog : 1-2 ml daily I/M, S/C.	Vials 10 ml, 30 ml.
LIXEN Water soluble powder Cephlexin 7.5% w/w	Broad spectrum antibacterial.	Livestock : 10 mg/kg b.wt as a drench or with food. 20 gm to be dissolved in required quantity of water for intrauterine use.	20 gm sachet.
MUNOMYCIN Forte Inj. Each vial contains. Procaine Penicillin 15×10^5 iu, Peni-cillin G. 5×10^5 iu strepto-mycin sulfate 2.5 g,	Builds resistance and prevents relapse, controls and cure bacte-rial diseases of livestock sensi-tive to penicillin and streptomy-cin.	Add 8.5 ml d.w. and give by deep I/M; cattle, Buffalo/ horse: 1-2 vials daily x 2-3 days or more.	2.5 g vials.
OSTOCALCIUM VET Each 5 ml contains: Tribasic calcium phosphate 0.24 g, Vit D_3 400 iu, Vit B_{12} 5 mcg	Rickets, poor growth, pica, pro-lapse, milk fever in cow, thin shelled eggs, prolapse and canni-balism in poultry	Cattles buffalo/horse: 50 ml bid orally Calves : 20 ml bid orally. Poul-try: 20-100 ml in drinking water per 100 birds daily.	500 ml, 1 litre bottle.
PIPERAZINE Liquid (45%) Each 100 ml contains : 45 g of Piperazine hydrate	Deworming of poultry and calves against roundworms and threadworm infestation.	Orally with drinking water or as drench Cattle, buffalo/horse: 115 ml. Calves, sheep/goat : 20-30 ml. Dog/cat: 2-5 ml (diluted). Poultry : 50 ml/100 birds.	Bottles of 115 ml and 500 ml.

Preparation	Indication	Dosage/Route	Presentation
PREPALIN Forte Inj. Each 2 ml contains: Vit A 600,000 iu, Chlorbutol 1% in oily vehicle	Infertility, night blindness, xe-rophthalmia, Keratomalacia, respiratory, urogenital and G.I. tract abnormality.	By I/M route For Infertility : cow/buffalo: 6 ml on 2 alternate days Hypovitaminosis A. Large animal: 12 ml/week Small animal: 6-12 ml/week Dog/cat : 2-6 ml/week in divided doses.	2 ml ampoule.
RANIDE (Rafoxanide 20%)	Against adult fluke and immature fluke.	Add 10 gm Ranide to 80 ml of water. Sheep: upto 20kg - 6 ml 21-30 kg - 9 ml 31-40 kg - 12 ml Cattle: upto 75 kg - 22.5 ml, 76-100 kg - 30 ml, 101-125 kg - 37.5 ml 126-150 kg - 45 ml 151-175 kg - 52.5 ml 176-200 kg - 60 ml 201-225 kg-67.5 ml 226-250 kg- 75 ml.	Sachet of 10 gm.
VETBACIN Contains: Bacitracin (as zinc) 500 iu, Neomycin sulfate 5 mg, soft paraffin base to 1 g.	Broad spectrum skin ointment, effective against both gram positive and gram negative bacteria and spirochaetes. Very good non-irritant ointment for wounds, abrasion, fistulae, furunculosis, otitis externa and skin surgery.	Apply a thin layer on the lesion as and when required.	Tubes of 15 g and 50 g.
VIBELAN Inj. Each ml contains: Vit B_1 25 mg, Nicotinamide 100 mg, Vit B_2 4.1 mg, D-Panthenol 5 mg, Vit B_6 2.5 mg, Ligno-caine HCl 5 mg	Co-therapy with antibiotics for rapid recovery. B- complex vitamin supplement.	By deep I/M Cattle, buffalo/horse: 10 ml daily X 3-4 days Dog/cat : 3-5 ml daily.	30 ml.
VIMERAL Each ml contains: Vit A 12000 iu, Vit E 48 mg, Vit D_3 6000 iu, Vit. B_{12} 20 mcg	For the treatment of crazy chick diseases and stress of transportation, vaccination etc. and vitamin supplement.	Cattle, buffalo/horse: 20 ml daily drench Calves : 10 ml daily drench Poultry : 5-10 ml/100 birds with drinking water.	30 ml 60 ml, 120 ml.
VITABLEND AD_3 Each g contains : Vit A 50,000 iu, Vit D_3 5000 iu	To increase milk fat, growth, production and body resistance.	Cattle, buffalo/horse: 5 g daily x 30 days followed by 2.5 g daily/animal or 200 g/ton cattle feed	20 g sachets and 1 kg.

Preparation	Indication	Dosage/Route	Presentation
VITABLEND WM Forte 1 ml contains: Vit A 1,00,000 iu	For increased egg production, hatchability, prevention of blood spots, and to develop body resistance against coccidiosis, coryza etc.	10 ml/100 birds with drinking water for 10 days.	100 ml bottle, 1 litre polythene bottle.
VITAPET	Skin and coat conditioner for dogs and cats -helps prevent rheumatism and arthritis -strengthens bones.	Puppies; Few drops Adult Dogs: 1 1/4 to 2 TSF Cats : 1 TSF to be given daily with food.	Bottle of 150 ml.

HERBAL PRODUCTS INDIA
5, Chandar Nagar
SAHARANPUR - 247 001

Preparation	Indication	Dosage/Route	Presentation
DYSENTRON (Antidiarrhoeals)	Acute or chronic diarrhoea of non-specific reasons. Acute or chronic dysentery, coccidiosis.	Cow, buffaloes, horses : 25-30 gm. Dogs & pigs (15 days to 2 month old) : 2-5 gm. Sheep, goats, adult pigs, colts, calves : 8-10 gm.	100 gm. 500 gm. 1 kg.
HEAT-X (Estrus inducer)	Anestrus due to non-functional ovary or non-specific reasons.	Cows, buffaloes, mares and heifers: 3 capsules. Goat, sheep, bitches: 2 capsules. It should be given orally with gur. If the animal does not evince heat within 24 hrs, the dose may be repeated.	6, 12, 24 capsules.
HERBITTOL (Skin ointment)	Antifungal, antiseptic, antipruritic, fly repellent.	Local application.	50 gm. 1 kg.
KAMDHENU BATISA (Appetite stimulant)	All digestive disorders including anorexia, dyspepsia, constipation, flatulence, colic etc. Ill health, general debility, exhaustion and stress condition.	Cows, buffaloes, horses : 40-60 gm. calves, colts. heifers, adult pigs: 10-15 gm. Dogs & piglets (15 days to 3 months) : 3-5 gm. Poultry & birds : 2-5 gm (mix with feed). To be given twice daily as a bolus or electuary.	100 gm, 200 gm, 500 gm, 1 kg.
LECTOCURE (Galactogogue)	Irregular lactation, failure of lactation, hypogalactia, low milk production in apparently healthy animals.	Cows, Buffaloes : 50 gm. Ewes, Goats : 10-15 gm.	500 gm, 1 kg.
LIVOMIN (Feed Supplement)	Growth promoter, liver tonic remedy for liver disorder, develops resistance to diseases, perfect feed additive for poultry & cattle.	Cows, buffaloes, horses: 50-70 gm. Sheep, goats, calves and colts: 15-20 gm. Poultry : mixed in feed. Broiler : 0.5%. Layers : 0.25%	1 kg.
PESTOKiL (Ectoparasiticidal)	Ectoparasitic infestation of lice, ticks, fleas, mites etc.	Dilute the medicine in 10 volumes of clean water, apply this solution liberally, let it remain for 48 hrs. If required repeat the application.	100 ml, 1 litre.

THE HIMALAYA DRUG CO.
Makali, Nelamangala
BANGALORE - 562 123

Preparation	Indication	Dosage/Route	Presentation
BONNISAN	Common gastrointestinal problems in newborn pups & chicks.	Pup: 1/4-1 tsp bid upto 3 months. Chicks : 5 ml per 50 chicks.	Bottle of 120 ml.
CYSTONE (Powder/tablets)	Urinary calculi, post-operative urolithiasis, crystalluria, haematuria.	Large animall 2-3½ gms thrice daily. Calves, foals, sheep, goat: 2 tabs thrice daily. Dogs: Large breeds: 3 tabs daily small breeds : 1-2 tabs daily for 7 days. In urinary calculi for 6 months & in haematuria for 4-6 weeks.	Powder: 10 x 50 g pack. Tablets: pack of 100 & 1000 tablets.
DIAREX (Tablets)	Non-specific diarrhoea.	Large animall: 16-20 tabs thrice daily. Calves, foals: 4-6 tabs thrice daily. Sheep, goat, pigs: 2-4 tabs thrice daily. Dogs: 1-2 tabs thrice daily.	Pack of 100 tabs.
GASEX (Tablets)	Tympanitis and frothy bloat.	Dose is same as for Diarex.	Pack of 100 tabs.
GERIFORTE (Tablet/Syrup)	For sustained fitness in ageing: stallions, stud bulls, circus animals, cattle, pet dogs.	Large animall: 10-15 tabs bid. Dogs: Large breeds: 2 tabs twice daily. Small breeds: 1 tab twice daily.	Pack of 100 tabs. Syrup-200 ml bottle.
LIV-52 (Drops, Syrup, Powder, Tablets)	As a tonic: in poor appetite, stunted growth, loss of condition, dullness of coat, post-operative recovery, convalescence, torpid sluggish liver.	Large animals: 7g bid daily. Foals, calves, yearlings: 2- 3 g bid daily. Sheep, goat, pig 3-5 g daily. Dogs: 1-2 tabs bid daily. Puppies: 1-3 drops tid. Poultry (powder/drops) 1 g/kg feed. Lambs & piglets: 1/2-1g daily.	Powder: 100g x 10 pack. Drops: 30ml & 120 ml bottle. Syrup: 120 ml. Tablets 50 x 100 pack.
	As a treatment: in equine jaundice, azoturia, biliary fever, joint ill, navel ill in foals, bovine jaundice, haemoglobinuria, FMD, HS, red water disease, theileriasis, leptospirosis, liver flukes, worm infestation, toxicity of drugs, plants, insecticides etc.	L.A. 7g tid daily. Foals, calves yearling: 2-3 g tid daily. Sheep, goat, pig: 3-8 g daily. Lambs, piglets: 1-2g daily. Dogs: Adults 2-4 tabs bid daily. Small breeds: 5-10 drops tid. Poultry: 10-15 drops/bird daily.	
RUMALAYA (Cream, Tablets)	Rheumatic arthritis, infective polyarthritis, osteoarthritis, neuritis, fibrosis, joint ill in calves, foals, sprains & strained tendons & ligaments.	Large animall: 8-12 tabs tid daily. Calves, foals: 4-6 tabs tid. Sheep, goats, Pigs: 2-4 tabs tid. Cream is applied locally with hot fomentation.	Collapsible tube of 28 gm, tabs pack of 100.

Preparation	Indication	Dosage/Route	Presentation
SEPTILIN (Tablets, Syrup)	To promote phagocytosis, protects against bacterial infections, acute & chronic ENT infections, intractable dermatological conditions, inflammation & exudates, UTI, wound healing.	Large animall: 16 -20 tabs tid, In acute cases : 24 tabs tid. Calves, foals : 4-6 tabs tid. Sheep, goats, pigs : 2-4 tabs tid. In acute cases : 6 tabs followed by 4 tabs tid. Dogs, Large breeds : 2 tabs tid. Small breeds : 1 tab tid. Cats : 1 tab tid.	Pack of 100, syrup : 100 ml bottle.
SPEMAN (Tablets, powder)	Oligospermia.	Large animals: 7 ½-12 g in 2 divided doses for 3-6 weeks. Rams: 2-4g in 2 divided doses for 3-6 weeks.	Pack of 100 tablets.
	For semen collection.	Large animals: 7 ½-12 g daily in 2 divided doses for one week prior to collection. Rams: 2-4 g daily in 2 div. doses one week prior to collection.	
	Prostatic enlargement.	Dogs: Large breeds, 1 tab tid. Small breeds 1 tab bid.	
STYPLON (Tablets)	Epistasxis, haematuria, vaginal & post-operative bleeding.	Large animall 16-24 tabs tid. Calves, foal: 4-6 tabs tid. Sheep, goats, pigs: 2-4 tabs tid. Dogs: Large breeds: 2 tabs tid. Small breeds: 1 tab tid.	Pack of 100 tablets.
TENTEX Forte (Powder/Tablets)	To improve sexual desire, poor stud performance & delayed reaction prior to mounting.	Orally for improving libido: Large animall: 3-4 ½ g daily for 7-10 days before natural service. Rams and bucks: 1-2 g daily for 7-10 days before natural service. Impotence: Large animall: 3-4 ½ g daily for 30 days. Rams and bucks: 1-2g daily for 30 days. Dogs: 1 tab daily for 7 days.	Powder: pack of 10 x 10g, Tablet. strip of 10 x 10.

HINDUSTAN ANTIBIOTICS LIMITED
Agro-Vet Division, Pimpri
PUNE - 411 018

Preparation	Indication	Dosage/Route	Presentation
ALBENDAZOLE 2.5% suspension. Each 5 ml susp. contains: 125 mg Albendazole	GIT nematodes, lungworms, tapeworms, liver flukes.	Roundworm & tapeworm: Cattle, buffalo, sheep & goat: 5 mg/kg b.wt. Dog & cat: 10-25 mg/kg b.wt. Liver flukes: Cattle & buffalo: 10 mg/kg b.wt. Sheep & Goat: 7.5 mg/kg b.wt.	60 ml, 120 ml & 500 ml bottles.
DYNACIL - VET Each vial contains: Ampicillin sodium 1 gm/2.5 gm	Broad spectrum antibiotic.	2-7 mg/kg b.wt. Intramuscular/intravenous.	Vials of 1.0 gm & 2.5 gm.
HAMIDIN Each tab contains: Sulphadimidine 5 gm	Pneumonia, wound infections, foot-rot, streptococal mastitis, metritis, coccidiosis, joint ill of foals & swine, calf diphtheria, calf scour, influenza, secondary bacterial complications associated with R.P. in cattle, and canine & feline distemper in dog & cat respectively, H.S.	200 mg/kg orally followed by half this dosage daily for 3-5 days. It can also be used as uterine passaries.	5 gm tablets in containers of 10 & 50 tablets.
HAMYCIN - AVS Hamycin equivalent to 200,000 units/ml.	Braod antifungal activity especially against *Aspergillus fumigatus* also against *A. glaucus* and *A. niger* infection in poultry.	*Therapeutic:* 10 ml of suspension/l of drinking water daily for 10-15 days and then prophylactic medication can be continued *Prophylactic:* 5 ml of suspension/l of water.	100 ml bottles.
HATRIX Bolus Contains :Each 1.2 gm bolus has sulphadiazine : 1000 mg Trimethoprim : 200 mg	Indicated for mixed bacterial infections, calf scours, diarrhoea, septicaemia, metritis, oral necrobacillosis, necrotic rhinitis, infectious poly-arthritis, abortion, placenta retention, pneumonia.	Cattle/horse : 2-4 Bolus for 5 days.	Strips of 5 x 4 tablets.
LONGACILLIN - VET 6 Benzathine Penicillin G equivalent to 600000 units LONGACILLIN - VET 12 Benzathine Penicillin G equivalent to 1200000 units LONGACILLIN - VET 24 Benzathine Penicillin G equivalent to 2400000 units LONGACILLIN - VET 48 Benzathine Penicillin G equivalent to 4800000 units.	Long acting penicillin; strangle abcesses, sinusitis, naval infections, post-castration infection, foot-rot, black-quarter, cystitis, anthrax, swine erysipelas, leptospirosis.	5 mg (6650 units)/kg body wt. every week deep intramuscular.	Vials of 6, 12, 24 and 48 lac units.

Preparation	Indication	Dosage/Route	Presentation
OXYTRA Each tablet contains: Oxy-tetracyclin hydrochloride 500 mg	Broad spectrum antibiotic and effective against actinomycosis, anthrax, B.Q., foot-rot, H.S., bronchitis, pneumonia, equine-influenza, joint-ill, metritis, poultry : CRD, blue comb, coryza, fowl cholera, infectious synovitis.	_Oral_ _I.u._ Large animal: 1 tab/50 kg; 1-2 tab Small animal: 1 tab/10 kg; ¼-½ tab	500 mg tablets in container of 5 and 25 tablets.
PIPERAZINE Liquid 45% Each 5 ml contains: Piprazine hexahydrate 2.25 gm	Roundworms in all sp., pin worm, oxyuris, hookworms etc.	Poultry: Ascaridia: 1 ml/2kg b.wt. Capillaria: 2 ml/2 kg b.wt. Cattle: Roundworm, nodular worm: 4 ml/10kg b.wt. Horse: Roundworm, pin worm, oxyuris, small strongyle: 4 ml/10 kg b.wt. Pigs: Roundworms, nodular worm: 5 ml/10 kg b.wt. Sheep & goats: Nodular worm: 5 ml/10kg b.wt. Dogs & cats: Roundworm 1 ml/5kg b.wt. Hookworms: 1ml/3kg b.wt.	Bottle of 500 ml and cans of 4.5 lit.
PRIMICIN - VET Gentamicin sulphate 40 mg/ml	For infections by gram negative & gram positive bacteria, enteric diseases of neonates like scour & salmonellosis.	Large animal: 1-2 mg/kg Small animal: 2-4 mg/kg IM IV bid.	10 & 30 ml vials.
PROCILLIN - VET 20 Each vial contains : Procaine benzyl penicillin 15,00,000 units Benzyl penicillin sodium 5,00,000 units **PROCILLIN - VET 40** Each vial contains: Procaine benzyl penicillin 30,00,000 units. Benzyl penicillin sodium 10,00,000 units	Septic wounds, abscesses, anthrax, B.Q., foot-rot, navel ill, pneumonia, bronchitis, nephritis, cystitis, sinusitis, actinomycosis, mastitis, strangles in horse. Otitis-externa in dogs & cats.	Horse & cattle: 8,00,00 units/100 kg b.w. Sheep, goat & Swine 4,00,000 units/25 kg b.w. Dogs & cat: 1,00,000-4,00,000 units intramuscularly.	Vials of 20 lac and 40 lac units.

Preparation	Indication	Dosage/Route	Presentation
VETOPEN Inj. Of 0.5 g Streptomycin sulphate 0.5g, Procaine benzyl penicillin 30,0000 units, Benzyl penicillin sodium 1,00,000 units Inj. of 1.0 g has: streptomycin sulphate 1.0 gm Procaine Benzyl penicillin 3 lack unit. Benzyl penicillin sodium 1 lack unit. VETOPEN 2.5 Strepto penicillin 2.5gm Procaine Benzyl penicillin 15,00,000 units. Benzyl penicillin sodium 5,00,000 units.	Actinomycosis, H.S., abscesses, respiratory infection, acute mastitis, pleurisy, uterine infections, navel infections, jntestinal obstruction, brucellosis.	Cattle & horse: 6-12 mg/kg Swine: 7.5-15 mg/kg. Calves, Foals, Sheep and Goat: 20-40 mg/kg. Dogs : 30-200 mg/kg	Vials of 0.5gm, 1.0 gm and 2.5 gm.

HINDUSTAN CIBA-GEIGY LIMITED
Animal Health Division
Royal Ins. Bldg, 4th floor, 14, J. Tata Road
MUMBAI 400 020

Preparation	Indication	Dosage/Route	Presentation
COSUMIX PLUS 100 gm contains : Sulphachloro pyridazine 10 g. Trimethoprim 2 gm.	Prophylaxis & treatment of bacterial & stress related infections in calves, sheep, pigs & poultry.	For all species @ 200 mg/kg body wt. orally as a drench in livestock & in drinking water in poultry.	10 g, 50 g, 250 g pouches.
DYNAMUTILIN (Anti CRD drink for poultry) Each gm contains : Tiamulin hydrogen fumerate 450 mg	For treatment of diseases such as CRD, Mycoplasma infections, spirochetes etc.	Prophylaxis :- 1-2 g/L of drinking water for 3 days. Treatment : 2 g/L of drinking water for 6 days. Post vaccination :- 1-2 g/L of drinking water for 3 days.	30 gm & 200 gm bottles.
ENDEX 8.75% Drench. 100 ml contains : Triclabendazole 5 g Levamisole HCl 3.75 g	Broad spectrum anthelmintic/ flukicide, for sheep for parasitic bronchitis, parasitic gastroenteritis & fascioliasis.	2 ml per 10 kg body wt. as a drench for sheep.	60 ml & 250 ml bottes.
ENDEX Drench 19.5% (for Cattle) 100 ml contains : Triclabendazole 12 gm. Levamisole HCl 7.5 gm.	- do -	1 ml per 10 kg body wt.	30 ml poly bottles.
FASINEX (Triclabendazole)	For immature and mature liver flukes.	12 mg/kg: Cattle & buffalo. 10 mg/kg: Goat & sheep orally	Fasinex 5% susp. for sheep & goat; 250 mg bolus for sheep, goat & young animals. 900 mg bolus for cattle & buffalo.
LARVADEX (Cyromazine 1%)	Fly control, affects larvae & adult flies.	mix 500 gm. of 1% Larvadex premix per tonn of feed.	2 kg powder 10 kg drums.
LEVAMISOLE HYDRO-CHLORIDE 10% w/w	As a feed premix, improve growth, production & reproduction	7.5 mg Levamisole HCl/kg body wt. or 75 mg of premix / kg body wt. Cows (270 kg): 20 gm of premix. Buffalo (540 kg) : 40 gm of premix. sheep, goat : 2 gm premix per 10 animal, Poultry : 200 mg premix / kg b wt. or cattle, sheep, pig: 7.5 mg/kg b.wt.	20 gm pouches.
LEVAMISOLE HYDROCHLORIDE 30% W/W	- do -	25 mg of premix per kg body wt. Poultry : 60 mg premix/kg bwt. Dissolve 100 gm premix in 200-300 litres of drinking water and provide to flock for one complete day.	20 gm pouch, 100 gm poly packs.

Preparation	Indication	Dosage/Route	Presentation
NEOCIDOL 20 EC (Diazinon 20%)	Mange, lice, ticks, blow flies in sheep, cattle, dog etc.	2-3 ml per litre of water for application on body or dip.	30 ml, 100 ml, 250 ml, 500 ml, 1 litre & 5 lits cans.
NUVAN 76% Dichlorvos	Insecticide (for control of flies)	Spray 50 ml Nuvan in 10 litre water for 500 sq.m. surface area.	100 ml, 250 ml, 500 ml and 1 litre.
PROTEXIN (Natural probiotic) Soluble powder	Maintenance of effective digestive system, in stress, as a growth promoter.	Calves, sheep, lambs : 1 g/ 25 kg bw. Poultry : 1g in 4 litre water for 5 day. Chicks : 1 gm/litre of drinking water for first 5-7 days.	10 gm, 100 gm.
PROTEXIN IN FEED	- do -	Chicks starter ration :- 100 gm/ ton of feed. Growers, broilers, Layers ration : 50 gm / tonn of feed	100 gm poly bottles.
ROXOLIN 300 PLUS 100 gm contains: Halquinol 12 %	High performance, non-antibiotic feed supplement for poultry, increases egg production, as a growth promoter.	Mix @ 500 g/tonn of feed for starter feed of broilers. mix @ 250 g / ton feed for finisher feed of boilers. For layers : 1 day old - 8 weeks : 500 g / ton 9 weeks - 16 weeks : 250 g / ton 17 week onwards : 500 g / ton	2 kg poly jars.
VETIMAST (Single dose intramammary) Each tube contains : Cephacetrile sodium 235 mg in 10 gm. suspension.	Clinical mastitis in lactating animals. For sub-acute, acute & chronic mastitis.	One tube per affected quarter (repeated in 24-48 hrs. in severe cases).	10 gm tubes with applicators.

HOECHST INDIA LIMITED
Hoechst House, Nariman Point
MUMBAI - 400 021

Preparation	Indication	Dosage/Route	Presentation
ALBERCILIN Each vial contains: Ampicillin sodium 2 gm	Broad spectrum bactericidal antibiotic.	2-7 mg/kg b.w. I/M or I/V.	2 gm vial.
AVIL (Pheniramine Maleate) 22.75 mg/ml	Allergic reactions, itching of unknown genesis & of various localisation, eczema, dermatitis, utricaria, skin oedema, insect bites, photodermatitis, rhinitis, tail eczema in horses, stomatitis, toxic hoofcorns, inflammation of hooves of cattle, serum sickness, paresis during pregnancy, puerperal toxaemia & secondary retention, pulmonary oedema in cattle, pulmonary emphysema in horses, anaphylactic shock, laminitis, bloat in ruminants due to histamine, atony of rumen & in treatment of acute septic metritis in conjunction with antibacterial therapy.	Large animal: 5-10 ml. Small animal 1/2-1 ml. IV, IM.	10 ml vial.
BERENIL (4, 4-diamidine-diazoaminobenzene-diacetur-ate)	Babesia infection, theileria infection, trypanosomiasis.	All species 0.8-1.6 gm per 100 kg body weight.	Bottle of 22.5 g and 5 g granules with 0.8 g plastic measure spoon.
BUTOX (Deltamethrin)	Ectoparasiticide	It is used as spray or dip. Ticks: 2 ml/l of water. Mites: 4ml/l of water. Lice: 1ml/l of water. Flies: 2ml/l of water.	1 litre, 50 ml.
CODRINAL Each gram contains: Hostacycline 0.05 g. Sodium salt of P-toluene-sulphonyl beta-methoxy-ethylurethane 0.55 g. Crystalline lactose 0.375 g Dried sod. bisulphite 0.025 g	Intestinal and caecal coccidiosis of poultry, pullorum disease, fowl coryza, pigeon paratyphoid, contagious coryza, bacterial infections secondary to certain viral disease of poultry.	4g codrinal in one litre of drinking water for 2-4 days. *For prevention:* 1g per litre of drinking water.	Bottle/sachet of 20 gm.

Preparation	Indication	Dosage/Route	Presentation
EVIPRIM Vet Co-trimoxazole. each bolus contains: Trimethoprim 0.4 g, Sulphamethoxazole 2.0 g	Broad spectrum bactericidal drug effective against primary bacterial infections as well as secondary due to viral disease; infection of urogenital tract, gastroentric tract, calf diarrhoea, respiratory infections, septicaemia, local and general infections.	Cattle, horse: 4 boli daily for 3 days. Calves, Sheep, Goat and Pigs: $^1/_2$-1 bolus daily for 3 days. For intrauterine : Cows and mares: 1-2 boli. Sows & ewes $^1/_2$-1 bolus.	Box of 4 (2 strip of 2 boli each).
FLAVOMYCIN-40 Each gm contains: Flavophospholipol 40 mg	In broiler, higher weight gain, improved feed conversion, shortening of the fattening period, reduction in mortality rate.	100 gm of flavomycin-40 per ton of broiler feed daily from day 1 to marketing age.	10 gm, 1 kg & 10 kg.
HOSTACORTIN - H Suspension (10 mg prednisolone in 1 ml suspension).	Anti-inflammatory, ketosis in cattle rheumatoid arthritis, bursitis.	Cattle, horses: 5-10-20 ml : Calves, pigs: 2.5-5 ml; piglets. Dogs, cats: 1-3 ml injection into joints and tendon sheaths: Large animal: 2.5-7.5 ml. Dogs, cats: 0.5 - 2.0 ml. Injection into bursae: 1-5 ml. Subconjunctival injection: 0.125-1.25 ml. Retrobulbar injection: -0.25-1.25 ml Infiltration: (as in periostitis): 1-5 ml.	10 ml vial.
HOSTACYCLINE (Water Solube) (5g tetracycline hydrochloride in 100g of Hostacycline water soluble).	Broad spectrum antibiotic to combat secondary infections associated with viral diseases, bacterial and ricketsial diseases.	*Poultry:* Prevention : 2.5g/4.5 litre of drinking water. Treatment: 5g/4.5 litre drinking water. Cattle, horses, sheep, goat, pigs dogs & cats: prevention: 2.5g/15kg boody wt. Treatment : 2.5-5g/15kg body weight.	100 gm Sachet.
LACTAID Contains: Calcium 1.86%. Proportion of Boric acid to calcium : 2.26 to 1	Milk fever, hypocalcaemia, during peak milk production etc.	Large animal: 200-350 ml I/V or S/C. Small animal : 60 ml. Dogs: 2.5 ml.	450 ml.
LACTAID PLUS Same as above, plus Dextrose 20%, magnesium hypophosphite 5%	Milk fever, magnesium tetany etc.	Large animal: 200-350 ml Small animal 60 ml.	450 ml.

Preparation	Indication	Dosage/Route	Presentation
3-NITRO HOECHST Each gram of 3-Nitro Hoechst 5% premix contains: 50 mg of 3-nitro 4-oxy-phenylarsonic acid	Feed supplement for poultry and pigs, stimulates rapid weight gain, increased feed efficiency increases egg production, improves general appearances and health.	Broilers & layers : to be added with feed @ 0.1%. Pigs (from the piglet stage to slaughter) to be added with feed @ 0.05%.	5 kg plastic jar. 25 kg drum.
NOVALGIN Analgin (Metamizole) 0.5 G/ml.	Reliefs pain in colics, labour, spastic conditions of cervix during parturition, rheumatic conditions, neuritis, neuralgia.	Horse: 20-60 ml. Cattle: 20-40 ml. Foal, calf : 5-15 ml. Sheep, goat: 2-8 ml. Pig: 10-30 ml. Dog, cat: 1-5 ml IV,IM.	Vials of 10 ml & 30 ml.
NOVOCAIN (2% Procaine hydrochloride).	Local, regional & epidural anaesthesia.	Epidural anaesthesia: Large animals for caudal extradural anaesthesia: Horses: 10-20 ml Cattle: 7-10 ml. Cranial extradural: Cattle: 40-60 ml. Dog: 2-11 ml. Infiltration anaesthesia: amount depends on the extent of the region of operation. Conduction anaesthesia: Horse/cattle:7-10-20 ml. Dog/cats: 2-3 ml.	Vial of 30 ml.
PANACUR: Bolus or powder 25% Each gram powder contains: fenbendazole 250 mg. 1.5g bolus contains: 1.5g of fenbendazole. 150 mg contains: 150 mg fenbendazole.	Broad spectrum anthelmintic against immature and mature stages of gastrointestinal nematodes and lungworms in cattle, buffaloes, sheep, horses, pigs and tapeworms in sheep & goats.	1 ml suspension per 3 kg b.w. (5mg fenbendazole/kg b.w.) in all species orally. Dissolve 6gm powder in 100 ml water. Bolus: Large animal: 5 mg fenbendazole/kg b.w. Dog & cat: 50 mg/kg b.w.	Panacur 25% powder 6g, 60g, 120g. bolus: 150 mg and 1.5g.
RECEPTAL (Synthetic GnRH) Each ml contains: 0.0042 mg buserelin acetate equivalent to 0.004 mg buserelin	Anoestrus, cystic ovaries condition, anovulation, delayed ovulation, induction of estrous cycle, improvement of estrous cycle, improvement of conception rate.	IV, IM, SC; for anoestrus: 5 ml in horse, cattle. For improved conception rate, anovulation & delayed ovulation : 2.5 ml in cattle, 10 ml in horse, 0.2 ml in rabbit; For cystic ovarian changes : 10 ml in horse, 5 ml in cattle.	10 ml vial.
STENOROL Each gm contais: Halofuginone 6 mg	Coccidiocidal in action, improve feed efficiency, growth rate, weight gain and lowers the mortality rate.	Mixed with feed @0.5kg/tonne of poultry feed.	bag of 1 kg.
TOLZAN - F (Oxyclozanide 3.4%)	Acute & chronic fascioliasis and amphistomes in cattle, buffaloes, sheep and goats.	Cattle, buffaloes: 10 mg/kg b.w. sheep, goat: 15 mg/kg b.w.	1 litre & 5 litres.
TONOPHOSPHAN (Sodium salt of 4-dimethylamino-2-methylphenyl-phosphinic acid) (20% solution)	Roborant & tonic in general metabolic disorders, debility and exhaustion, disorders of bone formation in combination with vitamin D, for tetany and paresis.	Acute conditions: Large animal: 5-10-25 ml Small animal: 1-3 ml SC, IM, Repeat at short intervals. Chronic conditions: Large animal 2.5-5 ml Small animal: 1-2 ml SC, IM on alternate days.	20% solution 5ml ampoules, 30 ml. vial

IMKEMEX INDIA LIMITED
304/305 Anna Salai
CHENNAI - 600 018

Preparation	Indication	Dosage/Route	Presentation
NILZAN Contains: 3% w/v Tetramisole HCl & 3% w/v oxyclozanide	Broad spectrum anthelmintic, Effective for treatment and control of nematodes, fascioliasis in cattle, sheep and goats.	Cattle, sheep, goat & buffaloes: 0.33 ml/kg b.w. orally	Bottle of 50 ml & 100 ml & polythene container of one litre.
ZANIL Suspension containing 3.4% w/v oxyclozanide.	For treatment & control of fascioliasis in cattle, sheep and goats. Also removes segment of Moniezia (tape-worm)	Cattle: 10mg oxyclozanide/kg b.w. or 30 ml/100 kg b.w. (Max 100 ml) orally. Sheep: 15 mg oxyclozanide/kg b.w. or as below: Body wt (kg) — Routine treatment — Acute fascioliasis upto 15 — 5ml — 15 ml 15-30 — 10 ml — 30 ml 30-45 — 15 ml — 45 ml over 45 — 20 ml — 60 ml Given with drenching equipment.	1 litre polythene container.

INDIAN DRUGS AND PHARMACEUTICALS LTD.
25, Gopala Tower, Rajendra Place
NEW DELHI-110 008

Preparation	Indication	Dosage/Route	Presentation
FORTIFIED PROCAINE BENZYL PENICILLIN: One vial provides:Procaine Benzyle Penicillin 3,000,000 I.U Benzyl Penicillin, 1,000,000I.U	Diseases caused by Penicillin sensitive bacteria.	By I/M injection Cattle/buffalo: 1-2 vials daily.	1 vial of 40 lacs units.
OTCIM Contains : Oxytetracycline 50 mg/ml..	Effective against gram positive and gram negative bacteria, reckettsia and some large viruses. Bacterial and protozola diseases of livestock and poultry.	By I/M, I/V or S/C injection Large animal:1-2 ml/25 kg. b. wt. daily x 3-4 days. Small animal: 1 ml/10 kg. b. wt. daily x 3-4 days.	Vial of 50 ml.
STREPTOMYCIN Inj. Contains: Streptomycin sulphate 1 gm. per vial.	Bacterial infection sensitive to streptomycin.	Large animal: 6-10 mg/kg b w Small animal: 20-40 mg/kg. b.wt.	Vial of 1 gm.
SULPHADIMIDINE Sodium Inj. Contains: Sulphadimidine sodium 33.3%.	Effective against gram positive and gram negative bacteria causing various diseases in animal.	30 ml/50kg. b.wt. initially followed by half the daily dose by I/V or S/C route.	100 ml & 450 ml.
SULPHADIMIDINE Tablets Contains: 5g Sulphadimidine per tablet.	Bacterial and protozoal diseases of livestock and poultry.	Large animal:1-2 tabs/50 kg. b. wt. initially followed by half the daily dose orally. Small animal: 1 g/5 kg. b. wt. followed by 0.5 g/5 kg. b. wt daily for 4-5 days orally. Intrauterine-Cow/buffalo-2-4 tab.	50 tabs.
SULPHAGUANIDINE (Tablet) Each tablet contains: Sulphaguanidine 5 gm.	Infections caused by gram positive and gram negative bacteria, calf scour, pneumonia and bacterial/coccidial enteritis.	Small animal: 1 gm/5kg. b.wt. following by 0.5 g/5 kg. b.wt. subsequently every 24 hours orally. Large animal: 2 tab/50 kg. b. wt. followed by 1 tab/50 kg. b. wt. daily orally.	50 tablets.
SULPHANILAMIDE (Powder)	Bacterial infection, wounds etc.	150 mg/kg b.wt. orally on the first day followed by 100 mg/kg. b.wt. orally on the subsequent days.	50 gm & 500 gm.
TETRACYCLINE (Powder) 1 g contains: Tetracycline HCl 50 mg.	Diseases caused by Tetracycline sensitive organisms.	Large animal: 2.5-5 g/ 15 kg. b.wt. daily orally Small animal: 2.5 g/2.5 kg. b.wt. daily orally Poultry: Preventive-2.5 g/4 litres water; curative-5 g/4.5 litres water.	100 gm.

Preparation	Indication	Dosage/Route	Presentation
THIACETAZONE and ISONIAZID Tablets Each tablet contains: Isoniazid 100 mg. Thiacetazone 50 mg.	For the treatment of tuberculosis.	Large animal: 50-100 tabs. daily. Small animal: 4-8 tabs. daily.	1000 tabs.
TRIBEXIN Pro-salt Each vial contains: 1.3 g Quinapyramine sulfate and 1.7 g Quinapyramine chloride.	For prevention and treatment of trypanosomiasis in animals.	By S/C injection only. Dissolve in 10 ml d.w., cattle, Buffalo/horse: 1.3 ml/45 kg. b.wt. (max. 10 ml). Camel: 1.3 ml/45 kg. b.wt. (max 12 ml). In disease-prone areas, repeat at every 3-4 months. Caution: sometimes salivation, restlessness and muscular tremors are noticed.	Vial of 3.0 gm.

INDIAN EXPLOSIVES LIMITED
Ennore
CHENNAI- 600 057

Preparation	Indication	Dosage/Route	Presentation
LOREXANE (Veterinary Cream) 0.1% pure Gamma isomer of benzene hexachloride, 0.1% proflavine hemisulphate & 0.45% cetrimide.	Active against blow fly maggots, common secondary bacterial invasion and dressing of all types of wounds of all types of animals.	Clean the area and let the area dry, smear the cream over the wound & nearby skin. Repeat the treatment once daily till complete healing takes place. For deep wounds the cream may be diluted with water.	Tubes of 20 & 100 g.
MYSOLINE Every tablet contains 250 mg Primidone	Epilepsy, epilepticform convulsions (fits), hysteria and encephalitis associated with canine distemper. Side effects – higher dose may cause neurotoxicity, slight ataxia & transitory incoordination.	Dogs: 50mg/kg b.wt. or 1 tab/5kg. b.wt. orally in 2 divided doses 12 hourly.	10 x 10 strips and 1000 tabs.
NILVERM Powder contains 30% w/w Tetramisole HCI.	Highly effective for treatment & control of nematodal gastroenteritis and lungworm infection in livestock & poultry.	100 g Nilverm powder is to be dissolved in 3 lt of clean warm water & given as below at the rate of 15 mg/kg. b.wt. (1.5 ml/kg.) orally. Cattle/Buff. (kg) — Dose ml (ml) — Sheep/goat (kg) — dose (ml) 100 — 150 — 15 — 15 150 — 225 — 15-25 — 30 200 — 300 — 25-35 — 45 250 — 375 — over 35 — 60 300 — 450 — (Max : 90 ml) Pigs: 15 mg/kg. b.wt. orally following overnight fast. Poultry: 100-150 mg nilverm/kg. b.wt. or 10g/4 lt water after 12 hrs of withdrawal of water.	100 g & 10 g sachets.
SAVLON (Vet. Concentrate) Contains: Hibitane (Chlorhexidine gluconate) 7.5% V/V & cetavlon (Cetrimide 15% w/v)	Antiseptic & detergent action. Active against gram positive & gram negative bacteria.	Used for disinfection of hospital, ward, equipment, stall, milking shed & farm equipment: 1:200 in water. Pre-operative hand wash: 1:30. Udder wash, milkers hands, dairy utensils: 1:150; Egg cleaning prior to incubation 1:150; Shampoo for dogs 1:5.	1 litre bottle.
TETMOSOL (Soap & solution) Soap contains 5% Tetraethylthiuram monosulphide with perfume & solution contains 25% w/w in alcohol.	For prophylaxis & treatment of all types of mange in animals. Highly lethal to fleas, lice, ticks & other ectoparasites & stimulates hair growth.	Produces good lather while giving bath to animals in order to wash dust & debris.	75 g cake, 50 ml bottle.

INDIAN HERBS
Sharda Nagar
SAHARANPUR (U.P.)

Preparation	Indication	Dosage/Route	Presentation
BLAZE	Dandruff, lice, for protection against ectoparasites (ticks, mites, fleas etc).	After complete wetting rub sufficient quantity of Blaze thoroughly, leave for 15-20 minutes & then wash with clean water.	100 gm bottle.
CAFLON	Cough, bronchitis, coryza, etc.	Large animal: 30-40 gm, Calves, sheep, goat, colts, pigs: 6-12 gm. Dogs, piglet: 2-4 gm. Poultry: 0.5%-1% w/w. mixed with feed.	Carton of 100 gm polybag of 1 kg.
COFECU	Mineral feed supplement (copper, cobalt and iron)	Cow and buffalo : 1 tab. Sheep, goat : 1/2 tab.	Vial of 20 tabs.
EGUP	To improve and optimise egg production in laying birds. To maintain peak production for long period To restore and optimise egg production or other reason.	30 gm per 1000 birds mixed in morning feed for 10 days.	30 gm Sachet.
GALOG	Irregular lactation and failure of lactation, hypogalactia.	Large animal: 50 gm. Ewes & does : 10-15 gm.	Carton of 300 gm polybag of 1 kg.
GALOG Bolus	Irregular lactation and failure of lactation, hypogalactia.	Cow and buffaloes : 3 boli Sows : 2 boli. Ewes and Does : 1 boli To be given once daily for 10-15 days.	Strip of 4 boli.
HIMALAYAN BATISA	Digestive disorders like anorexia, dyspepsia, constipation etc. General debility, stress and exhaustion.	Large animal: 40-60 gm. Calves, colts, heifers, Pig: 20-30 gm. Sheep, goat: 10-15 gm Piglets: 3-5 gm.	Carton of 100 gm. 200 gm, 400 gm polybag of 1 kg.
H.B. STRONG	For good digestion, better health and optimum production. As a co-prescription with antibiotics, anthelmintics etc.	Cow, buffaloes & horses: 10 gm Calves, colt, heifers, pigs: 5 gm. Sheep and goat : 2.5 gm.	Sachet of 10 gm.
HIMAX	Mange, skin infection, wounds, foot rot in sheep, foot lesions in FMD etc.	Local application.	Ointment 50 gm tube & tin of 1 kg. Lotion 100 ml bottle. Himax-D 25 gm tube
LIVOL	Jaundice, Hepatitis, aflatoxicosis, for increased body resistance, better livability, debility, convalescence, leg weakness, disease of liver. For improving feed efficiency.	Large animal: 40-60 gm. Calves, heifers, colts: 15-20 gm, Sheep & goat 8-12 gm. Dog and piglets: 3-5 gm.	Carton of 100 gm Poly bag of 1 kg, 5 kg.

Preparation	Indication	Dosage/Route	Presentation
LIVOL-PFS Concentrate	Counteracting the damaging effects of aflatoxins To improve growth, egg production and livability To improve digestion and restore feed consumption in stress conditions.	4-14 ml/100 birds per day for 10-15 days. 2-7 ml/100 birds per day to be given regularly 2-7 ml/100 birds per day for 7 days.	Bottles of 225 ml and 1 lit.
LOURELL	A herbal anti-dandruff, ectoparasiticidal cleanser, conditioner, hair nourisher for canine.	—	—
NEBLON	Acute or chronic diarrhoea and dysentery, scours, non-specific loose drooping in poulty, symptomatic relief from rinderpest.	Cow, buffalo, horse : 30-50 gm. Calves, sheep, goat : 6-10 gm. dogs & piglets : 2-3 gm. Poultry: 0.5% w/w mixed with feed for 3-4 days.	Carton of 100 gm Poly bag of 1 kg.
PESTOBAN	Ectoparasites (lice, ticks, fleas, mites etc).	Dilute the drug in 10 volumes of clean water and apply this lotion, allow the drug to act for 48 hours.	Bottle of 100 ml and 1 lit.
PRAJANA HS	Anoestrus due to non-functional ovary. Delayed maturity due to non-specific reasons in heifers.	Large animal: 3 capsules. Ewes & does : 2 capsules orally with gur or feed on the first day followed by another dose on the second day.	Carton containing 20 pouches of 6 capsules each. Vial of 6 capsules.
REPLANTA	Retained placenta, supportive therapy for uterine infection. Ideal uterine cleansing agent and tonic.	Large animal: 50-60 gm. Mares: 30-40 gm. Ewes, does-8-12 gm.	Carton of 100 gm Prolybag of 500 gm & 1 kg.
RUMBION	Anorexia, dyspepsia, ruminal stasis, debility, inappetance, irregular appetite.	Cow, buffaloes, horse: 2 boluses twice a day. Sheep and goat : 1 bolus for 2-4 days.	Pack of 4 boluses.
TAENIL	Tapeworm infestation in poultry, dogs and other animals.	Sheep and goat: 12-15 gm Dog, piglet : 4-6 gm Adult Pigs : 20-25 gm Poultry 2% w/w mixed with feed.	Carton of 100 gm, Polybag of 1 kg
TEEBURB	Ringworm, eczema, degnalla, mange, pruritus, wounds etc	Large animal: 2 capsules Dogs, pigs. sheep, goat, colt, calves: 1 capsule; Pups, cat, piglet : 1 cap. orally with feed twice daily untill complete cure is achieved.	Vial of 24 capsules.
TIMPOL	Gaseous and frothy bloat, colic, impaction	Large animal: 80 gm. Calves, colts, Heifers: 40 gm Pig, sheep, goat : 20-25 gm.	Carton 100 gm. polybag 1 kg

Preparation	Indication	Dosage/Route	Presentation
WOPELL	For eradication of GIT Helminths (nematodes and cestodes)	Large animal: 50-75 gm. Calves and Colts: (3-6 months) 10-12 gm : 15-20 gm. Sheep and goat : 12-15 gm. Adult Pig : 20-25 gm. Dog & piglets : 4-6 gm. Poultry : 0.5-1% w/w mixed with feed.	Carton of 100 gm Polybag of 1 kg.
ZEETRESS	To alleviate stress and restore normal physiological functions and immune status.	Broiler: 0-4 weeks : 5 gm/1000 birds 5th weak & onward - 10 gm/1000 birds Layers : 0-20 weeks : 5gm/1000 birds. 21 to 72 weeks : 10 gm/1000 birds To be given once daily in morning with drinking water for 10 days.	Sachet of 10 gm.
ZIGUP Syrup	Digestive tonic, metabolic stimulant, liver stimulant health tonic for canine.		
ZYCOX	Anticoccidial agent as well as antibacterial action.	0.6% Zycox with feed.	1 kg.

INDIAN IMMUNOLOGICALS
Head Office 11-4-657, Lakdi-Ka-Pul
HYDERABAD - 500 004

Preparation	Indication	Dosage/Route	Presentation
CAL. BOROGLUCONATE 25% Inj.	Acute & chronic hypocalcaemia, milk fever, drug induced liver damage.	Cows/buffaloes: 200-300 ml. Ewes, goat, sows: 30-50 ml. I/V or S/C	Multidose 450 ml bottle.
CAL. BOROGLUCONATE Inj. 25% with Magnesium and phosphorus	Milk fiver, hypomagnesaemia, hypophosphataemia.	Cows, buffaloes: 200-300 ml Ewes, goat, sows: 30-50 ml I/V or SC route.	Multidose 450 ml bottle.
DEXAMETHASONE SODIUM PHOSPHATE Inj. Each ml contains: Dexamethasone sodium phosphate - 4 mg.	Acetonaemia, arthritis, tendinitis, laminitis, bovine ketosis etc.	Cattle, buffaloes: 5-10 ml. Calves, sheep, goat: 1- 3ml Dogs: 0.5 - 1 ml	5 ml vial.
LITHIUM ANTIMONY THIOMALATE 6% Inj.	Nasal granuloma in cattle, papillomatosis.	Nosal granuloma: 15-20 ml by deep I/M 3 times at 1 week interval Papilomatosis: 15-20 ml I/M, 4-6 times at 48 hrs intervals.	Multidose 50 ml vials.
OXYTETRACYCLINE Inj. 50 mg/ml.	Systemic, RTI, UTI & GIT infections.	Large animals : 1.5-4 ml per 50 kg. b.wt. for 3-5 days. Small animals: 0.5-1 ml per 5 kg. b. wt. for 3-5 days I/V, I/M or S/C route	Multidose 30 ml & 100 ml vials.
SULPHADIMIDINE SODIUM Inj. Sulphadimidine Sod. 330mg/ml	Systemic & enteric infections, HS, bronchopneumonia, calf diphtheria, bacterial enteritis & actinobacillosis.	30 ml/50 kg. b.wt. initially followed by half of initial dose for 4-5 days	Multidose vials of 100 ml and 450 ml.
TROPHOVET Each vial contains: PMSG 1000 IU.	Anestrus condition in all animals, impaired spermatogenesis in male animals.	Cow (anestrus): 1500-3000 I.U. S/C or I/M, repeat after 2 weeks if necessary. Mare (anestrus) : 3000-6000 I.U. S/C or I/M. Sheep & goat (anestrus): 1000 I.U. repeat after 24 days if necessary. Bitch (estrus induction, sub normal estrus with non-acceptance : 50 to 200. I.U. S/C daily for 3 days. Impaired spermatogenesis: Bull : 1000-3000 I.U. twice weekly for 4 to 6 weeks. Ram/buck: 500-750 I.U. twice weekly for 4 to 6 weeks. Dog : 400-800 I.U. twice weekly for 4 to 6 weeks.	Vial of 1000 I.U.

Preparation	Indication	Dosage/Route	Presentation
VIT B COMPLEX Inj. with liver extract Thiamine HCl 10 mg, Riboflavin phosphate sod. 5 mg, Niacinamide 100 mg, Cyanocobalamine 10 mcg. Liver injection crude 0.66 ml.	Liver fluke disease, faulty degeneration of liver, anorexia.	Cattle/buffaloes: 10 ml for 3 days Calves : 5 ml for 3-4 days deep I/M route.	Multidose vials of 10 ml and 30 ml.
XYLAXIN Inj. Xylazine HCl 23.2 mg/ml.	Sedation & analgesia.	Cattle : 1.5 - 3.0 ml. Horses:25 - 50 ml. Dog: 0.75 - 1.5 ml. Cat: 0.1 - 0.75 ml. I/M route.	10 ml & 30 ml vials.

INDIAN PETROLEUM & CHEMICAL INDUSTRIES
(Vet. Division)
195/97, Crown Gate, Jagat Narain Road
LUCKNOW - 226 003

Preparation	Indication	Dosage/Route	Presentation
ADVET-AD Each gm contains: Vitamin A 50000 IU Vitamin D3 5000 IU Suitable base Q.S.	Prevents stress, weakness & debility, crazy chick disease, muscular distrophy in calves, improves reproductive efficiency.	Cattle & horses: 1-5 gms Calf, sheep, goat & pigs: 0.5-2 gm Dog: 0.25 - 1 gm Poultry : 2-5 gms/100 birds To be given daily with drinking water.	
ANTIBLOT Dimethicone (activated) 1% w/v Arachis oil 5% w/v In emulsion base Q.S. to 100%	All kinds of bloat, tympany and frothy bloat.	100 ml with equal vol. of water by drenching twice daily for cattle & buffaloes. 20 ml to Sheep & goats.	100 ml.
CAL-D-TONE B12 Each 5 ml. contains : Cal. Phosphate 240 mg Vit D3 400 IU, Vit B12 5 mcg Flavoured palatable base Q.S.	Calcium & phosphorus deficiency.	Cattle & horse : 50-100 ml. bid orally Calves: 20 ml. bid. Poultry: 20-100 ml./100 birds in drinking water Dogs: 5- 10 ml. bid orally or mixed with milk.	100 ml. and 450 ml..
ELECTROBLEND (WHO formula) Each pouch of 82.5 gm contains: Sodium chloride 10.5 gm Sodium bicarbonate 7.5 gm Potassium chloride 4.5 gm Dextrose 60.0 gm	In the treatment of electrolyte imbalance & fluid loss.	Dissolve approximately 5.5 gm in 200 ml. of boiled & cooled water.	Pouch of 82.5 gm.
FURACILLIN CREAM Each 100 gm contains: Nitrofurazone 0.2% in water miscible cream	Active against many Gram(+) & Gram (-) organism.	Externally used as ointment.	10 gm and 500 gm.
FURAVET Nitrofurazone 0.2% w/w 100 gm Suitable water soluble base Q.S.	Intestinal coccidiosis in poultry & necrotic enteritis of pigs.	Poultry: 0.1% in drinking water for 7 days or 0.24% in feed. Pigs: In feed at a conc. of 0.25% or 0.01% in drinking water.	100 gm.

Preparation	Indication	Dosage/Route	Presentation
FURAZOL Each 100 gm contains: Sulphathiazole 2 gm Acid Boric 5 gm Sterilised Talc Q.S.	Antiseptic dusting powder.	Local application.	15 gm.
GABEX (Ectoparasite dusting powder) Active gamma isomer of benzene hexachloride 0.625% Emulsion Gamma benzene Hexachloride 0.1% Proflavin 0.1% Emulsifying base to 100%	For control of tick & lice infestation.	Dust the powder or apply the emulsion on the affected part of animal and keep it for few hours.	50 ml., 300 ml., and 4.5 lit.
KITWORM Powder-50 Each gm contains: Mebandazol 500 mg	Broad spectrum Anthelmintic.	Cattle, horses, dogs and cats: 5-10 mg/kg. body wt. Sheep, goats & pigs: 5 mg/kg. body wt. Poultry: 0.5% in feed.	6 gm.
LYSOVET Each kg.. contains: Vit A 20,000,00 IU Vit D$_3$ 2,000,00 IU Vit B$_2$ 1000 mg Lysine mono HCl 50,000 mg	Feed supplement of Vit A, B, D$_3$, with lysine.	Mix 10-20 gm to total daily feed of cattle. For calves, sheep and goat: 2.5-5 gm to be given/day with wet meal.	
METHYDEX Iodine 4% w/w Methyl salicylate 5% w/w in ointment base	In sprains, lumbago, gout & arthritis.	Local application.	50 gm.
PECTOLINE (Powder) Each 5 gm. contains: Pectin 21.5 mg Beal powder 35.5 mg Ispagula 18.0 mg Chlorodyn 0.3 mg Kaolin to make 5.0 gm	Symptomatic treatment of enteritis, acute intestinal catarrh & diarrhoea.	Dogs: 0.5 - 5 gm Pigs: 15 - 30 gm Sheep : 30-60. Cattle : 50-250 gm.	100 gm.
RETABLEND A (WM) Each 2 ml. contains: Vit A 1,00 000 IU in water miscible base	Deficiency of Vit A.	Poultry: 1-10 ml./100 birds/day Cattle, horse: 0.5-2 ml. Calf, sheep, goat & pigs: 0.25-1 ml.	1 kg. bottle.

Preparation	Indication	Dosage/Route	Presentation
VETRAN Each 2 gm. contains: Sulphamethoxazole 800 mg Trimethoprim 160 mg	Respiratory, gastro-intestinal, uninary, systemic & pyogenic infection.	Cattle, sheep, goat, etc. 1gm/40 kg. body wt.	
VETSTRESS (Liquid) Each ml.. contains: Vit A 12000 IU Vit D_3 6000 IU Vit E 50 mg Vit B_{12} 20 mcg Suitable base Q.S.	For prevention of stress.	Cattle: 20 ml. daily Calves: 10 ml. daily Poultry: 5-10 ml./100 birds for 7 days every month.	
VETYPLEX Each 5 ml. contains: Vit B_1 3.75 mg Vit B_2 1.25 mg Vit B_6 0.62 mg Vit B_{12} 6.25 mcg Nicotinamide 37.5 mg D. Panthenol 1.25 mg Cholin chloride 5.00 mg In suitable base to 5.00 ml.	Poultry: As dietary supplement In calves: Effective feed utilisation	Poultry: 15-30 ml./100 bird/day in drinking water Calves: 50 ml./day in drinking water Cattle & horses: 100 ml./day as drench or in drinking water.	170 ml., 450 ml., 4.5 litre.
ZOLODINE *200* Furazolodine 20% ZOLODINE 50 Furazolodine 5%	By increasing feed efficiency & reduces the stress, it increases growth rate & increases egg productivity in poultry.	For antistress level: 50 gm Zolodine 200 per 100 kg. feed or 200 gm Zolodine 50/100 kg. feed. For treatment level: 200 gm Zolodine-200/100 kg. feed 800 gm Zolodine-50/100 kg. feed.	1 kg container.

INOVETYS PHARMACEUTICALS LTD
21-D, Prem Nager, Ashok Marg
LUCKNOW-226 001

Preparation	Indication	Dosage/Route	Presentation
PUPVIT Drops (Vitamins & mineral Supplement)	Stimulates growth, liver function, digestion, better skin coat, development of resistance to infections in pups.	Pups : 0.5-1.0 ml daily from 10th-15th day of age till 3 months of age.	15 ml.
VITAVIT-7 (Vitamins & mineral supplement)	Appetite stimulant, growth stimulant, skin & coat conditioning, prevents hair falling, promotes healing, and improves fertility.	Dogs : 10-20 ml daily for 10-20 days. Cats : 3 ml daily for 10-20 days. Calves & foals : 15 ml daily for 20-30 days. Poultry : 15 ml per 100 birds per days in drinking water.	120 ml.

INTERCARE LIMITED
7, Wood Street
CALCUTTA- 700 016

Preparation	Indication	Dosage/Route	Presentation
CHORULON Human Chorionic Gonado- tropin 1500 IU/vial.	**Cow & buffalo:** Repeated failure to hold to ser- vice, foetal resorption, early abortion	1500-3000 IU weekly for Ist four weeks after service I/M.	1500 IU/Vial with 5 ml. solvent.
	Anoestrus, silent heat, Cystic ovaries.	1500-3000 I.U. IM 1000-3000 IU IV. Repeat 8-10 days later if corpus luteum forms.	
	Nymphomania due to persistent follicles	1500-3000 I.U.	
	Oestrus-prolonged, failure of or delayed ovulation.	1500-3000 IU followed by a fur- ther dose 8 days later if corpus luteum is poorly developed.	
	Sheep & goat: Repeated failure to hold to ser- vice, foetal resorption, early abortion.	100-500 IU on day of or before service.	
	Mare: Anoestrus, suboestrus, follicles 2 cm diameter or more.	1500-3000 IU. Repeat in 3 days if required. Total inactivity first to be treated with serum gonado- tropin.	
	Lactation failure post partum.	1500-3000 I.U. Repeat every 24 hrs in combination witth syn- thetic oxytocin.	
	Nymphomania	1500-5000 I.U. IM, If pregnancy is required, inject on the day be- fore or of service.	
	Bitch: Repeated failure to hold to ser- vice, foetal resorption, early abortion.	200-500 I.U. on the day of service.	
	Lactation failure post-partum.	100-500 I.U. in combination with synthetic oxytocin. Repeat 24 hours later if necessary.	
	Nymphomania due to persistent follicles.	100-500 I.U.	
	Ovulatory failure	100-500 I.U.	
	Oestrus suppression.	100-500 I.U. on alternate days on three occasions.	
	Bull: Cryptorchidism & genital hypo- plasia (young animals).	1500-5000 I.U. twice weekly for 4-6 weeks. Doses may be trebled if necessary.	

Preparation	Indication	Dosage/Route	Presentation
	Deficient sex drive.	1500 I.U. twice weekly for 4-6 weeks.	
	Stallion: Cryptorchidism & genital hypoplasia (young animals).	1500-5000 I.U. twice weekly for 4-6 weeks. Doses may be trebled if necessary.	
	Ram, buck, boar: Cryptorchidism and genital hypoplasia (young animals).	500 I.U. twice weekly for 4-6 weeks, doses may be trebled if necessary.	
	Dog: Crytorchidism, genital hypoplasia, deficient sex drive, feminisation (either at puberty or associated with testicular neoplasia).	100-500 I.U. twice weekly for 4-6 weeks. Cryptorchidism doses may be trebled if required.	
FERTAGYL Contains : Gonadorelin 100 microgram/ml (identical to GnRH)	Controls production and secretion of LH and FSH by the pituitary gland.	Cattle: Therapy of cystic Ovarian disease : 5 ml IM Repeat breeder : 2.5 ml IM Improvement of fertility post partum : 2.5 ml IM.	Vials of 5 ml.
FOLLIGON Pregnant Mares serum gonadotrophin - 1000 I.U./vial.	Cow and buffalo: Anoestrus - True, ovaries inactive.	1500-3000 I.U. IM or IV, oestrus should follow in 2-5 days. Treatment may be repeated in 10-14 days. Mating should be deferred until second oestrus because of danger of super foetation.	1000 I.U. of vial with 5 ml. solvent.
	Mare: Anoestrus - True, ovaries inactive.	3000-6000 I.U. IM or SC, oestrus should follow in about one week. Ovulation is unlikely unless chorulon 1500-3000 I.U. IV is given.	
	Goat & sheep: Anoestrus - True, out of season mating.	1000 I.U. IM or SC, oestrus signs result in 24 hours later and last 3 days. Repeat 24 hrs. later with a dose of 750 I.U.	
	Bitch: Anoestrus - True, subnormal oestrus with non-acceptance.	50-200 I.U. SC. Treatment to be continued for upto 3 weeks unless symptoms appear. (Often in only 8-10 days.).	

Preparation	Indication	Dosage/Route	Presentation
	Bull & stallion: Impaired spermatogenesis.	1000-3000 I.U. IM. Repeat twice weekly for 4-6 weeks.	
	Dog: Impaired spermatogenesis.	400-1000 I.U. IM. Repeat twice weekly for 4-6 weeks.	
LARACARE 1 ml. ampoule contains: Nandrolone laureate Inj. (Vet.) 25mg, 50 mg	Chronic debilitating disease where casual & dietary measures are proving inadequate to correct defective protein metabolism, osteoporosis, delayed fracture and wound healing.	Dogs upto 10 kg. & Cats: 10 mg Dogs over 10 kg. : 20 mg. Mares & cows:- 100-200 mg Foal, calf, sheep, goat and pig:- 50-100 mg Administration - Subcutaneous or intramuscular injection. Injection should be given at 3 weeks interval.	25mg & 50 mg ampoules
METRIJET Each 19 gm disposable syringe contains : 500 mg, Oxytetracycline HCL 500 mg Furazolidone 500 mg, Clioquinol 05 mg, Ethinylestradiol	Cow : Endometritis, metritis, 19 gm syringe, pyometra.	Syringe contents given intrauterine by the help of catheter. Repeated 24-48 hrs later.	
PROSOLVIN Contains : Luprositol 7.5 mg/ ml (resembles PGF$_2\alpha$)	Cattle : Chronic endometritis, pyometra, mummified foetuses, subestrus induction of abortion, induction of parturition, estrus control, synchronisation of estrus Mares : Regresses corpus luteum, treatment following foetal death & resorption, Luteolysis of persistant corpus luteum, oestrus induction, Pyometra, endometritis treatment induction of parturition Pigs : Induction of parturition Sheep : Luteolytic effect.	Horse/pig/sheep : 1 ml (7.5 mg) IM Cow : 2 ml IM Heifer : 1 ml (7.5 mg) IM.	
RIFIJET injector : Each injector has : 50 mg Rifamycin SV in a base to 8 gm	Treatment of all types of mastitis caused by Gram (+) bacteria in lactating cows.	One syringe injected into each teat canal. May be repeated after 24 hrs.	Carton box of four injections.

Preparation	Indication	Dosage/Route	Presentation
RUMICARE Each 125 gm. contains: Calcium propionate 60 gms Methionine 5 gm Picorrhiza dry extract 250 mg Cobalt gluconate 40 mg Vit. B$_6$ 40 mg Dextrose anhydrous 53.5 gm	Bloat, digestive disorders due to decreased activity of reticulum & sudden dietary changes, intoxication, supportive therapy in disease caused by foreign bodies, hypoglycemic condition in cattle, calves, sheep & goats.	Therapeutic: Adult cattle:- 2 treatment with an interval of 12 hrs. Each treatment includes one sachet of 125 gm. Young animal:-1/2 sachet oid or bid, sheep / goat : 1/4 sachet oid Prophylaxis: Adult cattle: 1/2 Sachet Young cattle: 1/4 sachet/day for 2-3 days. Administer as a drench with 1/2 to 1 litre water.	125 gm sachet

INTERNATIONAL CHEMICAL CORPORATION (INDIA)
P.O. Box 115
AMRITSAR

Preparation	Indication	Dosage/Route	Presentation
ANALGIN Inj Contains: analgin 500 mg/ml.	Analgesic, antipyretic and antirheumatic	By I/M or I/V Large animal: 15-30 ml. Repeat 12 hourly. Small animal: 2-5 ml. Repeat if necessary	30 ml. vial.
FETIN 5 AND 20 % Contains : Furazolidone 5 g and 20 g per 100 g	Antibacterial as well as anti-protozoal, effective in gastrointestinal disorder of poultry and pigs, improves growth rate and egg production	With feed. Poultry: Proportion per 100 kg. feed (5%) (20%) Prophylaxis 100g 25g Therapeutic 600 g 150 g daily daily for 7 days 7 days (Pig /sow) General dose: 10-12 mg/kg. b.wt. daily x 5-7 days. Caution— prolonged use may cause testicular change, nervous disturbance and hyperasthesia.	100 gm.
FUE-FURAN Tab Contains: Nitrofurazone and Furazolidine	As antibacterial and coccidiostat.	10-12 mg/kg. b. wt orally or with feed	100 gm.
HEXACHLOROPHENE Tab Each tab contains: 100 mg Hexachlorophene or 1g Hexachlorophene	Liverfluke infestation in cattle, buffalo, sheep and goat.	10-15 mg/kg. b. wt. orally.	50 tab (100 mg), 50 tab (lg), Powder 3 kg.
ICCONTON Tab Each tab contains: Dried ferrous sulfate 2g, Antimony Pot. tartrate 2g	Digestive disorders, ruminal atony and low milk production.	Cattle/buffaloes: 2-3 tabs bid x 2-3 days orally. Heavy Animals: 5 tabs bid x 2-3 days Caution — Supply free water during treatment.	Bottle of 50 tab.
OXYTOCIN Inj Contains: Oxytocin 5 units/ml.	Uterine stimulant and for milk letdown.	By I/M route 50 mcg /kg. b.wt.	1 ml. x 100 amps.
PHTHALYLSULPHATHIAZOLE Contains: Phthalylsulphathiazole 5 g/tab	Active against gram positive and gram negative bacteria and some protozoa.	Orally, 100-160 mg/kg. b.wt. Ist day followed by 1/2 dose on subsequent days .	50 tabs pack.

Preparation	Indication	Dosage/Route	Presentation
STILBESTROL Inj. Contains: stilbestrol 10 mg/ml. Also stilbestrol 5 mg tablet	Estrogenic action to bring the animal into heat.	By I/M, S/C or I/U 20-40 mcg/kg. b.wt.	10 ml vial, 1000 tabs.
TETRAMISOLE HCL Each 100 g contains: 30 g Tetramisole HCL	Effective against roundworms infestation in livestock and poultry.	Cattle/buffalo: 15 mg/kg. b.wt orally. Pig/sheep/goat: 15 mg/kg. b.wt orally. Poultry: 20 mg/kg. b.wt orally. Caution— should not be used in animals with advanced liver or kidney diseases.	100 g pack.
LUPROMAZINE Inj Contains: Triflupromazine HCL 20 mg/ml.	Tranquilizer.	Dog/cat: As tranquilizer 2-4 mg/kg. b.wt I/M.	10 ml. vial.

JEPS PHARMA (P) LTD
C-207, Naraina Industrial Area, Phase -1
NEW DELHI- 110 028

Preparation	Indication	Dosage/Route	Presentation
ALBEN Tablet : Albendazole 150 mg Bolus : Albendazole 600 mg Suspension : Albendazole 2.5% & 5% Powder : Albendazole 5% & 15%	Broad spectrum wormicide against roundworms, Lung-worms, tapeworms & liver flukes.	For roundworms—7.5 mg /kg b.wt. for liver fluke—15 mg/kg b.wt.	Tab 150 mg, Bolus 600 mg. forte bolus 1.5 g, suspension 2.5 % w/v in 70 ml bottle & 1 litre jerrycan Suspension—5% w/v 70 ml bottle & 1 litre jerrycan. Powder 5% & 15% in 100 g pouch.
ANFRO PLUS Each bolus contains : Dried ferrous sulfate 2 gm. Antimony potassium tartrate 2 gm. Copper sulfate 50 mg Cobalt chloride 100 mg.	Ruminal stasis, anorexia, restoration of early milk production.	3-4 boli per day for one to two days.	Strip of 4 boli.
CLOZAN Tablet Oxyclozanide 200 mg w/w CLOZAN Bolus Oxyclozanide 1 g w/w CLOZAN Suspension Oxy-clozanide 3.4 % w/v	Treatment & control of liver flukes & amphistomes in cows, buffaloes, sheep & goats.	One tab/20 kg b. wt. one bolus/100 kg b. wt. Suspension : Cattle & buffalo: 30 ml/100 kg b wt. Sheep & goat 5ml / 15 kg b wt.	Strip of 10 tab Strip of 4 boli Suspension in 100 ml & 1 litre bottle.
FENZOLE Each bolus contains : Fenbendazole 1.5 g Powder contains : Fenbendazole 25%	Broad spectrum anthelmintic.	5 mg/ kg b. wt.	Bolus 1.5 g. Pouch of 6 gm & 120 gm.
GYNOLACTIN Bolus Contains: minerals, Selenium & vit E	Anestrus & infertility , restoration of early milk production & minimize dry periods.	One bolus on alternate days for 16-24 days.	Strip of 4 boli.
HYLACTIN (Vitamins & minerals)	Vitamin & mineral supplement, increases milk yield, enhances immunity.	Lactating & pregnant animals : 30-40 g/day Calves & heifers : 10-20 g / day	500 gm.
JEPLON Antiseptic liquid Contains : Chlorhexidine gluconate solution 1.5% v/v Cetrimide 3% w/v Isopropyl alcohol 3-4% v/v	Antiseptic liquid, powerful germicide & detergent.	First aid : 2 TSF/200 ml warm water. Personal hygiene : 2TSF/15 litre water. Bath : 4TSF/15 litre water. General antiseptic : 2TSF / 200 ml water.	1 litre bottle.

Preparation	Indication	Dosage/Route	Presentation
MEBVET Bolus : Mebendazole 500 mg Forte bolus : Mebendazole 2 gm. Forte powder : Mebendazole 50%. Powder : Mebendazole 10%	Broad spectrum anthelmintic.	10-15 mg/kg b. wt Large animals :- 2 g bolus/day for 2 days Small animals : 2 boli (500 mg) / day for 2 days.	Bolus of 500 mg & 2 gm.
POVIDIN Solution (5% Solution of povidine iodine)	Metritis, endometritis, pyometra, vaginitis, repeat breeding, retained placenta.	10-15 ml full strength intrauterine daily. Local application.	100 ml & 500 ml bottles.
TETZAN Tetramisole HCl 3% w/v Oxyclozanide 3% w/v	Broad spectrum anthelmintic.	0.33 ml/kg b. wt. Maximum dose: Cow & buffalo : 100 ml Sheep & goats : 20 ml.	100 ml & 1 litre bottle.

KARNATAKA ANTIBIOTICS AND PHARMACEUTICALS LIMITED,
Animal Health Division
Nirman Bhawan, 80 Fit Road, Ist Block Rajaji Nagar
BANGALORE - 560 010

Preparation	Indication	Dosage/Route	Presentation
ANALGIN Inj. (Vet) Each ml. contains: Analgin 500 mg.	All painful conditions of musculoskeletal system, pyrexia.	Large animal: 20-30 ml. I/M. Calf & Foal: 5-15 ml. I/M. Dog & cat: 1-2 ml. I/M.	30 ml. vial.
BENZAPEN BENZATHINE Penicillin Inj. (Vet). Each ml. contains Benzathine Penicillin 24 Lac units in 24 Lac vial and 48 Lac units in 48 Lac vial.	Anthrax, BQ, calf diphtheria, pneumonia, bronchitis, nephritis cystitis, foot rot, navel ill, wound, abscess, infection following parturition, castration, surgical operations, acute mastitis as supplement to udder infusion for prolonged blood level.	Large animal: 11,000-22, 000 units/kg. Once in 3-4 days I/M. Small animal: 3-6 Lac units once in 3-4 days I/M.	24 lac vial, 48 lac vial.
BEPEN - 20 Inj Benzyl Penicillin 20 L inj. (Vet) each vial contains benzyl Penicillin sod. 20 lakh units.	Anthrax, BQ, calf diphtheria pneumonia, bronchitis, nephritis, cystitis, foot rot, navel ill, wound, abscess, infections following parturition, castration, surgical operations, acute mastitis, as a supplement to udder infusion.	Large animal 4000-8000 units/kg. for 3-5 days. Small animal: 2,000- 4,00,000 units/kg. for 3-5 days I/M	20 lac vial.
CLOXACILLIN Inj. (Vet) Each Vial Contains: Cloxacillin sod. 1 gm.	Infections sensitive to penicillin and also penicillin resistant staphylococcus.	Large animal: 2-4 mg/kg. I/M. Small animal: 10 mg/kg. I/M.	1 gm vial, 500 mg vial.
DUOCIDAL Bolus (Vet) Each bolus contains: Sulfamethoxazole 2 gm, Trimethoprim 400 mg.	Bacterial diarrhoea, enteritis, coccidiosis, scour, colibacillosis, salmonellosis, bronchitis, pneumonia, polyarthritis, metritis, nephritis, blue tongue.	Large animal: 2-3 bolus/day for 3 days. Small animal: 0.5-1 bolus/day for 3-5 days.	4's strip.
DUOCIDAL Powder (Vet) Each gram contains: Sulfamethoxazole 500mg, Trimethoprim 100mg	Poultry — infectious coryza, fowl cholera, fowl typhoid, *E. coli* infection, coccidiosis, enteritis, bacterial diarrhoea.	Poultry: $^1/_4$ $^1/_2$ gm/litre of water. Livestocks: 0.5 to 1gm/100 kg. body weight	25 gm. 100 gm.
FURAZOLIDONE 200 (Vet) Each tablet contains. Furazolidone 200 mg.	Bacterial diarrhoea, enteritis, bacillary dysentery, scour, coccidiosis, salmonellosis, colibacillosis etc.	Large animal: 2-3 bolus bid 5 days.	10's strip.
FURAKAL BOLUS (Vet) Each bolus contains : Furazolidone 500 mg.	Bacterial diarrhoea, enteritis, bacillary dysentery, scour, coccidiosis, salmonellosis, colibacillosis etc.	Large animal : 2-3 bolus bid 5 days	4's strip.

Preparation	Indication	Dosage/Route	Presentation
GENTABIOTIC Inj (Vet). Each ml. contains: Gentamicin sulfate 40 mg.	Livestock & poultry—Colibacillosis enteritis, nephritis, mastitis, urethritis, metritis, CRD complex, salmonellosis, colihepatitis, gangrenous dermatitis and egg dipping.	Large animal: 1-2 mg/kg. b.wt. Small animal: 2-4 mg/kg. b.w I/U: 2 ml. in 20 ml. distilled water Poultry: 0.5ml./bird I/M Egg dipping 7 ml. in 493 ml. distilled water for 1000 eggs.	10 ml. and 30 ml. vials.
KALBEND (Vet) Suspension has: Albendazole 2.5% w/v. Tablet has: Albendazole 150 mg. bolus has: Albendazole 600 mg.	Total spectrum anthelmintic against roundworm, tapeworms, lungworms and flukes. Contraindicated during Ist month of pregnancy.	Livestock : Lungworm, tapeworm, roundworm and hookworm: Suspension: 6ml./30kg. b.wt. Tablet: 1 tab/30 kg. Bolus:1 bolus/120kg. Flukes: amphistome and fasciola Suspension: 12 ml./30 kg. Bolus: 2 bolus/120 kg. Poultry: Suspension: 500 ml./1250 birds above 6 weeks. 500 ml./2500 birds below 6 weeks.	Suspension 60 ml. 500 ml., 1000 ml., 5 litre Tablet strip of 10. Bolus strip of 4.
KALMEBEN 50% Powder (Vet). Each gm contains: Mebendazole 500 mg.	Livestock & Poultry—broad spectrum anthelmintic effective against roundworms, whipworms, lungworms, strongyles, oxyuris, hookworms, syngamus, capilaria.	Cattle & horse: 3-6 gm. Calf, sheep goat, pig: 0.5-1 gm. Poultry: 10-20gm/1000 birds.	50 gms and 100 gms.
KALMISOLE Bolus (Vet). Each bolus contains: Levamisole HCI 150 mg.	Livestock and poultry—broad spectrum anthelmintic effective against all nematodes and lungworms eg. haemonchus, ostertagia, trichostrongylus, cooperia, nematodirus, oesophagostomum, chabertia, bunostomum, ascaris, dictyocaulus etc. also immuno-potentiating effect.	Sheep, goat, calf, pig.: 150 mg/20 kg. b. wt.	4's strip.
KALMISOLE Forte Bolus (Vet). Each bolus contains: Levamisole HCl 1500 mg.	-do-	Large animal: 1.5 gm bolus /200 kg. b.wt.	2's strip.
KALMISOLE Powder (Vet) contains: Levamisole HCl 30%/w/w	-do-	Livestock: 0.5 gm in 30 ml. water for 30 kg. b.wt. Poultry: 50 gm/ 1000 birds in drinking water.	5 gm., 50 gm., 100 gm. and 250 gm.

Preparation	Indication	Dosage/Route	Presentation
KALPEN Forte PPF 20 Inj. (Vet) Each vial contains: Procaine Benzyl Penicillin 15 lac units. Benzyl Pencillin sod. 5 lac units.	Anthrax, BQ, calf diphtheria, pneumonia, bronchitis, nephritis, cystitis, foot rot, navel ill, wound, abscess, infections following parturition, castration, surgical operation, acute mastitis, as supplement to udder infusion	Large animal: 4000-8000 units/kg. for 3-5 days I/M. Small animal: 2,,00,000-4,00,000 units/kg. for 3-5 days I/M.	20 lac vial.
KALPEN Forte PPF 40 Inj. (Vet). Each vial contains: Procaine Benzyl Penicillin 30 lac units, Benzyl Penicillin sod. 10 lac units.	-do-	-do-	40 lac vial.
KAMPIBIOTIC Inj. (Vet) Each vial contains: Ampicillin sod. 1gm, 2 gm, 2.5 gm.	Anthrax, BQ, HS., pneumonia, nephritis, metritis, mastitis and infections sensitive to ampicillin.	Large animal: 4.5-11 mg/kg. sid. Small animal: 11-22 mg/kg. sid. I/M, 1/V for 3-5 days	1 gm, 2 gm and 2.5 gm vials.
KLOXAMP Inj. (Vet) Each vial contains: Ampicillin sod. 500 mg/1gm. Cloxacillin sod. 500 mg/1gm.	Anthrax, B.Q., H.S, pneumonia, bronchitis, mastitits, metritis, cystitis, nephritis, abscess and Penicillinase producing organism.	6-10 mg/kg. bwt. I/M 3-5 days.	1 gm vial. 2 gm vial.
MEBENDAZOLE 10% Powder (Vet). Each gm contains: Mebendazole 100mg.	Livestock & Poultry—Broad spectrum anthelmintic, effective against roundworms, pinworms, nodular worms, whipworms, lungworms, oxyuris, hookworms, synagamus, capilaria, strongyles.	Cattle, horse: 15-30 gm. Calf, sheep, goat, pig.: 2.5- 5 gm. Poultry: 50-100 gm/1000 birds.	20 gms, 100 gms and 500 gms.
PIPERAZINE ADIPATE Oral Powder Contains: piperazine 37%.	Large round worms in cattle, horse, sheep, goat, pig and poultry.	Livestock: 5 gm/24 kg. b. wt. Poultry: 450 gm/2000 adult birds, 450 gm/4000 chicks.	15 gms and 450 gms.
RIDALPIN Inj. (Vet) Each ml. contains: Analgin 500 mg, Pitofenone 2 mg, Fenpeverinium bromide 0.02 mg	Spasmodic and painful conditions of visceral organs, intestinal colic, musculo-skeletal pain	Large animal: 20-60ml. I/M Calf, foal: 5-15ml. I/M Dog, cat: 1-2ml. I/M	30 ml vial.
SULFAGUT Bolus (Vet). Each bolus contains: Sulfaguanidine 5 gm.	All types of diarrhoea caused by bacteria, enteritis, scour and other gut infections.	Large animal: 1-2 bolus/50 kg. b. wt. Small animal: 1 bolus/25 kg. b. wt. followed by half dose	2's strip.

Preparation	Indication	Dosage/Route	Presentation
SULFASYS Bolus (Vet). Each bolus contains: sulfadimidine 5 gm	Bacterial diarrhoea, enteritis, speticaemia, scour, bronchitis, pneumonia, foot rot, uterine infections	Large animal: 1-2 bolus/50 kg. b. wt. Small animal:1 bolus/25 kg. b. wt. followed by half dose I/U:1 bolus directly or powdered for douche.	2's strip.
TALSUR Inj. (Vet) Animal birth control injection contains: Ext. Mycobacterium Vaccae 100 mcg. per ml.. Protein measured as equivalent of bovine serum albumin.	Sterilisation and castration of stray bulls and street dogs.	Sterilization (Intracaudal) Bulls : 4-6ml. in each cauda epididymis. Dogs: 0.5-1ml.. Castration: (Intratesticular). Bulls: 6-10ml. Dogs: 2-3 ml.	10 ml. vial with disposable syringe and needles.
TETRAKAL Bolus (Vet) Each bolus contains: Tetracycline HCl 500mg.	Bacterial diarrhoea, enteritis, scour, bronchitis, pneumonia, HS, BQ, pharyngitis, actinomycosis, navel ill, actinobacillosis, wound, blue tongue, abscess, metritis, retention of placenta and as follow-up therapy to antibiotic injection.	Large animal: 4-6 bolus/day for 3-5 days. Small animal: 1/2-1 bolus. I/U: 1-2 boluses.	4's strip.
TETRAKAL Forte Bolus (Vet) Each bolus contains: Tetracycline HCl 1000 mg.	-do-	Large animal: 2-3 bolus/day for 3-5 days I/U 1/2-1 bolus	2's strip.

LYKA LABS LIMITED
Animal Health Division
A-2, Jitendra Industrial Estate, Opp. Sangam Cinema, Andheri - Kurla Road, Andheri (E)
MUMBAI - 400093

Preparation	Indication	Dosage/Route	Presentation
AMPILIN Inj. Vet. 2gm. vial provides: Ampicillin sodium equivalent to 2 g of anhydrous ampicillin	RTI, UTI, enteritis, all bacterial infection sensitive to ampicillin.	Dogs & cats: 5-10 mg/kg. body weight twice daily IM or IV.	Vials of 1 g & 2 g.
BAXIVET Inj. 2 gm vial provides: Ampicillin sodium equivalent to 1 gm ampicillin Cloxacillin sodium equivalent to 1 gm of cloxacillin	Pyrexia of unknown origin, septicemia, chronic wounds & abscesses, after surgery.	Dogs & cats: 4-10 mg/kg. body weight twice daily IM or IV.	Vails of 1 g & 2 g.
BIO BOOST Bolus Each bolus provides: Live yeast culture 3 g, Live lactobacillus sporogenes culture 20 million CFU, amino acids 2 gm, liver extract 5 mg	Anorexia, co-prescription with antidiarrhoeals, emaciation & debility.	Dogs & cats: 1/2 bolus once daily for 4 days.	Strip of 4 buluses.
BIOBOOST Powder Each 100 g provides: Live yeast culture 2.5g, Live Lactobacillus sporogenes culture 200 million CFU, Amino acids 2.5 g, Liver extract 50 mg, Excipient QS	Co-prescription with antibacterials to rejuvenate the microflora of intestinal tract. Persistent diarrhoea. Post vaccination to overcome stress & boost immunity.	Dog & cats: 5-10 g per day orally with milk or food.	Packs of 100 g & 1 kg.
CHLORAMPHENICOL SODIUM SUCCINATE Inj. 1 gm vial provides: Chloramphenicol sodium succinate equivalent to 1 g chloramphenicol	Enteritis, diarrhoea, UTI & RTI infections. All bacterial infections sensitive to chloramphenicol.	Dogs & cats: 20-30 mg/kg. body weight every 12 hrs IM or IV.	Vials of 1 g.
CHOLYMBI Each 50 gm provides: Choline Chloride (50%) 10 g Lysine HCl 10 g Methionine 10 g, Biotin 1 mg, Vit B_{12} 1.5 mg	Prevents hair falling, imparts lusture to hair and shining to skin. Build up/repairs tissues, prevents stunted growth.	Dogs & cats: 10 gm twice daily with milk, water or food.	Packs of 50 gm & 500 gm.
GENTAMICINE Cream 0.1% Gentamicin sulphate equivalent to 0.1% Gentamicin activity	Surgical wounds Otitis externa Infectious wounds Omphalitis.	Topical application.	Tubes of 50 g & 120 g.
OLPRO Combination of CHO, proteins, macro/micro minerals and Vit.	Pregnancy & lactation, debility, weakness, all stress conditions.	Dogs & cats: 2-4 teaspoonful per day with milk, soup or water.	Tins of 250 g.

MARC LABORATORIES PVT LTD
3, Vidhan Sabha Marg
LUCKNOW - 226001

Preparation	Indication	Dosage/Route	Presentation
BOVIREX Bolus. Each bolus contains: antimony potassium tartrate 2 g, ferrous sulfate 2 g, anhydrous copper sulfate 50 mg, cobalt chloride 100 mg.	Simple indigestion & anorexia.	Cattle & buffaloes: 3-4 boluses/day upto a maximum for 4 day. Heavy Ruminants: 4 boluses per day orally with feed or tracle for a maximum of 4 days.	Carton containing 48 boluses.
CALVIT -12 Each 5 ml contains: Cal. gluconate 416.5 mg. Cholecalciferol (Vit D3) 600 IU, proteolysed liver ext. 1.65 mg, ferric amm. citrate 83.5 mg, Vit B$_{12}$ 8.35 mg.	Hypocalcaemia, reduced growth, poor feed conversion, leg weakness, tetany, soft egg shell, reduced lactation, osteomalacial condition, poor hatching, anaemic condition.	Poultry: Chicks: 10 ml/day/100 birds. Growers & broilers: 20 ml/day/100 birds. Layers: 30-50 ml/day/100 birds. Cattle & horse: 50-100 ml/day. Calf, sheep & pig: 20-50 ml/day. Dog & cat : 10-20 ml/day with plain water or with milk & feed.	200 ml, 500 ml and 5 litre jar.
ERAWORM Bolus & suspension. Each bolus contains: albendazole 600 mg. Each ml susp. contains: albendazole 25 mg.	GIT round worms, lungworm, tapeworm, fluke infestation.	For roundworm/tapeworm/ lungworm. In Ruminants, horse & pig: 5 mg/kg b.wt. Dog & cat: 10-25 mg/kg b.wt. For flukes: Cattle/buffalo: 10 mg/kg b.wt. Sheep/goat: 7.5 mg/kg b.wt. orally with feed or tracle.	Each box has 20 boluses of 600 mg Susp. 60ml, 1 litre & 5 litre pack.
LIVOVET Each ml contains: Thiamine HCl 10 mg, Riboflavine 3 mg, Niacinamide 100 mg, Vit B$_{12}$ 10 mcg, liver inj. crude 0.66 ml.	Growth & development of young animals, anorexia & off feed condition, liver disorders, debility, neurological disorders, blood protozoan disease, eczemas and, Vit B complex deficiency.	Large animal: 5ml twice/week. Small animal: 0.5-1 ml twice/week I/M route.	Vial of 10 ml & 30 ml.
MARCOCILIN Each vial contains: Ampicillin sod. 1 gm or Ampicillin sod. 2 gm.	HS, BQ, enteritis, metritis, retained placenta, pneumonia, calf scours, brucellosis, salmonellosis, mastitis.	2-7 mg/kg b.wt. I/M or I/V	Vials of 1gm & 2 gm.
MARCODEX Each ml contains: Dexamethasone sod. phosphate 4 mg.	Ketosis, inflammatory conditions, arthritis, all types of shocks, pregnancy toxaemia and induction of parturition.	Cattle & buffalo: 4-20 mg daily. Calf, pig, goat, sheep: 2-4 mg daily. Dog & cat: 0.5 - 2 mg/day I/M or I/V	6 ml vial.
MARCOGENTA Each ml contains: Gentamicin sulphate 40 mg.	RTJ, UTI, metritis, repeat breeders, skin & soft tissue infection. Poultry: early mortality due to salmonellosis & pseudomonas species.	5-10ml in 20-40 ml of dw for intrauterine. Large animal: 1-2 mg/kg b.wt. Small animal: 2-4 mg/kg b.wt. I/M or I/V. 1 ml of marcogenta with 99 ml physiological saline soln. inject 0.5 ml /bird.	Vials of 2 ml, 5 ml, 10 ml, 30 ml.

Preparation	Indication	Dosage/Route	Presentation
MARCOGYL Bolus Each bolus contains: Furazolidone 0.5 gm. Iodochloro hydroxquinoline 1g, Kaolin 2 g, Belladona 12 mg.	Scouring, diarrhoea, enteritis etc.	Large Animal: 2-4 bolus bid. Calves: 1/2-2 bolus bid. Sheep & goat 1/2 bolus bid orally with feed or water.	Carton contains 25 boluses.
M. LORAX Gamma Benzene Hexa Chl. 0.1%, Proflavine Hemisulphate 0.1%, Cetrimide 0.45%.	For healing of all types of wounds.	Local application, clean the affected part & apply cream once or twice daily.	Tube of 25 gm & 100 gm.
MARCOPRIM Each bolus contains: Trimethoprim 400 mg, Sulphamethoxazole 2 gm.	Actinobacillosis, actino-mycosis, colibacillosis, strangles, coccidiosis & GIT, RTI, UTI.	Large animal: 4 bolus/day. Small animal: 1/2-1 bolus/day orally.	Pouch of 2 boluses 2.4 gm.
PYROXIN Bolus Each bolus contains: PCM 2 gm.	Analgesic & antipyretic action.	Large animal: 2-3 bolus bid Small animal: 1/4-1/2 bolus bid orally.	Carton contains 64 boli.
PENICURE-D Each 7 gm tube contains: Ampicillin sodium 100 gm, Cloxacillin sod. 200 mg, Dexamethasone 0.5 mg.	Mastitis.	One tube per affected quarter, repeat every 12 hourly for 3 times intramammary infusion.	7 ml tube.
PETOFEN Inj Each ml containts: Analgin 500mg. Petofen HCl 2mg, Fenverinum bromide 0.02 mg.	All painful conditions associated with spasm of small muscles, post-surgical and post-parturition agony, fracture, dislocation, injury to soft tissues, acute and chronic arthrits, colic and pain in G.I. tract.	Larger animal: 20 to 60 ml. Sheep/goat/calves: 2 to 15 ml. Dogs/cats: 1 to 2 ml. To be given slowly I/V or I/M.	30 ml vial.

MEDINEX LABORATORIES PVT. LTD.
27, Vithal Wadi
BHAVNAGAR 364 001

Preparation	Indication	Dosage/Route	Presentation
CRYSTAFOL PAREN-TERAL Vet Each ml supplies: 0.5 ml crude liver extract equivalent to 1 mcg Vit B_{12} activity, fortified with Vit B_{12} 100 mcg, folic acid 10 mg and Xilocinamide 100 mg	Recommended as vitamins supplement for all animals in the proplylaxis and treatment for all anaemia particularly where rapid replenishment of depleted tissue levels is desirable.	By I/M only Large animal: 2-5 ml twice weekly Small animal: 1-2 ml twice weekly or more Caution - Keep in a cool place and away from exposure to sunlight.	Vial 10 ml.
STADREN-V Inj. Each ml contains: carbozo chrome salicylate equivalent to 10 mg of Adrenochrome Monosemi carbazone and Benzyl alcohol (as preservative) 2.5%	To check external as well as internal bleeding, epistaxis, preoperative surgery, haemorrhagic gastritis, haematuria etc.	Large animal: 10 ml I/M Small animal: 2-5 ml I/M.	Vial 10 ml.

MERIND LIMITED
Animal Health Division
17, Cooperage Road, New India, Centre
MUMBAI - 400039

Preparation	Indication	Dosage/Route	Presentation
AMDON Amprolium hydrochloride 200 mg/g Furaltadone hydrochloride 200 mg/gm.	Coccidiosis & bacterial infections of poultry.	30 g/50 lt. water for 5-7 days.	30 g & 100 g.
AMFANIDE Each gm contains: Rafoxanide 200 mg	Against fasciola & Amphistomes in cattle, buffaloes & sheep.	7.5 mg of rafoxanide per kg body weight.	10 gm pouch.
AMPROLIUM Soluble Powder Amprolium hydrochloride 200 mg/g	Treatment & prevention of coccidiosis in poultry.	30-60g/50lt. water for 5-7 days.	30 g, 60 g & 150 g.
BIDOX Doxycycline hydrochloride 100 mg/g	Bacterial and mycoplasmal infection of poultry.	10 gm/20 lt. water.	10 g, 50 g, 250 g.
BOLIN Paracetamol 150 mg/ml Analgin 150 mg/ml Bolus: 1.5 gm each Paracetamol and analgin	Antipyretic, analgesic, antirheumatic & antispasmodic.	Cattle: 25-60 ml, sheep & goat: 3-10 ml IM or IV, Cattle : 1-2 bolus bid, Small animal : 1/2 bolus bid.	10 ml & 30 ml strip of 2 boli.
CALIFE - C Inj. Cal. Borogluconate inj.	Ketosis, milk fever, hypocalcaemia.	Cattle: 200-350ml Sheep:25-75 ml I/V or S/C.	Bottle of 450 ml.
CURAL Chlorpheniramine maleate 10 mg/ml	Anaphylactic shock, itching, dermatitis, urticaria, eczema, drug allergy. Insect sting, burns, pulmonary emphysema. Bloat in ruminants due to atony of rumen, stomatitis, Hypopepsia, metritis, rhinitis.	Cattle: 2.5-5ml Sheep & goat: 1-2 ml Dogs: 0.5 - 1 ml.	10 ml.
DEXAVET Dexamethasone sodium phosphate 4 mg/ml	Ketosis, inflammatory condition, anaphylactic & allergic condition.	Cattle, buffalo & horses: 2-6 ml Sheep, goat, calves: 1-2 ml IM or IV.	5 ml & 10 ml.
GENTIM Gentamicin sulphate 40 mg/ml	Bacterial Infection.	Large animal: 1-2 mg/kg b.wt. Small animal: 2-4 mg/kg b.wt. IM or IV.	10 ml & 30 ml.

Preparation	Indication	Dosage/Route	Presentation
MERICAL Liquid feed supplement Each 20ml contains: Cacl- ium 350 mg, Phosphorus 170 mg, Vitamin B_{12} 20 mcg Vitamin D_3 1600 I.U.	To improve milk yield in cattle, formation of strong bones in growing animals.	Cattle & horses: 100 ml daily Calves: 40 ml daily. Dogs: 20 ml daily.	100 ml, 500 ml bottle.
MERIMILK Liquid feed supplement with Vit. Calcium 350 mg Phosphorus 170 mg Vitamin D_3 1000 I.U. Vitamin B_{12} 120 mcg Vitamin A 10,000 I.U. Vitamin E 60 I.U.	To improve milk yield in cattle and general tonic.	Cattle & horses 100 ml daily Calves: 40 ml daily, Dog: 20 ml daily.	500 ml bottle with Vit. pouch.
MERINITRO/ROXARSONE (3-Nitro 4 hydroxy phenyl arsonic acid 50 g/kg).	To stimulate growth & feed effi- ciency. To potentiate action of coccidiostat.	1 kg/ton of feed	5 kg & 25 kg.
MERIQUIN Inj Each ml contain : 50 mg of Enrofloxacin	Cattle : Colibacillosis, Pasteurellosis Mycoplasmosis, Colisepticae- mia, Salmonellosis. Cattle : 1 ml per 2.0 kg b wt SC/IV		15 ml ampoule
MERIQUIN Oral Solution Each ml contains: 100 mg Enrofloxacin	Dog : Infection of respiratory, diges- tive and intestinal tract and in- fections of skin and ear.	Dogs : 1 ml per 10 kg b wt sc Poultry : 50 ml per 100 lit of drinking water for 3-5 days 100 ml bottle. Poultry : CRD, Colispticaemia, Pasteurel- losis, Coryza and Salmonellosis.	100 ml bottle.
MERITON (Liver extract, Vit B-com- plex & Lignocaine HCl)	Liver disorders, anorexia, anae- mia, impaired metabolism	Large animal: 10 ml Small animal: 1-2 ml IM or SC.	10 ml & 30 ml.
MERIVIT - 100 (Vit B_{12} 100 mg/kg)	To improve growth, weight gain, feed conversion & egg pro- duction.	Broilers: 220g/1000kg feed Lay- ers: 100g/1000kg feed Breeders: 150g/1000kg feed.	Pack of 5 kg & 25 kg.
OXYTETRACYCLINE Each ml contains : Oxytetracycline 50 mg	Broad spectrum antibiotics.	5-10 mg/kg b.wt.	100 ml.
PANFUGAL Fenbendazole 25% w/w Powder Tablet : Fenbendazole 150 mg.	Mature & Immature round worms, lung worms & tape- worms.	5 mg Fenbendazole/kg b.wt.	120 g powder, 1.5 gm bolus, 150 mg tablet.

Preparation	Indication	Dosage/Route	Presentation
PIPERAZINE HEXAHY-DRATE (Piperazine hexahy-drate 40.6 g in each 100 ml)	Worm infestation in poultry & livestock.	Cattle & buffaloes: 15-30 ml/30kg. b.wt. Calves: 5ml/10kg b.wt. Horses: 15ml/30kg b.wt. Dogs & cats: 2.5ml/10kg b.wt Birds (under 6 weeks): 30 ml/100 birds in 3-5 lt of water. (over 6 weeks): 60 ml/100 birds in 5-10 litre of water.	100ml, 400 ml & 4.5 L.
PRONIL - H (Diminazine aceturate 0.444g/g)	Trypanosomiasis, Babesiosis & Theileriasis.	0.8-1.6 g/100 kg b.wt. Deep IM or SC.	4.8 g, 11.25 g & 22.5 g.
REPLAMIN (Metasolates of Mg, Zn, Ca, Mn, Fe, Cu, Co with amino acid & NaCl	Nutritional chelated mineral supplement.	25 ml/5 L water.	500 ml & 1000 ml.
RIDEMA (Frusemide 50 mg/ml)	Diuretic for parenteral adminis-tration in oedema of all types.	Horse, cattle & buffalo: 5 - 10 ml. Dogs & cats: 0.25- 0.5 ml/5kg b.wt. Pigs: 1 ml/10kg b.wt. IM or IV	10 ml.
TELON - LA (Oxytetracycline 200mg/ml)	Active against gram + ve, gram - ve pathogens and certain Rickettsia & large viruses. Common systemic, respiratory & local infection.	Cattle : 20 ml Sheep: 5 ml Swine : 10 ml Deep IM (recommended dose rate is 20mg/kg b.w)	30ml.
TERIFIX-M Containing Calcium, phos-phorus, Magnesium and dex-trose	Ketosis, milk fever, hypocalcae-mia, hypomagnesemia, hypophosphatemia.	Cattle : 200-300 ml. Sheep : 25-75 ml 1/v or s/c	Bottle of 450 ml.
TRYPNIL (Quinapyramine sulphate 1.5g/2.5g Quinapyramine chloride 1g/2.5g)	Trypanosomiasis (Surra).	0.025 ml/kg b.wt. SC (2.5 gm vial should be dissolved in 15 ml DW & 15gm vial in 90ml DW)	2.5 g & 15 g

MICROLABS PVT. LTD.
303, 'A' Wing 3rd Floor, Queens Corner
Apartments 3-Queens Road, BANGALORE-560 001

Preparation	Indication	Dosage/Route	Presentation
AVICOX Contains: Nitrofurazone 25% and Furazolidone 3.6%.	As a preventive measure against all type of coccidiosis in layers.	Layers/Replacement : 500 g/ton feed upto 14 weeks and 375 g/ton feed thereafter. Broiler : 500 g/ton feed from day old till slaughter.	5 kg, 25 kg.
BACITRIN Contains : 10% W/W Zinc bacitracin.	As feed additive to improve feed efficiency and to reduce mortality, culls and rejection.	Layers: 500g/ton feed regularly or 1 kg/ton feed for 7 days every month. Broiler/starters upto 6 weeks : 500 g/ton feed/day. Finisher (till slaughter) 1 kg/ton feed.	5x1 kg plastic bag, 5x5 kg plastic bag, 25 kg tin.
FURALAY-200 Contains : 20% Furazolidone.	For better growth, production and feed efficiency and to reduce mortality and culls.	Chicks/growers: 500 g/ton feed. Layer: 250 g/ton feed regularly or 500 g/ton feed for one week every month. Broiler : 500g/ton feed from day old to 8 weeks.	25 kg drum.
FURANITRO One tab provides: Nitrofurazone 100 mg, Furazolidone 14.5 mg.	For prevention and control of coccidiosis in poultry.	Orally with drinking water of poultry. Prevention - 1 tab/4 litres x 10-12 weeks. Curative - 1 tab/litre of water x 7 days.	Pack of 50 tabs.
MICROSOL Contains: Furaltadone 20% w/w.	CRD, air sac diseases, colibacillosis, bacillary white diarrhoea, infectious synovitis and other bacterial disease of poultry.	1 g/litre of drinking water x 3-5 days.	50 g, 500g.
MORTIN-VET Contains: Trimethoprim 2% w/w, Sulphamethoxazole 10% w/w in water soluble base	Broad spectrum chemotherapeutic agent active against most of gram positive and gram negative bacterial infections in poultry and livestock.	With drinking water or electuary Poultry : 1g/litre drinking water x 5-7 days. Cattle/horse/sheep/goat: 1.2-5 g/100 kg b.wt. bid x 5 days. Dog/cat : 12.5 mg/kg. b.wt. bid x 5 days.	Tin of 50 g and 500 g.
WORMAL (Powder) Contains: 30% w/w Levamisole HCl.	Effective against most of the gastro intestinal nematodes and lungworms of livestock and poutlry.	Orally with drinking water. All animals : 7.5 mg Levamisole HCl/kg. b.wt. or 50g powder/liter drinking water and use as below : Sheep/goat (15-25 kg) : 5-10 ml (25-35 kg) : 15-20 ml (max). Cattle : (50-100 kg): 40 ml (100-200 kg) : 80-100 ml (max) Poultry : 10g/50 litre drinking water/500 layers/1000 chicks.	Tins of 50 and 500 g.

MORVEL LABORATORIES (P) LTD.
251, G.I.D.C. Estate, MEHSANA - 384 002 (Gujarat)

Preparation	Indication	Dosage/Route	Presentation
ALERT Vet Inj. Pheniramine maleate 22.95 mg/ml.	Drug allergies, anaphylactic shock, eczema, dermatitis, urticaria, insect-bite, pulmonary oedema, emphysema, toxemia, bloat, serum sickness, asthama, etc.	By I/M or I/V route. Large animal: 5-10 ml or more. Small animal: 0.5 - 1 ml or more. Repeat after 8-12 hrs if necessary.	Vial 10 ml.
ANSED Vet Inj. Each ml contains: Analgin 375 mg, Diphenhydramine 20mg.	Pain, fever, spasm, rheumatism, allergy with pain, vaginal prolapse, respiratory disorders with pain and pyrexia.	By I/M or I/V route. Large animal: 5 10 ml or more Small animal: 0.5 - 1ml or more Repeat after 8-12 hrs if necessary.	Vial 30 ml.
ATROPINE SULPHATE	Parasympatholytic, organophosphorus poisoning etc.	By S/C, I/M or I/V route a) parasympatholytic: Cattle, horse, buff.: 30-60 mcg/kg b.wt. Pig: 20-40 mcg/kg b.wt. Sheep & goat: 80-160 mcg/kg b.wt. Dog & cat 30-100 mcg/kg b.wt. b) Organophosphorus poisoning: All species: 1 mg/kg b.wt. Repeat if needed.	Vial 10 ml.
BEEPEX Liquid Each 5ml contains: Vit B_2 1.25 mg, Vit B_6 0.62 mg, Vit B_{12} 6.25 mcg, Nicotinamide 37.50 mg, D-Panthenol 0.65 mg, Choline chloride 10.0mg, Lysine mono hydrochloride 10.0 mg.	Poultry: Stimulation of growth, increase egg production, prevent post-vaccination reaction, dietary supplement for effective feed utilization.	Poultry: 15-30 ml/100 birds of drinking water. Calves: 50ml daily. Cattle & horses : 100 ml daily.	500ml bottle, 5 litre poly jar.
BEEPEX - Vet Inj. Each ml contains: Vit $B_1$25mg, Vit $B_2$4.1 mg, Vit $B_6$2.5 mg, Nicotinamide 100 mg, D-panthenol 5 mg.	Co-therapy with antibiotics, B-complex deficiency diseases, vitamin supplement.	I/M use only. Large animal: 10 ml daily. Small animal: 2- 5 ml daily.	30 ml vial.
BELIVE - Vet Inj. Each ml contains: Vit B_1 25 mg, Vit B_2 3 mg, Vit B_6 5 mg, Vit B_{12} 30 mcg, Niacinamide 100 mg, D-panthenol 5 mg, Choline chloride 15mg Crude liver extract 0.66 ml.	Anorexia, liver disorders, fatty, degeneration of liver, sluggish liver.	I/M route only. Large animal: 5-10 ml daily. Small animal: 1-2 ml daily.	10 ml vial.

Preparation	Indication	Dosage/Route	Presentation
BION - 12 - VET Each ml contains: Vit B$_1$ 30 mg, Vit B$_6$ 13.75 mg, Vit B$_{12}$ 500 mcg.	Anorexia, fatigue, debility, neurological disorders, dermatitis, pregnancy, lactation.	I/M use only. Large animal: 10 ml daily. Small animal : 2 - 3 ml daily.	10 ml vial.
BLOT Emulsion of dimethicone.	Bloat.	Large animal 100ml orally.	100 ml.
CALCIVET Each ml contains: Calcium levilunate 76.4 mg., Vit D$_3$ 5000 I.U. Vit B$_{12}$ 50 mcg.	Late pregnancy, early lactation, hypocalcaemia, debility, weakness.	I/M use only. Cattle/buffaloes-Pre-parturition: 10-15ml thrice a week. Post-parturition: 15-20 ml thrice a week. Debilitated animal: 10 ml thrice a week. Small animal: 1-5 ml thrice a week.	30ml vial.
GENTAMOR Inj. of gentamicin 40 mg/ml.	Gram negative and gram positive organism, U.T. & R.T. infections, repeat breeders.	I/M, I/V. Large animal: 2-4 mg/kg b.wt. Small animal 1- 2 mg/kg b.wt. Intra-uterine: 2ml diluted with 20-30ml of distilled water in repeat breeders.	2ml vial, 6ml vial, 30 ml vial.
MEPARIN Each ml contains: Analgin 125 mg, Phenylbutazone 125mg.	Pain, fever, rheumatism, non-visceral traumatic inflammatory disorders.	Deep I/M. Large animal: 10-15 ml. Small animal : 2-5 ml.	30 ml vial.
MORCAIN Lignocaine HCl. 21. 33mg, Adrenaline bititrate 0.01 mg.	Minor surgery e.g. removal of cysts, suturing, tooth extraction.	Dosage depends on the indication and the area to be anaesthetised.	30 ml vial.
MORDEX Each ml contains: Dexamethasone phosphate (as sodium salt) - 4mg.	Ketosis, arthritis, allergy, anaphylaxis, surgical shock, pregnancy toxaemia, systemic or local inflammation.	I/M, slow I/V. Large animal: 2-5 ml daily. Small animal: 0.5-1 ml daily.	5ml vial, 2ml vial.
MORGAN Each ml contains : Analgin 500 mg, Pitofenone HCl 2 mg, Fenpiverinium bromide 0.02 mg.	Spasm of GIT, colic, other painful conditions.	I/M, I/V. Large animal: 10-15 ml. Small animal: 1-2 ml. Never mix with other drugs in the same syringe.	30 ml vial.
MORPIN Each ml contains: Analgin 500 mg.	Analgesic, antipyretic, antirheumatic.	I/M, I/V. Large animal: 10-15 ml. Small animal: 2-8 ml.	30 ml vial.

Preparation	Indication	Dosage/Route	Presentation
MORPRIM Each 3 ml contains: Trimethoprim 160 mg, Sulphamethoxazole 800mg	Broad spectrum chemotherapeutic agent. UTI, RTI, GIT infection, mastitis, diarrhoea.	I/M. Normlly 3ml for 64 kg b.wt.	5 ml vial. 30 ml vial.
OMOCAL B-12 Each 5 ml contains: Tribasic Calcium phosphate 0.24 g Vit D_3 400 I.U. Vit B_{12}5mcg	Livestock: milk fever, growth supplement. Poultry: rickets, thin-shelled eggs, prolapse, cannibalism.	Oral : Cattle & horses: 50ml or more bid daily. Calves, sheep, goat: 20ml bid daily. Dogs: 5-10 ml twice daily. Poultry: 20-100 ml per 100 birds.	500ml bottle, 100ml bottle.
OXYMOR Each ml contains: Oxytetracycline 50mg.	Gram positive and gram negative bacteria, H.S., B.Q., joint ill etc.	I/M, S/C, I/V. Large animal: 1-2 ml/25 kg b.wt. Small animal: 1ml/8kg b.wt.	20 ml vial, 50 ml vial, 100 ml vial.
PIPERAZINE Piperazine hydrate.	Roundworms of livestock & poultry, nodular worms of swin and pin worms and strongylosis of horses.	Cattle, horse: 15ml/30kg b.wt. Calves: 5 ml/10 kg b.wt. Dogs & cats: 2.5 ml/10 kg b.wt.	5 litre.
PULP DEPOT 1 ml contains: Hydroxy progesterone caproate 250mg in oil base.	Repeat breeder, anoestrus, antipartem prolapse of vagina habitual abortion.	I/M. Habitual Abortion in early pregnancy: 750mg after 1.5 month of pregnancy. Repeat 4 or 5 times at 10 days interval.Repeat breeder with weak corpus luteum: 500-750mg followed per week for 3 weeks. Prolapse of uterus: 750mg for two days. Induction of estrus: 500 mg if no response, repeat after 10 days.	500mg ampoule, 750mg ampoule.
REMOT Frusemide 50mg/ml	Diuretic.	Large animal: 5-10 ml. Small animal: 0.25-0.5 ml/5kg b.wt.	10 ml vial.
SICVEL Each ml contains: Triflupromazine HCl 20 mg.	Psychomotor overactivity, preoperative agent with local or general anaesthesia, prolapse of vagina or uterus.	I/M, I/V. Large animal: 1 - 2ml Small animal: 0.25- 0.5 - 1 ml.	5ml ampoule.
VITAMIX AD₃	For deficiency of Vitamins	Mix 10 gm in 100 kg of feed.	10 gm.
WINNER LIQUID Each ml contains: Vit A 12,000 I.U., Vit D_3 6,000 I.U., Vit E 48 mg, Vit B_{12} 20 mcg.	Livestock: Stress of transport, vaccination, calving, deworming, decreased productivity. Poultry: Stress as above, debeaking, change in climate, feed, crazy chick disease.	Cattle: 20 ml daily. Calves:10ml daily. Poultry: 5- 10ml daily/100 birds.	30 ml, 120 ml, 500 ml.

P.C.I. PHARMACEUTICALS LTD.
20-203, Satyam Cinema Complex, Ranjit Nagar
NEW DELHI-110 008

Preparation	Indication	Dosage/Route	Presentation
CHEMOZINE Bolus Each bolus contains: Suphadiazine 1.0g Trimethoprim 0.2g.	Infection due to gram positive and gram negative organism.	Orally: 1bolus/80kg b.wt. twice daily I.U: 2-5 bolus.	5x4's' bolus.
CHEMOZINE Powder Each gram contains: Sulphadiazine - 100 mg Trimethoprim - 20 mg	For both gram positive and gram negative bacterial infection.	Orally with water, 1g/8kg bwt twice daily.	50 g, 250 g.
DIPRAVET Each ml contains: Analgin 0.5 g	Analgesic, antipyretic, antirheumatic	Cattle, buffalo and horses: 20-30 ml i/m or i/v Dogs & Cats: 2-3ml i/v, i/m.	10 ml, 30 ml vial.
GENTAVET Each ml contains: Gentamicin sulphate-50 mg	Broad spectrum antibiotic, used for both gram positive and gram negative bacteria.	Cattle, buffalo/ horses: 2-4mg/kg bwt. by i/m or i/v 24 hourly. Dogs & cats: 2-4 mg/kg bwt by i/m route.	2 ml, 5ml, 10ml vial.
HELMOSOL Mixture (1.5% Each 100 mg contains: Levamisole HCl 1.5% w/v	All types of round worms & lungworms	Cattle, buffalo, horses, sheep & gaot: 7-10 mg per kg bwt. orally.	120 ml, 500ml, 1 litre 5 litre.
MICROVET Inj. Each ml contains: Oxytetracycline- 50 mg	Effective in both gram positive and gram negative bacteria and certain large viruses.	Cattle, buffalo, horses: 4-5 mg kg bwt I/M or I/V by slow route. Dogs and cats: 5-10 mg/kg bwt I/V.	30 ml, 50 ml vial.
PHENIVET Inj. Each ml contains: Chloramphenicol 125 mg	Broad spectrum antibiotic, useful in salmonella infection and other bacterial infections.	By i/m injection only, Large animal:1-2g once or twice a day. Small animal: 10-30mg/kg b.wt. Once or twice daily.	10 ml, 30 ml.
PHENIVET SUCCINATE Inj. Each vial contains: Chloramphenicol sodium succinate-1g	Broad spectrum antibiotics. Effective against salmonella infection & other bacteria.	By i/m injection—Cattle and buffaloes: 1-2g daily	1 g vial.
SYNTHOVET Inj. Each vial contains: Ampicillin sodium-250 mg, 500mg, 1 g	Broad spectrum antibiotics, effective in both gram positive and gram negative bacteria.	Cattle, buffalo, horses: 5-7 mg/kg b.wt.i/m. Sheep. goats: 5 mg/kg bwt - i/m. Dogs and cats: 10mg/kg bwt-i/m	250 mg, 500 mg, 1 g.

PEARL CHEMICAL INDUSTRIES (PVT.) LTD.
42, Strand Road, CALCUTTA- 700 007

Preparation	Indication	Dosage/Route	Presentation
CESTOPHENE Each tablet contains: Dichlorphen - 0.5g	Tapeworm infestation in animals.	Dogs: 0.2 g/kg b.wt. Cats: 0.1-0.2 g/kg b.wt Sheep and goat: 0.5 g/2.5 kg b.wt Calves: 0.2 g/kg b.wt Route: Orally. Repeat treatment after 3 weeks.	10 tabs., 100 tabs. bottle.
MULTIMIN AB_2D_3K Each gram contins: Vitamin - A 40,000 I.U. Vitamin - B_2 20 mg Vitamin - D_3 5000 I.U. Vitamin - K 5 mg	Deficiency of vitamins, night blindness, etc.	1 kg/5 ton of feed.	1 kg.
MULTISOL BOVINE Each 5ml contains: Vitamin A 2,50,000 I.U. Viamin D_3 10,000 I.U. Vitamin E 150 mg	To improve fertility, growth rate, and productivity and repeat breeding.	5 - 10 ml/animal daily for 7 days orally.	35 ml 100 ml.
SULPHADIMIDINE Solution Contains 16% sulphadimidine W/V	Gram positive and gram negative bacteria and coccidiosis in poultry.	*General treatment*: 30 ml per 5 litre of drinking water for 4 days. *Coccidiosis*: 15ml/5 litre of water for 4 consecutive days.	450 ml.

PEE FARMA (INDIA)
Animal Care Division
Head Office, C-44, Rajendra Nagar
BAREILLY - 243 122 (U.P.)

Preparation	Indication	Dosage/Route	Presentation
DIGESTO Stomachic & General tonic powder.	Anorexia, dyspepsia, impaction, constipation, colic, flatulence, general debility, exhaustion and stress in animal.	Poultry: (mixed with feed) in 1% ratio Piglets (15 days to 2 month old): 3.5 gm Sheep & goats: 10-15g Adult pigs, calves, colts & heifers: 30 g Horses, cows & buffalo: 50g.	200g, 500g, 1 and 2.5 kg pack.
FURA - 20 (Furazolidone 20% w/w)	More egg production, increases growth rate, weight gain, increases fertility & hatchability.	In layers feed from point of lay till the end of lay; in broilers from day old to marketing: 250 gm of fura-20 in 100 kg of feed.	500g and 1 kg.
PASHUMIN Mineral mixture with amino acids (methionine and lysine).	Animal and fish feed supplement.	Cow, buffaloes: 30 gm daily S.A.: 10-15 gm daily.	500gm & 1 kg.
TRACE MIX (Cattle) (Trace mineral for cattle).	To produce more milk, increase body resistance & to provide strength to the bone.	One kg trace mix in 100 kg feed. Feeding rate - 30g/day	1, 2.5 & 25 kg bags.
TRACE MIX (P) (Trace minerals for poultry) Managanese, Iron, Iodine, Copper, Zinc, Cobalt.	To increase egg production, increase body resistance.	50g Trace Mix in 100kg feed. In stress: 100 gm in 100 kg of feed.	1, 2.5 & 25 kg.
TRACE MIX (S) (Broiler Special) Manganese, Iron, Iodine, Copper, Zinc, Cobalt.	Increases meat production.	Mix 500 gm Trace Mix (S) in 1000 kg feed.	1, 2.5 & 25 kg bags.
VEEMIX (A B_2D_3) Each gm contains: Vit A 40,000 I.U. Vit B_2 25 mg Vit D_3 6,000 I.U.	For deficiency of vitamins and night blindness.	Mix 100 gm in 1000 kg of feed for cattle, sheep, goats pigs and horses. Layers & Growers: 200gm in 1000 kg of feed.	1, 2.5 & 5 kg.
VEEMIX - FORTE Each gm contains Vit A 3,25,000 I.U. Vit D_3 50,000 I.U.	Vitamin A and D supplement.	Mix 15 gm in 1000kg of feed for cattle, horses, sheep goats & pig; 25 gm in 1000kg feed for layers & growers.	500 gm & 1 kg.
VEEMIX K (Vit AB_2D_3K) Each gm contains: Vit A 82,000 I.U. Vit B_2 50 mg Vit D_3 12,000 I.U. Vit K_3 10 mg.	Def. of vitamins & night blindness, curled toe paralysis, petaechial haemorrhage in GIT due to coccidial & helminthic infestation.	Mix 100 g in 1000 kg feed.	500g & 1 kg poly bags.

Preparation	Indication	Dosage/Route	Presentation
VITMIX - Concen. (Vitamin mineral feed supplement for poultry and livestock).	Better health and production in animals and birds.	Per kg feed add poultry, Starters, Finishers, breeders 50g Layers & growers : 25 gm. Goat, horses, cattle and pigs: 25g Pig Starters: 50 gm.	1, 2.5 & 5 kg.
VITRICAL (Calcium, phosphorus, Vit D_3 and Vit B_{12}) Nutritional value (per 100 ml) Calcium 2000 mg Vit D_3 8000 I.U. Phosphorus 1200mg Vit B_{12} 100mcg.	To improve milk yield in cattle, formation of stronger bones in growing animals.	Chicks & broilers: 20ml daily/5 litre drinking water for 100 birds. Growers: 50ml daily/7 litre drinking water for 100 birds Layers: 100ml daily/10 litre drinking water for 100 birds Cattle & horse: 100 ml daily. Sheep, goat and pigs: 20ml twice daily. Cats & dogs: 10-20 ml twice daily.	450 & 900 ml poly pack bottles

PETCARE, DIVISION OF TETRAGON CHEMIE (P) LTD.
No. 90, 3rd Cross, 2nd Main Road, Ganganagar
BANGALORE - 560 032

Preparation	Indication	Dosage/Route	Presentation
EXTODEX [Amitraz 5% w/v in Each ml and Emulsifiable carrier Q.S.]	Sarcoptic and Demodectic Mange.	6ml/L. of water and make a dip concentrate. Small dog:- 1-3 l. Large dog:-3-5 l. Bathe the animal with warm water and soap and pat dry with towel. Apply the dip conc. all over the animal using sponge. Do not towel dry or rinse after application.	6ml Vial, 60 ml.
NOTIX SCRUB [1-Naphthyl-N-Methylcarbamade 5% and Detergent base Q.S.]	External parasites.	Wet the dog with adequate water. Sprinkle a small part of Notix scrub, work up a luxurious lather. Rinse thoroughly to degrease the skin. Repeat the procedure once again leaving the lather on for 7-10 min. Prevent the dog from licking the application. Rinse lightly. Pat dry with a towel. Brush the coat, when fully dry.	15 gm pouch.
NOTIX SCRUB Liquid (1-Napthyl-N-Methylcarb-amade 10% and detergent base)	External parasites.	-do-	30 gm and 150 gm in liquid form.
NOTIX TALC [1-Napthyl-N-Methylcarbamade 5%, Talc. Q.S.]	External parasites.	Dust over the dog and rub it down to the skin. Begin at the head and work back. Ensure to include feet, in between toes and under the tail.	150 gm container.
NUTRIBIX ROLLS Each 10 gms contains: Protein 1000 mg Fat 250 mg Methionine 150 mg Lysine 50 mg Choline 100 mg Vit B$_2$ 9 mcg Niacin 14 mcg Calcium Pantothenate 40 mcg Vit A 5000 IU Vit D 1000 IU Vit B$_{12}$ 5mcg	Nutribix is a conveniently roll shaped delicious snack, containing whole digestable egg protein. Nutribix is ideally formulated as a crunchy tonic for dog and is a gum and teeth exerciser.	Give as often as liked. There is no danger of overdosing. Use it as reward during training.	400 gms.

Preparation	Indication	Dosage/Route	Presentation
NUTRIBIX ECONOMY TREATS [Protein 20%, Fat 4%, Calcium 1%, Phosphorus 0.8% Energy 2700 KCal/kg.]	Tonic.	Give as often as you like. There is no danger of over dosing. Use it as reward during training. Treat dog with Nutribix for good behaviour.	250 gms.
NUTRICOAT Each 5 gms contains: [Lanoleic acid, Linolenic acid, Oleic acid 3000 mg Lecithin 50 mg Vit B_6 400 mcg Vit A 1000 IU Vit E 10 IU Vit D_3 100 IU Zinc 4.5 mg Selenium 0.2mcg Biotin 45 mcg.	Helps to correct all types of skin & coat condition like dull coat, flaky skin, excess shedding and scratching caused by deficient diet.	Pour directly into the month or mash into feed. 1 teaspoonful (5gms) per day for a dog of approximately 10 kg b.wt. 2.5 gms (1/2 teaspoonful) for wirehaired dog and 10 gms (2 teaspoonful) for pregnant or nursing bitches.	150 gms.
NUTRIPET FOOD BOOSTER Each 30 gms provides: Live yeast culture - 7.5×10^9 viable cell, Vitamin A (Retinol) 1100 IU, Vit B_1, Vit B_2, Vit B_3, Vit D_3, Vit E, Choline chloride, Calcium chloride, Iodine, Copper, Iron, Mg, Mn, Phosphorus, K, Na, Se, Zn, Total protein - 22%	Nutripet Food Booster is the complete Vitamin Mineral- protein feed supplement for dogs. It is rich in protein content.	Growing puppies:-15 gm. twice daily. Small dogs under 10 kg : 20 gm per day. Large dogs and hounds over 15 kg-30 gm/day. Mash thoroughly into the diet of your pet.	150 gm.
NUTRIPET PET - MEAL [Protein 24%, Fat 4.5%, Calcium 1.5% Phosphorous 1% Energy 2800 KCL/kg. Vit. A, Vit. D_3, Vit. E & Vit. B complex factors & essential minerals added as per nutritional requirement]	Nutripet pet meal is nutrionally balanced, precooked, ready to eat, wholesome food that dogs and growing puppies need. It ensure healthy growth.	Small/growing puppies-100 gm 2 times a day. Small/toy breeds- 250 gms/day Medium sized dogs:- 400 gm/day Large dogs and Hounds:-upto 750 gms - 1 kg.	1 kg, 5 kg.
PRAZI PLUS Each bolus contains: Albendazole : 300 mg Praziquantel : 25 mg	Helminth infestations as roundworms, hookworms, whipworms, tapeworms of all animals. Also effective for nematodes & flukes in cattle, sheep & goat.	Dogs/cats: 1bolus/10 kg b.wt; cattle/ sheep/goat: 1 bolus/10 kg wt.	Package of 1x10's

PHARMANZA (INDIA)
70/1, G.I.D.C.
KANSARI - 388 630, Dist. Kheda

Preparation	Indication	Dosage/Route	Presentation
FURAN-U Bolus Contains : Nitrofurazone 60 mg, urea 6 gm.	Retained placenta, cervicitis, metritis, vaginitis.	2 boluses. intrauterinc. Repeat after 24 hrs.	Strip of 4 boluses.
KALROL-D_3 Bolus Contains : Tricalcium Phosphate, Vita D_3 and B_{12}	Tonic and growth stimulant for all animals.	Large animal : 1 bolus daily Small animal : $^1/_4$-$^1/_2$ bolus daily	5 boluses strip.
KALROL - D_3 Liquid contains : Vita D_3, B_{12} and Tricalcium Phosphate	Tonic and growth stimulant for all animals.	Large animal : 50-10 ml bid Small animal : 2.5 - 5 ml bid orally,	500 ml bottles.
MICOTRIM - D Tablets/Bolus Contains : Sulphadimidine 0.5 gm/5 gm	Bacterial enteritis, bacterial pneumonia, metritis, coccidiosis, foot rot, calf scour. H.S.	Large animal : 2 bolus bid Small animal : 1 bolus bid.	Strip of 4 boluses, Box of 50 tabs.
MICOTRIM-U Bolus Contains : Sulpha methoxazole 0.5 gm Trimethoprim 0.1 gm Urea : 6 gm.	Retained placenta, cervicitis, metritis, vaginitis and urinary tract infections.	2 boluses given intrauterine. Repeat after 24 hrs.	Strip of 4 boluses.
MILCONZA Tablet (Herbal)	Improves and maintains milk production.	10 tablets to 20 tablets daily.	10 x 100 tablets in plastic jar.
MILCONZA Forte bolus (Herbal)	Indicated in habitual and irregular let down of milk. Improves milk production.	1-2 bolus bid.	Strip of 4 boluses.
MINVET Powder Contains : Cu, Co, Mg, Fe, Zn, I, Cal, Phos, L-Lysine, DL- Methionine.	Mineral supplement for optimum growth and productivity.	20-30 gms per days to adult animal. Poultry: Mixing rate 2% of feed.	1 kg bag.
PRAZOLA DS Capsule : Mrigakshi, Dharam Pattan, Shringawar Vadehi	Anoestrus due to inactive overies or non-specific reasons.	3 capsules daily for 3 days if no heat repeat after 10 days.	6 caps sachets. 6 caps x 20 sachets box.
RUMINOL Bolus Contains : Antimony Potassium tartrate : 2 gm, Ferrous Sulf : 2 gm	Simple indigestion and ruminal atony.	Large animal : 3 to 4 bolus for 1-2 days	Strip of 4 boluses and Jar of 50 boli.

Preparation	Indication	Dosage/Route	Presentation
RUMINOL-C Bolus Contains : Antimony Potassuim Tartrate : 2 gm, ferrous Sulf : 2 gm, Copper Sulf : 50 mg Cobalt Chloride : 100 mg	Off feed, indigestion, ruminal stasis, dyspepsia, anorexia and impaction.	2 to 4 boluses daily for 3-4 days.	Strip of 4 boluses.
UTRONZA Tablets. (Herbal)	Retention of placenta, metritis, endometritis, vaginitis, ecbolic, genito urinary infections. cervicitis.	10-20 tabs bid.	10 x 100 plastic jar.
WORMIZA Powder/Bolus Bolus Contains: Mebendazole 500 mg Powder: Wormiza 50% Wormiza 10%	For gastrointestinal infestation of roundworms. tapeworms and hook worms.	Bolus : Large animal: 5-10 mg/kg b wt Small animal: 5 mg/ kg bwt. Powder (50%) Suspend 10 gm in 125 ml water Give 2 ml/15 kg bwt Poultry : 10 gm per 500 birds.	Strip of 4 boluses. Powder : 100 gm and 20 gm packs.

PFIZER LIMITED
Animal Health Division
Express Towers, Nariman Point
MUMBAI - 400 021

Preparation	Indication	Dosage/Route	Presentation
AMOXISOL Contains : Amoxycillin trihy-drate : 50% w/w (Water soluble)	Coliform infection. Gumboro infection bronchitis, laryngotracheitis, CRD, coryza. Fowl cholera, fowl typhoid pullorum disease, necrotic enteritis and wingrot.	Poultry : 40 mg Amoxisol per kg body wt. Given in drinking water every day for 3 to 5 days.	50 gm bottle.
ANOREXON Forte Each bolus contains: (Cobalt sulphate 100mg, ferrous sulphate 200mg, Thiamine 50 mg; Vit B_{12} 40 mcg, choline bitartrate 18.2 mg).	Primary and secondary anoxexia and reduced feed intake.	1-2 bolus/adult cattle or bufalo per day for 2-3 days.	Strips of 2 boli.
BANMINTH (Morantel citrate) Tab: 118.8mg morantel base Bolus: 594 mg morantel base, oral solution 3%, soluble powder 9%	For immature & adult gastro intestinal nematodes in all species.	Cattle, buffalo, calves, sheep, goats, horses, mules & donkeys (for horses solution is not recommended) 5.94 mg morantel base/kg, Banminth Tab 1tab/20kg for smaller animals & calves. Banminth forte bolus 1 bolus/100kg for L.A. Banminth soln. 4 ml/20kg for sheep, goat & other animals. Banminth soluble powder: dissolve 100gm powder in 1 litre this is sufficient for 50 sheep of 30kg each.	Tablet : 10 strips of 10 tabs, each : Bolus: 5 strips of 4 boli each Solution: Bottle of 500ml and cans of 5 litre, Powder : Sachet of 20 gm and 100 gm.
BIFURAN Feed supplement Contains : Nitrofurazone : 25% w/w Furazolidone : 3.6% w/w	To promote growth, weight gain and feed conversion efficiency in chicks and growers by keeping coccidiosis away during growing period.	500 gm of Bifuran supplement in 1000 kg. feed during first 8 wks of life then 400 g of Bifuran in 100 kg feed from 9th wk to point of lay.	5 kg bucket.
BIFURAN Tablets Contains : In each tab Nitrofurazone : 100 mg Furazolidone : 14.5 mg(Water soluble)	Prevention and treatment of Caecal and intestinal coccidiosis in poultry.	Curative : 1 Tablet of Bifuran in 1 lit of drinking water for 7 days. Preventive : 1 tab in 4 lit of drinking water.	Bottle of 50 tablets.
COXISTAC Contains : Salinomycin 6%	For control of coccidiosis in broilers. Improves intestinal health, weight gain and feed efficiency.	Broilers : 1 kg Coxistac in 1000 kg feed	5 kg bags.

Preparation	Indication	Dosage/Route	Presentation
DIADIN Tab. Each bolus contains: (Sulphadimidine 5 gm)	Any condition where sulfonamide therapy is needed eg. H.S., Footrot, strangles, joint ill, metritis etc.	2 Tab/50 kg body wt or 200 mg/kg.	Tins of 50 boluses.
DISFECT - S Polyalkyl monohydric phenols 40% w/w, Dodecyl Benzene sulphonic acid 24% w/w, Metacresol (40%) 5% w/w Base Q.S.	Used as disinfectant of equipments, hospital premises, as foot dips and wheel dips at farms. Effective against all families of virus, bacteria and fungi.	Level of disfects varies from 50ml-200ml per 20 litres of water.	100ml bottle 1 & 5 litre Jery can.
DISTODIN (Oxyclozanide) bolus 1 gm each. Tab 200 mg each	For fascioliasis and amphistomiasis.	Cattle : 10 mg/ kg b.wt. or 1 bolus/100 kg body weight 5 tab/100 kg body weight Sheep : 15 mg/kg b.wt.	10 strips of 4 boli in a carton. 10 strips of 10 tab. in a corton.
FURASOL Powder contains : Furaltadone hydrochloride 20% w/w	For poultry diseases as coliform infections, bronchitis, infectious laryngotracheitis. Salmonella infections, infectious synovitis, Black head and Caecal coccidiosis.	Poultry : 1 gm of Furasol per lit of water for 10 days. Birds under 2 wks of age : 0.5 gm furasol per liter of water.	Sachet of 30 gm. Sachet of 450 gm.
FUREA BOLUS Each bolus contains: Nitrofurazone 60mg, Urea 6 gm	Uterine infections associated with retained placenta, metritis, cervicitis, vaginitis.	2-4 bolus intrauterine repeat after 24 hrs.	Strips of 6 boli.
NEFTIN-200 Each Neftin-200 contains: Furazolidone 200 mg	To improve egg production, hatchability, growth rate and weight gain in poultry.	250 gm Neffin-200 in 1000 kg feed.	1kg and 5 kg.
NUTRICAL Each 5ml contains: Calcium 100mg, Phosphorus 50 mg, Vit D_3 400 IU Vit B_{12} 5 mcg	For calcium & phosphorus supplementation, prevents rickets, osteomalacia, osteoporosis. Ensure better productivity & skeletal growth.	Cat & dog: 10-20ml bid; Calves, sheep, gaot : pig: 20-50 ml bid. Cattle, horse : 50-100ml bid Poultry: Chick & broiler: 20ml/100 bird in 5 It water, Grower : 50 ml/100 bird in 7 litre of water. Layer: 100 ml/100 bird in 10 litre of water.	1 litre & 5 litre.
NUTRILAY Contains : Vita A, D_3, E, K, B_2, B_6, B_{12}, Calcium Pantothenate, Nicotinamide, Choline Chloride, Calcuim, Cobalt, Copper, Iodine, Iron, Manganese, Selenium and Zinc.	To promote growth rate, increase weight gain improve egg production and to prevent laying slumps.	Poultry 2.5 kg of Nutrilay per 1000 kg feed for growth promotion and improve egg production. 1.5 to 2.0 kg Nutrilay per 1000 kg feed during laying slumps, retarded growth.	2.5 kg bags.

Preparation	Indication	Dosage/Route	Presentation
NUTRIMILK Vit A, D, E, Niacinamide Ca, P, Co, Cu, I, Fe, Mn, Se, Zn	Retarted growth, low fertility, abortions, low milk production, post calving complication, milk fever etc.	1 kg of nutrimilk in 100 kg of feed, common salt shoud also be added; or 25-50 gm per cow/buffaloes per days. 15-25 gm per calf/sheep per day.	1 kg bags.
RUMENTON Each Tab. contains : Antimony pot. tartrate 2gm and ferrous sulphate 2 gm	Simple indigestion, Acute impaction.	2-3 tab/Adult cattle & buffalo per day for 2 or 3 days.	Tins of 50 tablets.
STAFAC - 20 (20gm virginiamycin per kg of Stafac-20)	For promoting growth rate, weight gains & feed conversion efficiency in calves, pigs and fish. For improving quality & quantity of milk yield in milch cows & buffaloes.	Mixing rate of Stafac-20 per 100kg of feed Fish:1-2 kg from fingerlings to harvest. Pig: 500 gm from day old to marketing. Calves: 1-2 kg from day old. Milch, cow & buffaloe:1-2 kg throughout lactating period or 7.5-15 gm in feed per cow/buffalo/day.	10x100 gm sachets 5x5 kg polybabs.
TERRAMYCIN Injectable solution (Oxytetracycline 50 mg/ml)	Used as a broad-spectrum antibiotic.	2-10 mg/kg b.wt. by I.M. I/V or S/C.	30 ml and 100 ml vials.
TERRAMYCIN/LA (Oxytetracycline 200mg/ml)	Used as a prolonged antibiotic action.	1 ml/10kg b.wt. I.M. Poultry : 0.25 ml/kg bwt S/C	30 ml vial. 50 ml vial.
TERRAMYCIN Formula Tablets. Each tablet contains:(Oxytetracycline 500mg)	As an antibiotic specially to Oxytetracycline sensitive organism.	Oral route:1 tab./100kg b.wt.; for Genital tract use: cows & mares 2-4 tab in uterus; Ewe, sow, bitch 1/2-1 tab. in uterus.	Strips of 4.
TM - 100 Terramycin feed supplement (100gm Oxytetracycline in 1 kg feed supplement).	To improve feed efficiency, to increase growth rate, to increase milk production.	In livestock: 100-400gm/ton of feed In poultry: 500g- 1kg/ton of ration.	5 kg pack.
TERRAMYCIN (Oxytetracycline + Vit A, K, E, B_{12}, D_3, B_2, B_3, B_5).	To enhance egg production. It reduces mortality.	1 T.S.F. in 45 lt of drinking water in normal condition (2 gm Tarramycin egg formula/100 birds). 1 TSF in 9 lt of water when pullets first came into production (10 gm of Terramycin egg formula/100 birds). 1TSF in 4.5 lt of water in the presence of disease (20 gm of Terramycin egg formula/100 birds).	100 gm.

Preparation	Indication	Dosage/Route	Presentation
TERRAMYCIN liquid Each ml contains: Oxytetracycline HCI 50 mg	For treatment & control of wide range of bacterial infection of reproductive tract & local cutaneous.	10-30 ml diluted with equal quantity of sterile water intrauterine; can be used topically.	60 ml bottles.
TERRAMYCIN With antigerm 77 Each TSF (4gm) contains (Oxytetracycline 200mg + benzethonium chloride (antigerm 77) 200 mg.)	In treatment & prevention of disease, disinfection of water, for maintenance of egg production. It minimize laying slumps.	1 T.S.F. in 4.5 litre of drinking water.	Tins of 125 gm.
VALBAZEN Powder 5% Albendazole, Bolus: 150mg, & 600mg Albendazole, Suspension : 2.5% Albendazole	A total spectrum anthelmintic for treatment and controls of all stages of gastrointestinal nematodes, lungworms, tape worms and fluke infestations in all animal.	*For Roundnworm & tapeworm* Spp. Powder Bolus Suspension Sheep, 150 mg horse, pig, camel: 2gm/20kg 1/30kg 1ml/5kg Cattle, buff. 15g/100kg 1/20 kg 3mk/10 kg dog, cat: 6g/10kg 1/5kg 12ml/10kg Deer: 2g/50kg 1/75kg 6ml/75kg For Flukes Sheep 3g/20kg 1/2/10kg 3ml/10kg Cattle, Buff. 3g/10kg 1/10kg 6ml/10kg	Powder 30gm , 300 gm, Tablet 150 mg, bolus 600 mg Suspension 60ml bottle, 1 litre.
VISOL - B Contains : Vita B_2, B_6, d-Panthenol, Niacinamide, B_{12}, Choline chloride, L-lysine and DL-Methionine (Liquid supplement)	For better growth and to increase productivity in chicks, growers, layers & breeders.	15 ml to 20 ml per 100 birds, daily in drinking water.	1 lit and 5 lit cans.

PIYA PHARMACEUTICALS WORKS
Mohan Nagar
GHAZIABAD (UP)

Preparation	Indication	Dosage/Route	Presentation
CLOPIMIX 25% Premix Clopidol 125g/500g.	Coccidiostat of poultry and promotes feed efficiency.	With feed at the rate of 500 g/1000 kg of poultry feed.	Buckets with 10 bags of 1 kg.
FURANITRO Each tablet contains: Nitrofurazone - 100 mg, Furazolidone - 14.5 mg.	Effective against coccidiosis in poultry.	With drinking water daily for 10-12 weeks as preventive. Curative-1 tab/litre of water for 7 days.	Pack of 50 tablets.
GASS CUTTER Tablet Each tablet contains: Streptomycin Sulphate- 250 mg, Neomycin Sulphate-100 mg, Vitamin A - 25000 I.U.	Calf scours and avitaminosis A	Cattle, buffalo, horses : 8 tablets twice daily for 3 days. Calves, sheep, goats:- 4 tabs twice daily for 3 days. Dogs: 1-2 tab daily for 3 days.	Bottle of 20 tabs.
KALAYAN MULTIMIN Forte Each tablet contains: Multivitamins and Multiminerals.	To prevent legs paralysis, curled toe, stomatitis, thin-shelled eggs, and to promote optimum growth, egg production and function of thyroid gland.	With feed: 1 kg/400 kg layer feed. For starters: 1 kg/200 kg feed.	Polythene Jar - 2 ½ kg.
KALYAN B Complex Syrup Each 5 ml contains: Vit. B_1 - 3.75 mg, Vit. B_2 - 1.25 mg, Vit B_6 - 0.6 mg, Vit. B_{12} - 6.25 mcg, Niacinamide-37.5 mg, Panthenol - 1.25 mg.	A feed supplement for better feed efficiency, growth and egg production in poultry. As general tonic for horse and cattle.	Orally or in drinking water. Poultry: 15-30 ml per 100 birds with water daily. Horse, cattle, buffalo 100 ml as drench or with drinking water.	Bottle - 460 ml.
NILAMISOL Each gram contains: Tetramisole HCl 30%.	Broad spectrum anthelmintic for cattle, buffalo, sheep, goats and pigs.	Orally dissolve 10g/300 ml water and give @ 1.5 ml/kg. b.wt. (max. 450 ml). Pigs: 1 g Nilamisol/22.5 kg. b.wt. Poultry: 10g Nilamisol per 4 litre drinking water for 100 birds.	Pouch of 10 g, 100 g.
OXYCYCLINE Tablet Each tablet contains: Oxytetracycline HCl-500 mg.	Broad spectrum antibiotics effective against the diseases caused by gram positive and gram negative bacteria, rickettsia and some large viruses in domestic animals and poultry.	Oral Large animal : 1tab/50-80 kg. b.wt. Small animal-1 tab/10 kg. b.wt. for 3-4-days	4 x 4 strips.
OXYZON Suspension Contains: Tetramisole 3% w/v, Oxyclozanide 3% w/v.	Broad spectrum anthelmintic for nematodes, fascioliasis and tapeworms.	Cattle, buffalo, sheep, goat @ 0.33 ml/kg body wt.	1 litre.

Preparation	Indication	Dosage/Route	Presentation
PIYABEE Each gram contains: Vit. B_1 4 mg, Vit. B_2 8 mg, Vit. B_{12} 40 mcg, Niacin-60 mg, Cal. pantothenate - 40 mg, Vit E - 40 mg, Folic acid - 4 mg.	Vitamin B complex supplement, better feed conversion, growth, production and hatchability anaemia and poor feathering in poultry.	200 g - 250 g/ton poultry feed.	Tin of 1 kg.
PIYABLEND AD$_3$ Type 50/5. Each gram contains: Vitamin A 50,000 I.U., Vitamin D$_3$ 5000 I.U.	For rapid growth, better feed utilization, more milk and egg production, protection from parasite infestation and good skin and health in cattle.	20 gram/100 kg cattle feed in the absence of greens; 10 g/100 kg cattle feed with greens.	1 kg.
PIYADIAL (ORS) WHO Formula. Pouch of 82.5 g contains: Sodium chloride 10.5 g, Sodium bicarbonate 7.5 g. Pot. Chloride 4.5 g. Dextrose 60 g	For correcting electrolyte imbalance in diarrhoea, burns, fever and exhaustion.	Orally: 5.5 g/200 ml boiled and cooled water to be given according to need.	Carton of 10 sachets.
PIYAFIN Each tablet contains: Dichlorphen - 0.5g.	Taeniasis in dogs, cats, cattle, sheep and poultry.	Orally: Sheep, cattle, goat-0.5g/kg b.wt. Dogs: 0.2 g/kg b.wt. Cats: 0.15g/kg. b.wt. Poultry- 0.3 g/kg. b.wt.	10 and 100 tablets.
PIYAMENTON Each tablet contains: Ant. Pot. Tartrate-2g. Ferrous sulphate - 2 g.	Rumenotoric, impaction, and atony of rumen.	Orally: Large animal: 2-3 tabls daily for 2-3 days. Small animal: 1/2-1 tab daily for 3 days.	Tin of 50 tablets.
PIYAMIX A+B$_2$+D$_3$+K 1 g contains: Vitamin A - 82,500 I.U., Vitamin B$_2$ - 50 mg, Vitamin D$_3$ - 12000 I.U., Vitamin K - 10 mg.	Better growth rate, more production, resistance to infection, good hatchability and protections from blood loss during severe coccidiosis.	100 g/ton of poultry feed daily.	1 kg.
PIYA MYCETINE 1 g contains: Chloramphenicol powder 250 mg, Vit B$_{12}$-0.5 mcg, Vit. B$_2$-0.25mg, Niacin - 5 mg.	For colibacillosis, enteritis, pasturellosis, actinobacillosis. salmonellosis, pneumonia, nephritis and cystitis in livestock and poultry.	Orally: 100g/10 litres of drinking water for 5-7 days.	Carton of 10 pouches of 25 g.
PIYANITRO Each bolus contains: Nitrofurazone 60 mg, Urea 6g.	Prevention and management of uterine infection, metritis, retention of placenta, cervicitis, vaginitis, infertility and repeat breeding.	2-4 bolus into each horn. Repeat after 24 hrs. for 2-3 times.	Pack of 4 boluses.
PIYAPHENE Each tablet contains: Hexachlorophene - 100 mg.	Liverfluke infestation in ruminants.	Orally: Calf, sheep, goat 1-2 tablets. Repeat after 21 days. Lambs 1/2 tablet.	Jar of 50 tablets.

Preparation	Indication	Dosage/Route	Presentation
PIYAPLEX WM FORTE Each ml contains: Vitamin A 1,00,000 I.U.	Vitamin A feed supplement for poultry and livestock during stress, outbreak of coccidiosis, vaccination, transport and moulting.	Orally: Poultry. 2-5 ml/100 birds in drinking water.	100 ml and 1 litre.
PIYASOL-P Each 5 g contains B-complex (B_2, B_6, B_{12}, Calcium pantothenate, niacin)	For better hatchability, growth of chicks, egg production, to prevent curled toe paralysis, polyneuritis, mortality in chicks, growth promoter and prevents dermatitis.	Orally: Poultry 15g/200 chicks in drinking water daily.	250 g jar, 1.5 kg tin.
RAINIL Oxyclozanide - 3.4% w/v.	Immature and mature flukes, amphistomiasis and Moniezia.	Orally: Sheep and goat 0.5 ml. per kg body weight, or 15 mg/kg b.wt.	1 litre.
TETRAMISOLE HCl Soluble powder Tetramisole HCl 30%.	Broad spectrum anthelmintic, for roundworms and lungworms of livestock and poultry.	Orally: Dissolve 10 g powder in 300 ml warm water (1.5 mg, Tetramisole HCl per 1.5 ml). Cattle 150 ml/100 kg b.wt. (max. 450 ml). Sheep and goat 1 to 1.25 ml/kg body wt. (max.60 ml). Poultry- 10g/4 litre of water during morning. Pigs-1 g powder/22.5 kg. b.wt.	10 gm, 100 gm
TRIMO - VET 1 g contains: Trimethoprim-2% w/w, Sulphamethoxazole-10% w/w.	Broad spectrum, chemotherapeutic for bacterial diseases, coccidiosis, in animals and poultry.	Orally: All animals and poultry-8 g/litre drinking water for 5-7 days or 12.5g/100 kg. b.wt. with water or as electuary for 5 days.	Tins-50 g plastic jar-500g.
VETAPINE Each ml contains: Vitamin A-12000 I.U., Vitamin D_3-6000 I.U., Vitamin E-48 mg., Vitamin B_{12}- 20 mcg.	To promote resistance, coccidiosis, CRD, infectious bronchitis, prevent blood spots in eggs and haemorrhages in poultry. For better growth in animals.	Orally: Chicks: 1 teaspoonful/100 birds. Broilers: 1 1/2 teaspoonful / 100 birds. Layers: 2 teaspoonful / 100 birds. in drinking water daily. Cattle, buffalo, horse: 2-3 tsf. daily orally.	Bottle of 100 ml and 500 ml.
VITAPLEX AB_2D_3 1 gm contains Vitamin A - 40,000 I.U., Vitamin B_2 - 25 mg, Vitamin D_3- 6000 I.U.	Faster growth, early weight gain, more production, resistance to parasitic and other diseases, to withstand stress.	Orally: 200 g/ton of poultry feed.	1 kg.
ZONAMIX Each gm contains: 250 mg of 3,5-dinitro- O-toluamide (DOT).	Potent coccidiostat, controls all forms of coccidia in poultry. Severe exposure and understress. Average growing condition, no stress. Better than average condition.	*Dosage per ton of feed* Chicks (upto 6 weeks) 500 g. Growers (6-14 weeks) - 300 g. Discontinue at 14th week. Chicks - 330 gm. Growers (Upto 10th week) 250g (10-14th week) 160g. Chicks (upto 3 weeks) - nil. (3-6 weeks) 350 g. 6-10 weeks - 160g Discontinue after 10 weeks.	40 g, 500g, 1 kg.

RADIX PHARMACEUTICAL
S.C.O. 845, Kalka Road, Manimajra
CHANDIGARH

Preparation	Indication	Dosage/Route	Presentation
CALVET Inj Calcium borogluconate 25% w/v	Hypocalcemia, milk fever, lactation tetany, liver damage.	S/C or I/V route. Cattle and horse: 200 to 350 ml or more. Calves, sheep, goat, pigs: 60 ml, Dogs, cats: 2 to 5 ml.	450 ml bottle.
DEXGYL Inj. Metronidazole 2 mg in 5% Dextrose soln.	Gastrointestinal disorders. Dextrose, in addition, provides necessary calories.	I/V only. 20 mg of metronidazole/kg b.wt.	540 ml bottle.
DEXTROSE Inj (5%, 10%, 20%)	Haemorrhage, shock, post-operative surgical care, hypoglycemia, ketosis, acetonemia, pregnancy toxemia, supportive nutrition.	I/V only. Cattle/buffalo: 400 ml or more. Goats/ewes: 50 ml or more Dogs: 10-15 ml or more Piglets : 4 ml or more.	500 ml bottle.
DEXTROSE *5% and* Sodium Chloride 0.9%(Inj) Sterile anhydrous dextrose-5%. Sodium chloride-0.9%	Same as above.	Same as above.	Bottle of 500 ml.
KALDEX-M Calcium 1.86% w/v Proportion of boric acid to calcium in the injection 2.26:1. Magnesium hypophosphite 5% w/v. Anhydrous glucose-20% w/v	To prevent milk fever, hypocalcemia, hypomagnesaemia, Eclampsia, Grass tetany Azoturia, Acetonaemia, Osteomalacia, Uterine inertia, Carbon-tetrachloride poisoning.	I/V or S/C route; Cattle, buffalo, horse: 200-450 ml. Sheep, goat, pig: 30-50 ml, Bitches: 2-5 ml	Bottle of 450 ml.
LIGNOCAINE Inj. 2% inj.	Local, regional and epidural anaesthesia.	*I/M route: obstetrical corrections:* Large animal: 10-15 ml locally. Small animal: 2-5 ml locally. *Caudal extradural anaesthesia.* Horse: 10-20 ml. Cattle: 7-10 ml. *Cranial extradural anaesthesia* only in cattle: 40-60 ml *Laparotomy in dogs* 2-10 ml. *Diagnosis of lameness.* Horse and cattle: 10-20 ml. Dogs and cats: 2-3 ml.	Vial of 30 ml.

Preparation	Indication	Dosage/Route	Presentation
MEBEN (Powder, Tablet, Suspension) Mebendazole 5 gm powder 500 mg. 1 tablet 100 mg, 5 ml suspension 100 mg	Mature and immature forms of roundworm, lungworms, and tapeworm, and all major parasites of G.I. tract of livestock and poultry.	Poultry: Powder: 1-2 tsf/100 birds; Suspension: 130 ml/100 birds. Dogs: Powder: 1/2-1 tsf in 2 divided doses x 3 days. Suspension: 1/2-1 tsf bid x 3 days Tablets: 1/2-1 bid x 3 days Cattle, buffalo, horses: Powder: 20 to 40 g, Suspension: 100-200 ml. Tablets: 20-40. Calf, sheep, goat, pigs: Powder: 10-20g. Suspension: 50-100 ml. Tablets : 10-20 Mix with feed or drench.	100 pack.
MICRODINE Solution Povidone Iodine - 5% equal to 0.5% w/v of active iodine.	Non-irritant, multipurpose microbicidal, effective against bacteria, fungi, protozoa, yeast and viruses, infertility associa- ted with mild endometritis, post-partem endometritis, used on skin, mucous membrane, abrasions, burns, dermatitis and mastitis.	Topical application Mastitis-10-20 ml intramammary intrauterine. Large animal - 10-40 ml.	100 ml 500 ml.
OXYTOCIN Inj. Oxytocin 5 unit/ml	Uterine stimulant, for milk let down.	I/M route For all animals-50mcg/kg b.wt	1 ml x 100 ampoules.
PECTOZOL Suspension Each 5 ml contains: Light Kaolin-500 mg, Pectin-75 mg, Furazolidone-25 mg, sodium chloride - 35 mg, Potassium Chloride-15 mg Sodium Citrate - 30 mg.	Specific and non-specific diarrhoea, dysentery, calf- scours.	Dogs & cats: 10-25 ml twice daily, Sheep, goat, calves: 30 ml to 60 ml twice daily	60 ml, 400 ml bottle.
RADIPRIM Powder Each 5 g contains: Trimethoprim 400 mg, Sulfamethoxazole 2000 mg.	Broad spectrum chemotherapeutic agent. Effective against most of gram positive and gram negative bacterial infections of alimentary, respiratory, urinary and genital tracts of livestock and poultry.	Orally in drinking water Poultry: 0.5g/litre of water x 5-7 days Growers, layers: 1g/litre of water x 5-7 days Dogs: 2.5-5g bid x5 days. Large animal: 12-15 g/100 kg b.wt. bid x5. days pig, sheep, goat: 6-8 g Intrauterine: Cow, buffalo, mares: 10- 15 g in 50 ml sterile water for 3-5 days.	100 g pack.

Preparation	Indication	Dosage/Route	Presentation
RADIPRIM Suspension Each 5 ml contains: Trimethoprim 40 mg, Sulfamethoxazole 200 mg,	Same as Radiprim powder.	Poultry: 1 ml/litre of drinking water for 7 days. Dogs: 1 tsf tid x 5 days	50 ml, 400 ml bottle.
RADOXY Inj. Each ml contains: Oxytetracycline- 50 mg.	Infection caused by gram positive and mycoplasma organism.	S/C, I/M, I/V Injection Catttle, buffalo, sheep, goat: 2.5 - 5mg/kg b.wt. Horse, dogs, cats, pigs: 5-7 mg/kg b.wt. 24 hourly. In severe cases increase the dose to 10 mg/kg body wt.	30 ml. 100 ml vial.
RAPROVIT Each 15 ml contains: Protein hydrolysate (equivalent to 96 mg, of nitrogen) - 600 mg. Ferrous gluconate-300 mg. Vitamin B_{12} - 15 mcg. Vitamin B_6 - 3mg. Niacinamide - 5 mg. Folic acid - 1.0 mg.	A general tonic with proteins, iron and vitamin B- complex supplement for proper digestion and better growth. Useful in hypovitaminosis and anaemia.	Dogs and cats:1-2 tsf bid x 15 days	200 ml bottle.
RNALGIN Inj. Each ml contains: Analgin 0.5 g.	Effective analgesic, antipyretic, antispasmodic, and antirheumatic agent in all animals.	I/M, I/V route. Horse: 20 to 60 ml. Cattle, buffalo: 20-40 ml. Pigs: 10-30 ml. Sheep and gaot:2-8 ml. Dogs and Cats: 1-5 ml Foals and calves: 5-15 ml.	30 ml vial.

RAJSHREE DRUGS
BARAUT - 250 611

Preparation	Indication	Dosage/Route	Presentation
BLOTEX Powder	Tympany or Bloat in ruminents	Cattle & buffalo: 100 gm. Sheep & goat : 40 gm. To be given after dissolving in 200 ml of mustard oil for cattle & buffalo and in 50 ml for sheep & goat, 2-3 times in a day.	100 gm., 1 kg., 10 kg.
COFODEX Powder & Bolus	Cold, cough, bronchitis, pharyngitis & pneumonitis.	Powder: Cattle & buffalo : 50 gm. sheep & goat : 20 gm should be mixed with molasses & given as electuary. Bolus: Cattle, buffalo: 2-4 boluses bid. Sheep & goat: 1-2 boluses bid.	Powder 10 gm, 1 kg, 10 kg. Bolus : 20 & 100 boluses.
CP-VET Bolus	Burning micturiation, urinary tract infection, cystitis, anurea, polyurea.	Cattle & buffalo: 2 bolus tid. Sheep, goat, dog: 1 bolus tid. Should be given at least for 10 days.	20 boluses.
DECARIN Powder	Roundworms, hookworms, tapeworms, liver fluke, amphistomes infestation.	Cattle & buffalo: 50 gm for 3 days. Sheep & goat : 20 gm for 3 days.	100 gm. 1 kg, 10 kg.
DIGEPLAN Powder	Indigestion, anorexia, ruminal, stasis, imbalance in ruminal pH, dyspepsia, flatulence etc.	Cows & buffalo : 40-50 gm bid. Sheep & goat : 20 gm bid.	100 gm, 200 gm, 500gm, 1 kg.
DIROL Powder	Acute and chronic diarrhoea amoebic & bacillary dysentery, colitis, coccidiosis, rinderpest, scours and summer diarrhoea.	Cattle & buffalo : 40-50 gm. Sheep & goat : 20-25 gm. To be given twice or thrice daily in rice gruel.	100 gm. 1 kg, 10 kg.
DIROL D.S. Bolus	- do -	Cattle & bufffalo: 2-4 boluses bid. Sheep & goat : 2 boluses bid.	20 boluses, 100 boluses.
HERBOLEEN Liquid	Retained placenta, pyometra, metritis, delayed involution of uterus, delayed puberty, lower milk yield.	Cattle & buffalo : 100 ml. Sheep & goat: 50 ml. To be given twice a day for one week. For retained placenta: First give 150 ml and then 100 ml every hour for 3 times.	500 ml, 1 litre. 5 litre.
LACTOLET-M Bolus	Low milk yield, irregular lactation, difficulty in galactopoiesis, lactogenesis or galactokinesis.	Cattle & buffalo: 2 boluses. Sheep & goat : 1 bolus. To be given once or twice daily for 10 days.	20 boluses.

Preparation	Indication	Dosage/Route	Presentation
LACTOTONE Powder	Same as Laclolet—M bolus	Cattle & buffalo : 50 gm. Sheep & goat : 20 gm. To be given once daily for 10 days.	250 gm, 1 kg, 10 kg.
LIVOMEX Bolus & Powder	Anorexia, hepatitis, jaundice, hepatomegaly, liver cirrhosis.	Bolus/ Powder; Cattle & buffalo: 2 boluses bid/40- 50 gm bid. Sheep & goat : 1 bolus bid/ 10-15 gm bid to be given till full recovery of diseased animal.	Bolus : 20 boluses Powder : 1 kg, 10 kg.
ORACAL AD$_3$ Syrup	Hypocalcemia, hypophosphatemia, Vit A & D deficiency, rickets, osteomalacia, reduced milk yield, prolopse of uterus in bovine. Poultry—early mortality, rickets, stunted growth, thin shelled eggs, higher culling rate, early moulting, poor weight gain.	Cattle & buffalo : 100 ml once or twice a day. Sheep & goat : 25 ml once or twice a day. Dog: 5-10 ml twice a day. Poultry: 20-100 ml/100 birds in drinking water.	Bottle of 500 ml.
PROLAPE-CURE Powder	Prolapse of uterus & vagina.	Cattle & buffalo: 150 gm. To be dissolved in 1 litre of water and given as drench.	450 gm.
PROMIN Bolus	Ruminal stasis, loss of appetite, liver dysfunction, disturbed ruminal microflora.	Cattle & buffalo : 4 boluses sid or bid. Calves, sheep & goat : 1 bolus bid.	Strip of 4 boluses.
ROPAK Ointment	Wound, burns, cracks in nipples, mange, ring worm, maggots, degnala etc.	After cleaning the effected part apply ointment, 2-3 times in a day.	50 gm, 100 gm, 1 kg.
SPORIN Liquid	For inhalation in cough, pneumonia, pleurisy, pharyngitis & bronchitis.	Add 2 to 5 ml Sporin in 2 litres of boiling water & let animal inhale vapours of it. Give 2 to 3 inhalation in a day.	30 ml, 450 ml.

RAKESH PHARMACEUTICALS
C-1/158, G.I.D.C. Estate, Kalol (N.G.)
AHMEDABAD-382 725

Preparation	Indication	Dosage/Route	Presentation
APPEVET Bolus Ayurvedic preparation	Digestive, stomachic, tonic, improves peristalsis, and enhances the activity of ruminal microflora.	Oral route 5 to 6 boli twice a day.	50 bolus.
ESTRONA Cap. Ayurvedic preparation.	Induces ovulatory heat, regulates estrous cycle, uteriseptic and antinflammatory.	Oral route cow and buffalo: 2 cap daily.	10 boluses, 100 boluses.
ESTRONA Forte (bolus) Ayurvedic preparation.	Induces ovulatory heat, regulates estrous cycle, uterine antiseptic and anti-inflammatory.	Oral route cows and buffalo: daily one bolus for 10 days.	10 boluses, 100 boluses.
LACTOVET Powder Ayurvedic ingredients with mineral mixture.	Improves health, high production rate.	Cows and buffaloes: 50 gram daily. Mixing rate 2.5% of feed for poultry.	500 g, 25 kg. bag.
LIVOMA Tab. Ayurvedic preparation.	Liver disorders.	Oral route 10 tablets bid.	1000 tablets.
MILKOPLEX Bolus Ayurvedic preparation.	Galactagogue, specially in the psychologically disturbed milch animals.	Oral route Cows and buffaloes: 1 to 2 bolus bid.	20 boluses, 200 boluses.
MILKVET Tab. Ayurvedic preparation.	Non-hormonal, lactogenic, galactagogue product.	Oral route cows and buffaloes: 10 to 20 tabs bid.	1000 tablets.
MINAREX Bolus Each bolus has:- Calcium 27%, Cu- 30.10%, P-14% Mn-00.12%, NaCl-22%, Co-00.02%, Fe-00.6%, Mg-00.4%, I_2-00.1%, Base-Q.S.	For better health and productivity.	Cattle and buffalo: 2 to 4 boluses per day.	50 boluses.
MINAREX Powder Ca-24%, Cu-0.1%, P-9%, Co-0.02%, Mn-0.12%, Fe-0.6%, I_2-0.01%, NaCl-30%,	To improve health and productivity in livestock and poultry.	28 gram per day for adult cattle. Mixing rate: 1.5% of feed for poultry.	1 kg bag and 25 kg bag.
PROCTIVE Bolus Ayurvedic preparation	Protects from prolapse of uterus and vagina during pregnancy. Nourishes well the fetus during pregnancy.	Oral route 4-6 boluses daily.	30 boluses.
RUMENTONIC Powder Ayurvedic preparation.	Digestive, stomachic, alterative, carminative, laxative and tonic.	Oral route cattle and buffalo: 80 to 100 gm. sheep and goat: 25 to 30 gm.	200 gm, 400 gm, 1 kg, 10 kg.
UTEROVET Tab. Ayurvedic preparation.	Cleansing draught, genito-urinary antiseptic, and analgesic. Indicated in retention of placenta, metritis, repeat breeder.	Oral route cows and buffalo: 10-20 tablets bid.	1000 tablets.

RANBAXY ANIMAL HEALTH CARE DIVISION
11th Floor, Ansal Tower, 38 Nehru Place
NEW DELHI - 110 019

Preparation	Indication	Dosage/Route	Presentation
ALBAC 15% (Zinc Bacitracin 15% w/w)	Growth promoter for poultry.	Upto 4 wks of age : 33-333 gm per tonne feed. 5-16 wks of age 33-133 gm/tonne feed. 17 wk onwords 33-100 gm / tonne feed.	
BIOTRIM Injection (Vet) (I/M) each ml contains: Sulphadiazine 400mg, Trimethoprim 80mg.	Infections of respiratory tract & urogenital tract H.S., B.Q., bronchopneumonia, mastitis, metritis, pyometra, bacterial diarrhoea, repeat breeding due to infections, retained placenta, secondary complications of equine influenza, F.M.D., R.P., blue tongue brucellosis.	1 ml/30 kg body weight by deep I/M injection for a period of 3-5 days.	10 ml. & 30 ml. ampoules.
BIOTRIM IV Each ml contains: Sulphadiazine 200 mg, Trimethoprim 40 mg.	- do -	Daily injection of 1 ml/15kg body weight byI/M or slow IV routes for a period of 3-5 days.	30 ml vials.
BIOTRIM Oral Each ml contains: Sulphadiazine 200 mg, Trimethoprim 40 mg.	- do -	1 ml per 2-4 liters of drinking water for 3-5 days.	100 ml.
BIOTRIM Bolus Each bolus contains : Sulphadiazine 1000 mg Trimethoprim 200 mg	- do -	4 boluses at 12 hrs interval for 3-5 days.	Strips of 4's
BMD-100 Bacitracin Methylene Disalicylate 10% w/w)	Poultry : Better feed conversion & wt. gain. Improves egg production, hatchability & shell quality, for treatment of necrotic enteritis. Cattle, buffalo : Better feed conversion & milk production, prevention of liver abscesses, prevention of bloat. Swine : Better feed conversion & wt gain, prevention of swine dysentery.	Poultry: As growth promoter for better F.C.R. 50-250 gm per tonne feed. In control of necrotic enteritis : 250-500 gm per tonne of feed. Cattle, buffalo : 150-300 gm per tonne of feed during lactation. Swine : @ 100-150 gm per tonne feed.	5 kg packs & 25 kg bags.
CALDIVET Liquid. Each 5 ml contains: Calcium gluconate 200 mg, Cholecalciferol 500 I.U., Cyanocobalamine 5 mg., Cobalt 5 mg.	Milk fever, Osteomalacia, Osteoporosis, Hoof deformation, Alopecia, Dermatitis, Infertility, Anoestrus, Agalactia, Rickets, Fracture, Lameness, Anaemia, Stunted growth & related disorders.	Caldivet is given orally bid for 3-5 days at following rates : Cattle, buffalo : 50-75 ml. Bulls, horse, Camal : 75-100 ml. Calves, sheep, goat & pig : 20-50 ml. Dog : 5-10 ml.	500 ml plastic bottles.

Preparation	Indication	Dosage/Route	Presentation
CALDIVET B$_{12}$ Liquid Each 5 ml contains : Calcium lactate 250 mg, Calcium Gluconate 200 mg, Cholecalciferol 500 I.U., Cyanocobalamine 10 mcg, Chloline Chloride 200 mg,	Stunted growth, perosis, Osteomalacia, Rickets Anaemia, Cannibalism, thin shelled eggs, drop in egg production, fatty liver syndrome, Aflatoxicosis & related disorders of musculo skeletal system in poultry.	Caldivet -12 is given per 100 birds for 7-10 days as follows : Chicks : 10-12 ml. Growers : 20-50 ml. Layers : 50-100 ml.	5 litres jar.
CALMEX-M Liquid Each 450 ml contains : Calcium 1.86% w/v, Boric acid 4.2% w/v, Mag hypophosphite 5% w/v, Dextrose anhydrous 20%w/v, Chlorocresol 0.1% w/v.	Milk fever, lactation tetany & acetonemia.	250-400 ml by slow I/V injection.	Bottle of 450 ml.
CANOVITE-C Each gm contains: Vit A 3500 IU, Vit B$_1$ 4.0 mg, Riboflavin 0.5 mg, Vit B$_6$ 3.0 mg, Vit B$_{12}$ 1.5 mcg, Vit D$_3$ 175.0 IU, Vit E 10.0 IU. Niacinamide 3.5 mg, Folic acid 0.1 mg, Cal. pantothenate 3.0 mg, Manganese sulfate 0.35 mg, Potassium iodide 0.15 mg, Ferric ammonium citrate (Iron) 0.10 mg., Mag. gluconate 0.1 mg.	Palatable oral vitamin and mineral supplement for dog and cats.	1 gm/5kg body weight daily.	50 gm aluminium lacquered tube.
CHECK-O-TOX A blend of organic salts like propionates, Benzoates, Sorbates, Acetates.	Antifungal, prevents formation of Aflatoxins, Ochratoxin, etc in feed (livestock & poultry).	1-2 kg /tonne feed.	1 kg pouch.
ENROCIN Inj. Each ml contains : Enrofloxacin 100 mg.	Broad spectrum antibacterial activity.	5 mg/kg b.wt. I/M.	15 ml ampoule.
ENROCIN Oral Each ml contains : Enrofloxacin 50 mg	-do-	Prevention : 5 mg/ kg b.wt. per 2-4 litres of drinking water for 7-10 days. Treatment : 10 mg/kg b.wt. per litre of drinking water for 3-5 days.	
FAMITONE Each 5 ml contains: Vit A 250000 IU, Vit D$_3$ 25000 IU, Vit E 150 IU, Vit C 500 mg.	Stress, Vitamin deficiencies.	5-10ml/100 birds daily for a week every month in drinking water. 10-15 ml Famitone daily for one week to weak and debilitated cattle.	100 ml, 500 ml & 1 litre plastic bottles.

Preparation	Indication	Dosage/Route	Presentation
FENBEZOL Powder (Vet) Each gm contains: Fenbendazole 250 mg, excipient Q.S.	Effective against the round worm infections in different species.	1gm/50kg (5 mg, fenbendazole/kg body weight).	6gm pouches & 120 gm plastic bottles.
FLOCLOX - D Each syringe contains: Cloxacillin benzathine equivalent to 500 mg, of Cloxacillin.	Sub-clinical mastitis (during dry period). Dry cow mastitis due to new infections during dry period.	Infuse one syringe of Floclox-D per quarter of the udder after the final milking of the lactation. The teats should be cleaned with a good disinfectant before the administration of Floclox-D. Repeat the procedure 3 weeks prior to calving.	3 gms syringe.
FLOCLOX - L Each syringe contains: Cloxacillin sodium equivalent to 200 mg Cloxacillin.	Effective in treatment of clinical mastitis.	Infuse one full syringe each into the infected quarter after stripping off the milk at 24-48 hours interval.	3 gm syringe.
HIVIT Inj (Vet) Each ml contains: Vit A 2000 IU., Vit D_3 2000 IU., Vit E acetate 4 mg, Niacinamide 10 mg, Thiamine HCl 10 mg, Pyridoxin HCl 5 mg, Riboflavin 1 mg, D. panthenol 1 mg, Vit B_{12} 10 mcg, Botin 10 mcg, Calcium 10 mg	Debility & exhaustion, Infertility. Prevention & treatment of neonatal disorders. Prevention of retained placenta. Prevention of milk fever and downer cow syndrome.	1 ml/10-15κg body wt. by S/C, I/M or slow I/V injection, 3- 5 injection may be given on alternate days.	30 ml vial.
LEMASOL 75 Inj (Vet) Each ml contains: Levamisole HCl 75 mg.	To potentiate the action of vaccines (H.S., FMD, R.P. etc). To strengthen body defence mechanism & prolong duration of immunity. To hasten post-operative healing. To reduce morbidity/ mortality in an outbreak. To reduce calf/lamb mortality & neonatal diseases.	1 ml per 30 kg body weight by S/C route repeat if need at an interval of 48 hours.	10 ml & 30 ml vial.
LEMASOL - P Levamisol HCl 30%.	For control & removal of adult, immature & larval stages of roundworms of poultry. It can also eliminate the fowl eye worm & the gape worm. Lemasol-P is also ovicidal in its action.	20-25 mg,/kg. body weight, dissolve 100 gm lemasol-P in 200-300 litres of drinking water & provide this water to the flock for one complete day. Repeat at 2-3 months interval.	100 gm.
LEMASOL Powder (Vet) Levamisol HCl 10% w/w & 30% w/w.	Roundworm infestation leading to loss of production.	75 mg, Lemasol (7.5mg, Levamisole HCl) per kg body weight.	20 gm & 100 gm

Preparation	Indication	Dosage/Route	Presentation
LIVERTONE Each 5 ml contains : Riboflavine 1.25 mg, Pyridoxine HCl 0.62 mg, Cyanocobalamine 6.25 mcg, D-Panthenol 1.25 mg, Niacinamide 3.75 mg, Choline Chioride 5.00 mg, L-lysine Hydrochloride 500 mg, DL-Methionine 5.00 mg.	Prevention & treatment of hepotodegenerative diseases like aflatoxicosis, Fatty liver, curled toe paralysis, perosis, early chick mortality.	15-20 ml per 100 birds daily in drinking water.	
PAQUIN Each 30 gm contains: Sulphaquinoxaline sodium equivalent to sulphaquinoxaline 7.5 gm (25% w/w)	For the prevention & treatment of coccidiosis. It is also effective against pasteurella spp. & salmonella spp.	Paquin should be given in drinking water at the rate of 30gm/25 litre of water; the treatment should be given for 3 days followed by a break of 2 days and again another course of 3 days (3-2-3- schedule).	30 gm.
POLYMIX MULTIVIT Plus Each Kg Contains Vit A 50, 000, 000, I.U., Vit D3 12, 000, 000, I.U., Vit E 75, 000, I.U., Vit K 12.5 gm, Nicotinamide 45 gm, Folic acid 2.5 gm, Nicotinic acid 100 gm, Pantothenic acid 32.5 gm, Selenium 55 mg, Biotin 6 mg, Choline Chloride 100 gm, Unidentified growth factors 120 gm, BHT 130 gm.	Improves wt. gain in broilers & egg production in layers, Improves performance & hatchability in breeders. Prevents diseases associated with vitamins & mineral deficiency in livestock & poultry.	150-200 grams per ton feed or as needed to complete the feed.	25 kg bags.
ROSCILLIN Inj (Vet) Ampicillin sodium 2.5 gm.	Antibacterial.	Dissolve the contents of 2.5 gm vial in 15 ml of D.W. & administer at the rate of 7 mg/kg. body wt. daily by S/C, I/M or I/V route for 3-5 days. In very acute condition treatment may be given twice daily.	2.5 gm vials.
ROSCILLIN Oral Powder. Each 30gm contains Ampicillin as ampicillin trihydrate 3 gm.	Antibacterial for poultry, calves, foals & pigs.	40-120 mg, (4-12mg of Ampicillin) of roscillin oral powder per kg. body wt. twice daily for a period of 3-5 days for calves, Foals and pigs. Administer Roscillin oral powder in drinking water at the rate of 1gm/litre twice daily for 3-5 days in poultry.	30 gm.

Preparation	Indication	Dosage/Route	Presentation
ROSCILOX (Vet) 2 gm inj. contains: Ampicillin sodium equivalent to 1 gm ampicillin. Cloxacillin sodium equivalent to 1 gm cloxacillin.	Bactericidal	6-10mg per kg body wt. daily by I/M or I/V route for 2-3 days.	2 gm vial.
STRONIC Inj (Vet) Thiamine HCl 25mg, Riboflavin 5 mg, Niacinamide 50mg, Cyanocobalamin 50 mcg Pyridoxine 5mg, Liver crude extract having Vit B_{12} activity not less than 2 mcg of cyanocobalamin.	Anorexia, Pyrexia. Rumen atony. Supportive therapy. Anaemia. Hepatitis. Jaundice. Diarrhoea. Post-operative condition.	1 ml per 30 kg body wt. daily by I/M route for 3-5 days.	10 ml & 30 ml vials.
TEK-TROL Liquid Contains: ortho-phenylphenol 12% Ortho-benzylpara-chlorophenol 10%, Para-tertiary-Amylphenol 4%	Heavy duty cleaning, wetting, penetration of soil & organic matter, For disinfaction of almost all areas, eg. transport vehicle, poultry shed, beeder barn, hatchary, chick boxes, foot pans, feeders cages, calf pens, stables foaling sheds, hospital, laboratories, Kennel, etc.	Usage : Tek-Trol concentrate is dilluted @ 4 ml per litre of water & is applied for disinfection by either spray, soak sponge or mop. Subsequently, rinse the surface with water.	Plastic jar of 3.78 lts.
TETRADOX (Doxycycline 2% Formulation)	Prevention of common diseases associated with bacteria like *E. coli*, Salmonella, Streptococcus Hemophilus, Klebsiella, Corynebacterium spp, etc in poultry, swine, livestock.	Layers : 250 gm/tonne feed a week- a month. Broilers : 125-250 gm per tonne feed from day 1 till day of marketing. Pullets : 125-250 gm/ tonne feed, till onset of lay. Pig : 250-500 gm/tonne feed. Livestock :500 gm/tonne feed.	5x5 kg bags.

RHONE POULENC (INDIA) LIMITED
(MAY & BAKER PHARMACEUTICALS)
Rhone Poulenc House, Worli
MUMBAI - 400 025

Preparation	Indication	Dosage/Route	Presentation
ACETYLARSAN Diethylamine acetarsol-23.6%	General tonic in debility, malnutrition, anaemia, helminthiosis, chronic skin afffections.	Horses & cattle (4 months to 1 years): 5 ml. Adult: 10 ml IM or SC route 3-6 times at 48 hrs interval.	Boxes of 5x10ml ampoules.
ANTHIOMALINE Lithium antimony thiomalate 6%	Nasal granuloma in cattle and papillomatosis.	Papillomatosis: Cattle & horses 15 ml 4-6 times at 48 hr interval Dog: 1 ml inj, raising by 0.5 ml increments upto 2.5 ml on alternate days. Nasal granuloma: Cattle: 20 ml at weekly interval 2-3 times deep IM route.	50 ml containers.
ANTRIMA Bolus Sulphadiazine & trimethoprim	RTI, GIT, UTI & Genital tract infections.	30 mg/kg body weight orally. I/Uterine: Cows and mares: 2.4 to 4.8 gm. Sows & ewes: 1.2 to 2.4 g.	4 x 1.2 g, 4 x 2.4 g.
BIO SPUR Each kg contains: Lactobacillus sporogenes 30,000 million spores, Alpha amylase enzyme 5 g	Improves growth rate, weight gain, nutrient utilizations, meat & egg yield, reduces mortality in broilers, layers & breeders.	Broiler, chicks, growers: 500 gm per ton of feed. Layers: 1 kg/ton of feed.	Plastic Jar of 1 kg, Drum of 25 kg.
CALBOROL Cal. Borogluconate sol. 25%	Hypocalcaemia. Milk fever, Liver damage prevention due to drugs.	Cattle & horses: 200-350 ml Sheep, goat, pig: 60 ml. Dogs: 2-5 ml SC or IV.	Multidose containers of 450 ml.
IMEQUYL Each ml of 20% imequyl solution contains: Flumequine 0.20 g, Benzyl alcohol 0.01 ml, Excepients qs 1.00 ml	Colibacillosis, Salmonellosis, Coryza, Avain cholera, Complication due to CRD, Bumble foot/Bact. arthritis (Staphylococci).	12 mg flumequine/kg body weight in the whole drinking water for 3-5 days. Oral route.	Bottles of 50 ml & 100 ml with measuring cup.
METRONIDAZOLE Inj. (Vet) Metronidazole 5 mg,/ml	Cattle/Buffalo-metritis, Pyometra, endometritis, abortion, repeat breeding, wound infection. Horses: Hoof/Frog infection including abscesses & thrush, sinusitis, balanitis, balanoposthitis. Small animals: Abscess, wounds, otitis externa, gingivitis, anal sacculitis.	Intra uterine: 25-50 ml every alternate day for 3 days. Topical: quantity according to lesion. IV: 4 mg/kg body weight daily for 7 days.	100 ml bottles.

Preparation	Indication	Dosage/Route	Presentation
MIFEX Cal. borogluconate, Magnesium, Phosphorus, Dextrose	Milk fever due to hypocalcaemia or associated deficiencies of magnesium and/or phosphorus.	Cattle : 200 to 350 ml SC or IV route	Multidose 450 ml containers.
PROMETHAZINE HCl Promethazine HCl 5%	Eczematous conditions, urticaria, allergic rhinitis, insect bites, gaseous bloat, laminitis, serum sickness, anaphylactic shock.	Horse & cattle: 15-20 ml per 450 kg body weight, Sheep & pig: 2.5 to 5 ml. Dog & cats: 0.5 to 1 ml IM route only.	Boxes of 10 x 5 ml ampoules.
PROVIMIN Forte Bolus Lactobacillus sporogenes 20 million spores, protein hydrolysate 500 mg, Zinc sulphate 0.6 mg, Copper sulphate 0.6 mg, Magnesium sulphate 1.5 mg, Manganese chloride 1.5 mg, Cobalt chl. 1.5 mg, Iodine 0.5 mg, Liver extract 5 mg, Selenium 0.1 mg, Yeast extract 50 mg	Non-specific anorexia, anaemia, debility, revives health, growth & production, recovery from mineral deficiency.	*Animal Acute Chronic* Small: 1-2 bolus 1/2-1 bolus Large: 2-4 bolus 1-2 bolus As long as required oral.	Strip of 4 boluses.
SULPHADIMIDINE Sodium Inj. 33 1/3%	Bact. pneumonia, Metritis, septicaemia, bact. enteritis, foot rot in cattle, coccidiosis in cattle & sheep.	30 ml/50 kg initially followed by half of this dose once daily.. Dogs: one half of initial dose given twice daily, maintenance half of the above dose daily.	Multidose containers of 100 ml and 450 ml.
TEGERON Cream Terpineol 3%	Provides protection to veterinarian's hands during rectal and vaginal exam. Protection against dermatitis associated with cleansing of *Brucella abortus* infected cows.	Topical application on hands and arms.	Tube of 100 gm.

ROCHE PRODUCTS LIMITED
28, Tardeo Road MUMBAI-400 034

Preparation	Indication	Dosage/Route	Presentation
ROVIBE Each gm contains: Vitamin B_1 - 4 mg, Vitamin B_6 - 8 mg, Niacin - 60 mg, Cal. pantothenate-40 mg, Vitamin B_{12}-40mcg, Vitamin E-40 mg	For improving egg production and hatchability, stimulates growth, prevents mortality, better resistance to stresses in poultry.	200-250g/ton of poultry feed daily.	1 kg
ROVIMIX A+B_2+D_3 Each gram contains: Vitamin A 40000 I.U. Vitamin B_2 20 mg, Vitamin D_3 5000 I.U.	For improved growth, resistance to parasitic infection, sustaining the stresses of medication, heat etc. improved hatchability and fertility and low mortality in poultry.	200-250 g/ton of poultry feed	1 kg.
ROVIMIX A+B_2+D_3+K Each gram contains Vitamin A-82,500 I.U. Vitamin D_3-12000 I.U. Vitamin B_{12}-50 mcg Vitamin K-10 mg,	Provides full stability, resistance to heat and pressure, full biological activity, improved growth and production and lowers the mortality.	Poultry: 200-250 g/ton of feed of poultry. The amounts may be increased according to need.	1 kg.
ROVIMIX AD3 Type 50/5 Each gram contains: Vitamin A 50000 I.U. Vitamin D 5000 I.U.	Vitamin supplement for horses. Improves the growth rate and lowers mortality in foals, increases fertility and provides better resistance to parasitic infections and improves feed conversion.	Orally with feed Foals: 0.25 g/ 100 kg b.wt. sid. Yearling : 0.5g/animal daily, Working and race Horses 1g/animal daily.	50 g, 500 g.
ROVISOL A (Oral type 100) Each ml contains: Vitamin A-1,00,000 I.U.	During stress, hatching seasons, outbreak of coccidiosis, after worms cure and moulting in poultry.	Chicks/broilers(1 week): 10 ml/100 birds daily with drinking water. 2nd-4th week: 15 ml/100 birds. Pullets: (5-8 weeks or more): 15 ml/100 birds with drinking water. Layers: 25 ml/100 birds with drinking water.	Bottle of 100 ml and 1 litre.
ROVISOL AD3 EC (oral) Each ml contains: Vitamin A 50,000 I.U. Vitamin D_3-5000 I.U. Vitamin E - 30 I.U. Vitamin C - 100 mg.	For better growth, more egg production, improved hatchability, protection from stresses, resistance to parasitic infestations and decreased mortality.	Chicks/broilers (1 week): 10 ml/100 birds with drinking water. Broilers and pullets (2nd week onwards): 15 ml/100 birds with drinking water. Layers: 25 ml/100 birds with drinking water.	Bottle of 100 ml and 500 ml.

ROUSSEL PHARMACEUTICALS (INDIA) LTD.
Agro-Vet Division, Dr. Annie Besant Road, Worli
MUMBAI-400 018

Preparation	Indication	Dosage/Route	Presentation
SOFRAKAY Suspension Vet. Each 5 ml contains Soframycin (Framycetin Sulphate)-50 mg, Light Kaolin-0.5g, Pectin-, 50mg, in flavoured base.	Severe gastroenteritis due to *E. coli*, *Salmonella*, *Shigella*, *Proteus*, *Pseudomonas* infection and other non-specific organism causing diarrhoea.	Orally for 3-4 days Calves: 10-20 ml tid. Foals: 10-20 ml tid. Dogs, cats, piglets: 5-10 ml tid	Bottle of 60 ml with 5 ml spoon.
SOFRAMYCIN Cream-Vet Soframycin (Framycetin sulphate) 1% in a cream base.	Infection of udder, teats, cuts, wounds, ulcer, burns, skin infection, impetigo and dermatitis.	Milkout the quarter completely after washing the udder properly. Infuse the content of one tube (15 gm) intramammary every 24 hrs. for 3-4 days. The treatment can be repeated after 48 hrs. in less severe cases.	15 g tube and 120 gm tubes.
SOFRAMYCIN Eye-Drop-Vet Framycetin sulphate 0.5% in a sterile aqueous solution.	Eye problems like conjunctivitis, blepheritis, corneal ulcers, injuries, burns, post- removal of foreign bodies and post-operative occular surgery.	Instill 2-3 drops 5-6 times daily for 2-3 days, then 2 drops twice daily.	5 ml vial.
SYNASTAT-VET Tablet Each tablet contains: Trimethoprim-160 mg Sulfamethoxazole-800 mg.	Braod spectrum antibacterial action. Effective in gastro-intestinal, respiratory and urogenital tract infection of both livestock and poultry.	Oral or intrauterine : Oral: Cattle, buffaloes, horses: 6-10 tabs daily Calves, sheep, goats, pigs: 2-4 tabs daily Dogs and cats: 1/2 tab daily Poultry : 1/2 tab/30 birds with drinking water. Intrauterine: cows and buffaloes and mares: 4-6 tab in 50 ml distilled water 24 hourly.	10 tab strips.

SALUS PHARMACEUTICALS
105, G.I.D.C.
HIMAT NAGAR-383 001 (Gujarat)

Preparation	Indication	Dosage/Route	Presentation
APETONE Bolus Each bolus contains: Cobalt sulphate 50 mg, Ferrous sulphate 100 mg, Yeast (Dried) 1 gm	Anorexia due to digestive disorders, stress and disturbed ruminal microflora.	2 boluses daily for 2 to 3 days.	100 boluses.
CALCIMIN PLAIN (F.F.) (Mineral mixture)	Growth promoter for calves, optimum milk production, prevents milk fever, repeats breeder.	Calves: 5 to 15 gm daily. Cattle and buffalo: 30 gm daily.	1 kg, 10 kg.
CALCIMIN Powder (F.F.) (Mineral mixture with Amino acid)	Optimum milk production during lactation, supportive treatment of rheumatism, Ephemeral fever, Fracture of bone etc.	Calves: 5 to 15 gm daily. Cattle and buffalo: 30 gm daily.	1 kg, 5 kg, 10 kg,
ENTRODONE Bolus Each bolus contains: Furazolidone 0.5 gm Metronidazole 0.3gm	Gut acting antibacterial and anti-protozoal preparation for the treatment of enteritis, metritis, vaginitis etc.	Large animal: 6 to 8 boluses per day orally Small animal: 0.5 to 1 bolus per day orally. Intrauterine: 1 to 2 boluses.	20 boluses.
FURAZOLIDONE Powder 5%	Broad spectrum local antibacterial for dressing and intrauterine use.	As per need and severity of infection.	20 gm, 100 gm.
FURAZOLIDONE Powder 20%	Calf scour; for prophylaxis and treatment in outbreak of poultry disease.	As per severity of infection.	20 gm, 100 gm
IMPACTONE Bolus Each bolus contains: Antimoney potassium tartrate-2 gm, Ferrous sulphate -2 gm	Ideal rumenotoric for impaction and rumen stasis.	1 to 2 boluses per day.	20 boluses.
METROZOL-U Bolus Each bolus contains: Nitrofurazone 60 mg Urea 6 gm	Prevention and treatment of uterine infections with retained placenta, metritis, cervicitis, vaginitis etc.	2 to 4 boluses intrauterine.	4 boluses.
OPIGIN Bolus Each bolus contains: Oxyphenbutazone 5 gm Analgin 2.5 gm	Antipyretic and anti-inflammatory in all cases of fever associated with painful syndrome and in the treatment of musclo-skeletal affections.	1 to 2 boluses daily till symptom disappear.	20 boluses.
PHOSPHAMIN-VET Bolus Each bolus contains: Copper sulphate 500 mg, Cobalt sulphate 40 mg, Ferrous sulphate 100 mg, Phosphorus 540 mg, Calcium 900 mg,	Delayed maturity, anestrus, subestrus, repeat breeder, pica, growth promoter, post-partum haematuria, prevents milk fever, rheumatism, ephimeral fever etc.	1-2 boluses daily.	20 and 100 boluses.

Preparation	Indication	Dosage/Route	Presentation
SALDIN Bolus Each bolus contains: Sulphadimidine 5 gm	Braod spectrum antibacterial chemotherapy.	2 boluses per 50 kg b.wt followed by half the dose daily (for oral and intrauterine use).	20 boluses.
SALMINTH Bolus Each bolus contains: Albendazole 1.5 gm	Broad spectrum anthelmintic.	Roundworms: Cattle, buffalo, horse, sheep goat: 1 bolus per 300 kg b.wt Flukes : Cattle: 2 boluses per 300 kg b.wt.	2 boluses.
SALPRIM Bolus Each bolus contains: Trimethoprim 0.4 gm Sulphamethoxazole 2 gm	Broad spectrum antibacterial preparation.	Large animal: 1-2 bolus per day. Small animal: 0.5-1 bolus per day (for oral and inrauterine use).	20 boluses.
SALWORM Powder (Tetramezole HCl 30%)	Broad spectrum anthelmintic.	Cattle, buffalo: 15 gm per 300 kg b.wt Sheep, goat: dissolve 10 gm in 300 ml water and administer as follows: 12 kg bwt - 15 ml 15-25 kg bwt - 30 ml 25-35 kg bwt- 45 ml over 35 kg bwt- 60 ml Poultry: Dissolve 10 gm in 4 lit. drinking water for 100 birds.	100 gm
VETCYCLINE Bolus Each bolus contains. Tetracycline HCl 500 mg	Broad spectrum antibiotic.	Large animal: 2-4 boluses per day. Small animal: 1-2 bolus per day. For oral and intrauterine use	20 boluses.
AYURVEDIC PRODUCTS (Salus)			
CYCLO-HERB Bolus Contains: Emmenogogue herbs	Anestrus, silent heat and delayed post-partum estrus.	1 bolus per day for 3 days; repeat after 20 days.	20 boluses.
DUGDHA Powder	For increasing milk yield, fat and SNF content of milk.	25 gm per day for 20 days then break of 10 days and again for another 20 days.	500 gm
EMDOKLIN Bolus Contains: herbs which increase uterine muscle contraction	Ecbolic for the treatment of retention of placenta, endometritis, pyometra etc.	3-4 boluses per day for 5 days	20 boluses.
METRO HERBS Bolus Contains: herbs having antibacterial effect	Endometritis causing repeat breeding, retention of placenta, metritis, pyometra etc.	2-4 boluses intrauterine	4 boluses.
MILKO HERB Bolus Contains: herbs having galactogogue action and tranquilising effect.	Agalactia, irregular or suppressed lactation, psycological agalactia (death of calf or first lactation or change in milker), as post-mastitis adjuvant therapy, increasing milk production. etc.	1-2 bolus per day for 10 days.	20 boluses.

SARABHAI CHEMICALS
Wadi - Wadi
BARODA - 390 007

Preparation	Indication	Dosage/Route	Presentation
AMPICILLIN Inj. Vet. Each 2 gm vial has Ampicillin sod equivalent to 2 gm of anhydrous Ampicillin.	Calf scours, enteritis pneumonia, ear infections, Pharyngitis, tonsilitis, metritis pyelonephritis, mastitis, Brucellosis, H.S. & secondary bacterial infections.	Large animal : 2-7 mg /kg b.wt. I/M or I/V Small animal : 5-10 mg/kg. b.wt. I/M or I/V.	Vials of 2 gm & 250 mg.
BELAMYL (B-complex, liver extract, Vit B$_{12}$ inj.)	Non-specific anorexia, liver disorder, debility and general weakness, eczemas, Parasitic anemia, growth and development of young animals, blood Protozoan disease, gastro-intestinal disorder with Vitamin B-complex deficiency, neurological disorders.	Large animal: initiate therapy with 4 ml and repeat 5 ml on every alternate day. Small animal: 0.25 ml-0.5 ml twice weekly. (I/M route only)	Vial of 10 ml., 30 ml.
BOVIRUM Bolus (Antimony pot. tartrate 2 gm, Ferrous sulphate 2 gm, Copper sulphate anhydrous 50 mg, cobalt chloride 100 mg).	Simple indigestion, anorexia.	Cattle & buffalo: 3-4 bolus/day. Heavy ruminants: 4 boluses/day, orally.	Strips of 4 boluses.
CURAMINTH Bolus Each bolus has Fenbendazole 1.5 g and 150 mg	Broad spectrum anthelmintic.	Cattle & buffaloses : 5 mg / 1 kg b.wt. Horses : 5-10 mg/kg.b.wt. Sheep : 5 mg / kg. b.wt. pigs : 5 mg / kg. b.wt. Dogs : 20 mg / kg b.wt. Poultry : 8 mg/kg. b.wt. Orally.	Bolus of 1.5 g strips of 2. Boluses of 150 mg strip of 10.
DICRYSTICIN-S (Large dose) (Streptomycin sulphate 2.5 gm, Procaine penicillin 15,00,000 units, Penicillin G. Sod. 5,00,000 unit).	Effective against wide variety of gram negative and gram positive bacteria, mixed infections and infections in which the organism cannot be readily identified.	Add 7.5 ml of D.W. to make 10 ml suspension. Large Animal: 2 ml/50 kg. b.wt. Small Animal: 1 ml/5kg. b.wt. I/M.	2.5 gm vial.
DOXYTERIN-DS Powder Each gm. of Doxyterin -DS Powder contains: Doxycycline HCl equivalent to Doxycycline 25 mg (2.5%)	Antibacterial in poultry, livestock and small animals.	Dosage: Poultry : Prevention : 1gm Doxyterin -DS per litre of drinking water for 4-5 days. Treament 2 gm Doxyterin-DS per litre of drinking water for 5 days. Livestock : 2-4 gm Doxyterin -DS per 50 kg. b.wt.	50 gm, 100 gm.

Preparation	Indication	Dosage/Route	Presentation
ESGIPYRIN - N (Phenylbutazone 150 mg. Analgin 150 mg. Lignocaine HCl 10 mg).	Pain, fever, rheumatic condition of joints, muscle and nerves.	Large animal: 5 to 15 ml I/M. Small animal: 1-5 ml I/M.	Ampoules of 5 ml.
F.P.P. 20 lacs & F.P.P. 40 Lacs. F.P.P. 20 lacs has Procaine penicillin 15,00,000 IU & Penicillin G.Sod 5,00,000 I.U. F.P.P. 40 lacs has procaine penicillin 30,00,000 I.U. & Penicillin G.Sod 10,00,000 I.U.	Treatment of infections caused by penicillin sensitive organisms.	Preparation : add 4 ml D.W. to F.F.P. -20 vial & 8 ml D.W. to F.F.P.-40 vials. Large & medium sized animals : 4,000 units/kg b.wt. at 24 hrs, interval Small animals : 2,00,000-4,00,000 units at 24 hr interval.	20 lacs & 40 lacs units vials.
GWALA Mineral Mixture: Calcium 28%, Phosphorous 12%, Iron 0.5%, Cobalt 0.013%, Manganese 0.12%, Zinc 0.18%, Iodine 0.026%, Copper 0.077%, DL-Methionine 0.19% & L-Lysine mono HCl 0.44%	To enhance the palatability of feed & increase feed consumption of lactating animals : Improves milk production & fat percentage, to improve fertility & conception rate. Provides all essential minerals & amino acids for balanced nutrition.	Add 1 kg/100 kg of feed concentrate. Individual feeding rates : Adult Cattle, buffaloes : 25 gm/day Calves : 5-15 gm/day.	1 kg packet.
HEXANIDE Suspension and Bolus Suspension contains 3.4% w/v Oxyclozanide. Bolus contains oxyclozanide 1 gm	Effective against both adult & immature liverflukes and amphistomes in cattle, sheep & goat.	Suspension : Cattle & buffaloes : 10 mg/kg b.wt. Sheep & goat : 15 mg/kg b.wt. Bolus : 1 bolus per 100 kg. b.wt.	Suspension 90 ml, 1000 ml. Bolus : Strips of 4 boluses.
MILKMIN Calcium 24%, Phosphorus 9%, Manganese 0.12%, Iodine 0.1%, Iron 0.6%, Copper 0.1%, Cobalt 0.02%, Sod. chloride 30%, Fluorine not more than 0.03%.	Feed additive.	Add 1 kg Milkmin to every 100 kg of feed. Adult cattle & Buff.: 28 gm/ animal. Calves: 5-15 gm.	1 kg packet and 25 kg bags.
MILKMIN (Type II) (Without salt)	Mineral feed concentrate for buffaloes, and cattles.	Average rate of 2-3% of the concentrate mixture under normal feeding condition.	Bags of 20 kg.
OXYSTECLIN Inj. (Oxytetracycline dihydrate 50mg/ml).	Broad spectrum antibiotic against gram positive and gram negative bacteria, spirochaetes, rickettsia, large viruses and certain protozoa.	Large Animal: 5-10 mg/kg b.wt. Small animal: 1 ml/10kg b.wt. Poultry: 4-10 mg/kg b.wt. (for IM, IV, SC routes).	Vials of 30 ml and 50 ml.

Preparation	Indication	Dosage/Route	Presentation
OXYTETRACYCLINE Long acting (Oxytetracycline 200 mg/ml).	Long acting broad spectrum antibiotic Effective against G+v and G-ve bacteria, spirochaetes, anaplasma, thilaria.	Cattle, buffalo, sheep, goat: 1 ml/10 kg b.wt. I/M, only.	30 ml vials.
PENDISTRIN - SH Procain penicillin 100,000 units, Streptomycin sulphate 100mg, hydrocortisone acetate 20 mg, sulphamerazine-500 mg, plastobase q.s. to make 6 ml	Acute and chronic mastitis caused by G+ve & gram-ve organism.	1 tube of pendistrin-SH in each quarter on every 12 hrs interval.	Tubes of 6 ml with applicator.
PROFIDONE-200 Powder Contains: Furazolidone 20 % w/w.	Increases egg production, improves feed efficiency, combats stress effectively, reduces mortality & culling, avoids early chick motality.	As an aid in increasing egg production, reducing mortality & culling & improving feed efficiency : 250 gm per tonne feed. For combating stress : 500 gm per tonne feed for 7 days. For avoiding early chick mortality. 2 kg per tonne feed for frist 10 days of life.	Plastic Jars of 5 kg.
SIQUIL (Triflupromazine HCl 20 mg/ml).	Increases tolerance of animal to pain, restrain of animal for examination, radiography & handling, pruritus. An antiemetic for motion sickness, management of nausea & vomiting associated with clinical disorder, failure of let down of milk; postoperatively to ease pain & prevents self mutilation, prolapse of uterus or vagina, preoperatively with local and general anaesthesia.	Dog: 1-2 mg/kg I/V 2-4mg/kg I/M Cattle:10mg/100kg I/V 20mg/100kg I/M Horse: 20-30mg/100kg I/V 100mg I/M (max) Pigs: 80mg/100kg IV 120mg/100kg I/M Sheep: 10 mg/100 kg (Max 40 mg) I/M.	Vials of 5 ml.
TETRACYCLINE HYDROCHLORIDE Bolus (Tetracycline HCl 500 mg).	Infection of digestive, respiratory and urogenital tracts of livestock.	Cattle, sheep, goat, horse, pigs: For prevention: 1- 2 bolus/day orally. For treatment: 4-6 bolus/day orally. For intrauterine: 1-2 bolus deep into the uterus. Lambs, kids, dogs: 1/2-1 bolus/day. Ewe & Sows: $^{1}/_{2}$-1 bolus/day.	Strips of 4 boluses.
SUGAPRIM Bolus (Vet) Each bolus contains : Trimethoprim 250 mg, sulphamethoxazole 1250 mg.	Effective against most G+Ve & G-Ve bacteria causing calf scours, neonatal septicaemia, non-specific enteritis, urogenital infections.	Oral : Cattle, horse, sheep, goat & pig : 1 bolus per 50 kg b.wt. Intrauterine : Cows and mares : 2-4 boluses, sows : 1-2 boluses.	Strips of 4 boluses.

Preparation	Indication	Dosage/Route	Presentation
SULFADIMIDINE Tablets (Vet). Each Tablet contains Sulfadimidine 5 gm	Bacterial pathogens sensitive to sulfadimidine therapy.	Large animal: 0.1-0.2 gm per Kg. b.wt. or 1-2 tab. per 50 kg followed by half this dose daily. Small animal: 1 gm per 15 kg. b.wt. followed by 0.5 gm/5 kg. b.wt. daily.	Pouches of 2 tablets.
SUPPLEVITE - M (Vitamin mineral feed concentrate).	Feed supplement.	For horse, cattle, sheep, goats & pigs: 1 kg powder to 400 kg feed or 25 gm/adults cattle. For layer: 1 kg powder/400 kg feed for starter and breeder: 1 kg powder/200 kg feed.	1kg (4 x 250gm) polythene bags, 2.5 kg jars and 5 kg bags.
SUPPLIMIN (Vet) (Poultry mineral feed concentrate without salt).	Mineral feed supplement.	Supplimin may be fed on an average rate of 2.5% of compounded poultry feed.	Bags of 20 kg.
VITAMINE AD$_3$E Inj. Each ml contains: Vit A as palmitate 2,50,000 IU, Vit D$_3$ 25,000 IU, Vit E 100 IU.	Vitamin deficiency, stress (advance pregnancy, high milk yield, parasitic infection), xerophthalmia. Night blindness, muscle dystrophy, epithelial keratinization, malformation of bone, reproductive disorders etc.	Route deep I/M only. For prophylactic use: Cattle: 1-6 ml, Sheep: 0.5-2 ml, Pig:o.5-2 ml Horse: 1-2 ml, For treatment: Cattle: 2-10 ml, Sheep: 1-2 ml, Swine: 1-3 ml, Horse: 2-4 ml. Repeat in 3 to 4 weeks as needed.	Vials of 10 ml.
VETALOG Inj. (Triamcinolone acetonide 6 mg/ml).	Bovine ketosis & arthritis in cattle, traumatic arthritis, tendosynovitis and related disorder, management of dermatological disorder, pruritus and allergic reaction in dog & horse; pregnancy disease or pregnancy toxaemia in ewe.	In bovine ketosis: 2.5 mg, to 10mg, I/M; In arthritis or tendosynovitis: 6-18 mg, intra-articularly or intra-synovially. Horse & cattle: 12-20 mg, I/M or S/C for allergic condition. Dog & cats: 0.1-0.2mg, per kg I/M or S/C route for allergic conditions.	Vial of 5ml.
VETCLOX - PLUS. (Cloxacillin+Ampicillin). (Cloxacillin sod. 200 mg, Ampicillin sod. 75 mg, in each tube).	To treat the mastitis caused by unidentified organism, resistant staphylococci, streptococci, *E. coli, Corynebacterium pyogenes*.	One tube in each affected quarter repeated at every 12 hours.	10 ml tube.
VETKAL - B$_{12}$ Each 5 ml contains: Calcium phosphate 0.24 gm, Vit D$_3$ 400 I.U., Vit B$_{12}$ 5 mcg.	Livestock: To improve milk production and formation of strong bones in young growing animals. Poultry: Improves egg quality, production and hatchability.	Orally Cattle & horses: 100 ml bid. Calves: 20 ml bid. Dogs: 10-20 ml bid. Poultry: Chicks: 20ml/100 birds. Growers: 50ml/100 birds. Layers: 100ml/100 birds.	500 ml and 5 litre.

Preparation	Indication	Dosage/Route	Presentation
VITCLIN-112 Powder Each gm has Tetracycline HCl 112 mg.	Poultry : B.W.D., Blue Comb, C.R.D., Infectious Coryza fowl cholera, fowl typhoid, spirochaetosis hexamitiasis, infectious sinusitis, secondary bacterial infections. Livestock: prevention & treatment of anthrax, B.Q., H.S, pneumonia, leptospirosis, acute metritis, foot-rot, C.B.P.P., calf scour, and prevention of secondary & post-operative infections.	Prevention : Poultry Livestock 5 gm/20 l 2.5 gm/30 kg b.wt of drinking as electuary water Treatment : 5 gm / 10 lts 5 gm/30 kg b.wt. of drinking water as electuary	100 gm pouch.
ZOBID Inj. (Vet). Each ml of Zobid contains Diclofenac sod. 25 mg, Benzyl alcohal 40 mg & water for injection Q.S.	Alleviation of acute pain and inflammation.	1 mg/kg b.wt. by deep I/M route only.	30 ml vial.

S.G. PHARMACEUTICALS LTD.
Shree Niketan, Shiv Sagar Estate, Dr. A.B. Road, Worli
MUMBAI-18

Preparation	Indication	Dosage/Route	Presentation
ACITROM Each tablet contains: Acenoncoumarol- 1mg, & 4 mg	Thrombosis, embolism.		10x1 mg, tablets 10x4 mg tablets.
ESGIPYRIN-N Each 5 ml contains : Phenylbutazone 750 mg, Analgin 750 mg, Lignocaine HCl 50 mg,	Fever, Pyrexia, Pain, rheumatism, arthritis, myositis & neuritis.	Cattle, buffaloes, horses: 2.2-4.4 mg./kg bwt. 1/m Dogs: 2.2 mg./kg bwt. Maximum is 5 ml/day given by deep i/m route.	5 ml ampoule.
GESICAIN Veterinary Inj. Contains: Lignocaine HCl 2%	Local anaesthesia in dental operation, tail docking, castration, dehorning, laparotomy, caesarian, operation, gynaecological manipulations.	Large animal: 10-15 ml Small animal: 2-5 ml locally	30 ml vial.

THEMIS CHEMICAL LTD.
11/12, Udyog Nagar, Ind Estate, S.V. Road, Goregaon (West)
MUMBAI 400 062

Preparation	Indication	Dosage/Route	Presentation
BIOGRAND-10 Contains: Nitrovin - 2%	Ensures natural defence against internal infections, acts as probiotic, stimulates growth of lactobacilli, prevents invasion of pathogenic bacteria, Lactobacilli secrete lactalin, acidolin, and acidophyllin which inhibit pathogenic enteric bacteria.	Oral route. Cattle, buffaloes, horses: 10-20 g daily. Calves, sheep and goats: 5-10g daily or add 1kg/1000 kg of cattle feed.	1 kg.
CICIN Inj. (Vet) Each ml contains: Gentamicin sulphate equivalent to gentamicin base 40 mg.	Broad spectrum antibiotic, used in metritis, endometritis, enteritis, urinary and respiratory tract infections, osteoarthritis, otitis in dogs, skin wound in livestock and collibacillosis, Staphylococcosis and mycoplasmosis in poultry.	I/M, I/V route or intrauterine Large and small animals: 2-5 mg/kg bwt twice on first day, then once daily. In large animals, intrauterine: 2.5-6 ml/30-100 ml distilled water. Repeat on the second day. Poultry: 3-5 mg/kg bwt. I/M twice daily.	10 ml, 30 ml vials.
ERYSTRIM Each 100 gm provides: Erythromycin thiocyanate-15 gm, Sulphadizine - 15 gm Trimethoprim - 3 gm	Broad spectrum antibacterial for mycoplasma, gram positive and gram negative bacterial infection in poultry and livestock.	In drinking water Dissolve 100g/100 lit. water and provide to chicks during 1-5 days of life and repeat after six days for five days. Pullets and layers: give medicated water for 3 days. Animals: 1g/20 kg bwt. every 8 hourly.	100 g pack.
GROMAX Cyproheptadine with Vit. B_{12}	A water soluble feed additive for broilers for efficient feed conversion, maximum weight gain and to overcome stress.	With feed: Daily dose for 1000 chicks. 1-14 days old - 1 tsf (5g) 15-28 days old-2 tsf (10g) 29-48 days old-4 tsf(20g)	Jar of 500g.
KETMIN-50 Inj. Each ml contains: Ketamine HCL-50 mg	Very rapid, non-irritant, non-narcotic anaesthetic agent. Used in fracture correction, tooth extraction, cleaning of abcesses, radiography, castration, spaying, laparotomy and caesarian operation.	I/M or I/V route Dogs: Following 15 min. of preanaesthetic viz Atropine sulphate @ 0.6 mg/kg b.wt. I/M and Largactil 1 mg/kg b.wt. I/V (by slow method), inject Ketamin @ 10 mg/kg b.wt. Cattle: @ 3-5 mg/kg b.wt. I/M or I/V. Calves: @ 5-8 mg/kg b.wt. Horse: Inject Xylazine @ 1.1	

Preparation	Indication	Dosage/Route	Presentation
		mg/kg b.wt. and use Ketamin @ 2.2 mg/kg b.wt. by I/M route, 5 minute later. Wild cat: 2-4 mg/kg b.wt. Monkey: First give Diazepam 1 mg/kg bwt I/M followed by Ketamin @ 8 mg/kg bwt 10 minutes later Reptiles: 50-100 mg/kg b.wt.	
LACTOBOOST Each 500 g contains: Ca-22% Mn- 0.012% Fe-0.5% P-11% Co-0.013% Cyanocobalimin-0.5% I₂-0.26% Acid insoluble ash-2.5% Cu-0.77% Moisture-5%	Boosts milk production as well as energy in dairy animals.	Large animal: 10-20 g daily or 500g/ton feed Small animal: 6-10g daily or with feed. N.B.: Add 110g sodium chloride to 500 g lactoboost prior to mixing or using .	500g sachet.
LYMCHO Each Kg provides: L-Lysine 400 g, DL- Methionine 200 g Choline Chloride-400g	Feed additive for better growth, weight gain, production and resistance against stresses in poultry.	With feed @ 500g/ton feed of routine use.	1 kg.
NEFUR AND NEFUR-HC Nefur: Each kg contains: Furazolidone (Vet)-44g Nefur-HC: Each kg contains: Furazolidone (Vet)-224g.	Ideal feed supplement which protects poultry from enteric infection, controls chick mortality, improves feed conversion, growth rate and production.	With feed: Chick, growers: Nefur-9 kg/ton feed Nefur-HC-1.8 kg/ton feed Period-Ist-10 days. Broilers: Nefur-1.125 kg/ton feed Nefur-HC-0.125 kg/ton feed Period-upto 8th week. Layer: Nefur-2.25 kg/ton feed. Nefur-HC-0.450 kg/ton feed Period- 7 days in a month or Nefur -1.25 kg/ton feed; Nefur HC-0.225 kg/ton feed. Period continuous use.	100 g Pack, 5 kg jar of Nefur 5 kg jar of Nefur-HC.
REGECOCCIN Premix contains: Clopidol-25%	For prevention as well as treatment of caecal and intestinal coccidiosis in broilers, layers and breeders.	With feed: Prevention : 500 g/ton feed daily till marketing of broilers and till 16 weeks of age in layers. Treatment: 1-1.6 kg/ton feed for 2-4 days.	5 kg jar, 10 kg bucket.

Preparation	Indication	Dosage/Route	Presentation
SUMETROL Inj. Each 5 ml contains: Trimethoprim-80 mg Sulphamethoxazole-400mg	Broad spectrum bactericidal agent. Effective against respiratory, urinary and intestinal infection caused by a variety of pathogens.	By I/V or I/M route Cattle, buffaloes, sheep, goat and horses: 2.5ml/16 kg b.wt by I/V or I/M. In severe cases @ 2.5 ml/10 kg b.wt daily. Dogs and Cats: 2.5 ml/8kg b.wt. by I/M or S/C daily.	30 ml vial.
THEMINEURON Inj. Each ml contains: Thiamine HCl 50 mg. Pyridoxine HCl 25 mg. Cyanocobalamin 500 mcg. Benzyl alcohol 1.5%	Anorexia, disturbed metabolism, and general weakness.	I/M or I/V route Cattle, buffaloes, horses: 5-10 ml daily for 3-5 days. Calves, sheep and goats: 3-5 ml daily. Dogs: 1-2 ml daily	10 ml vial.
VERMITAN (Tab/Bolus/Suspension and Powder) Contains: Albendazole-150 mg/tab, 1.5g/bolus, 2.5g/ml (w/v), and 15 g/100g powder respectively.	Roundworms, liver flukes, tapeworm and hook worm infestation.	Oral route: Cattle, buffalo, horses: Roundworm-5 mg/kg bwt. Liverfluke-10mg/kg bwt. Sheep and goat: Roundworms: 5mg/kg bwt Liver fluke-7.5 mg/kg bwt. Dogs and cats: Hook Worms and tapeworms - 10-15 mg/kg bwt. Poultry: Roundworm and tapeworms 5-10mg/kg b.wt. Repeat after 21 days.	4 x 25 boluses 1 x 12 boluses 60 ml and 1 lit suspension 15 gm, 100 gm and 500 gm powder.
VITATOR C LMB Each 50 g provides: L-Lysine-25 g, D, methionine-12 g, Biotin-0.8 mg Vit. B_{12}-0.08mg	Anorexia, delayed wound healing, dermatitis, hair falling, and poor health.	Orally Large animal: 20 g daily Small animal: 10 g daily	Pack of 50g, 500g, and 5 kg.
VITATOR 100 Each kg contains: Vitamin B_{12}-100mg	Enhances growth, feed conversion, egg production hatchability, weight gain, and livability in poultry & protects from stress.	Mix @ 150-250g/ton feed	1 kg bagx10.

T.T.K. PHARMA PVT. LTD.
66 Luz Church Road
CHENNAI-600 004

Preparation	Indication	Dosage/Route	Presentation
CHLORIL Inj (Vet) Each ml contains:- Chlorpheniramine maleate- 10 mg.	Anaphylactic shock, pruritus, urticaria, dermatitis, insect bite, eczema, and the diseases caused by over production of histamine.	I/M route Cattle and buffaloes: 25-50 mg. Sheep, goats, pigs: 10-20 mg. Dogs: 5-10 mg.	10 ml, 30 ml vial.
EPIDOSIN Inj. (Vet) Each ml contains: Valethamate bromide-10 mg.	As a cervical dilator during normal labour to help easy expulsion of the fetus, to combat dystocia, to overcome hard cervix, to prevent cervical and vaginal tear and other related gynaecological problems.	I/M injection only Buffaloes, cattle, mares: 100-150 mg. Sheep, goats, pigs: 50 mg(5 ml) Dogs: 25-50 mg.	5x5 ml ampoules.
FLEMATIC Skin Oil Contains: extract of Deodar oil and other selected vegetable oils.	Highly effective in dermatitis, eczema, and other skin disorders, all ectoparasite like fleas, ticks, mites and lice. Revives the hair growth and is absolutely safe.	Apply on the skin before bath. For ectoparasites, apply the oil liberally on affected area and give bath 60 minutes later. For better body coat and prevention of ectoparasites, weekly one application is advised.	90 ml.
LIVOBEX Inj (Vet) Each ml contains: Thiamine HCl-10 mg. Riboflavin - 3 mg Vit B_6 5 mg. Niacinamide - 100 mg. Cyanocobalamin - 25 mg. Crude liver extract - 0.66.ml	Non-specific anorexia, general weakness, anaemia, gastrointestinal disorders, Vit. B complex deficiency, haemoglobinuria, and convalescent period.	By I/M route only Cattle, buffaloes and horses: 3-5 ml daily. Sheep, goat, pigs: 1-2 ml daily, Dogs: 0.5-1 ml daily for 3-5 days or more.	Vials of 10 ml and 30 ml.
OSSOPAN Vet Granules Each 5g contains: Calcium - 165 mg Phosphorus-75 mg.	Hypocalcaemia, mineral supplement, during lactation, osteoporosis, fractures, rickets, etc.	Cattle, buffaloes, horses: 20-40 g or more/day Sheep, goats, pigs: 20-30 g or more/day. Dogs:- 5-10g or more/day. Poultry: 1-2g/kg feed.	100 g. 500g.
RIPASON Inj. Each ml contains: Antigen free, water soluble anti-cirrhotic extract of liver-0.026 g.	Non-specific anorexia, acute hepatitis, latent disorders of liver, anaemia, ascites, convalescence, stunted growth etc.	I/M route: Cattle, buffaloes, horses, sheep, goat:-8-10 ml. Pigs: 3-5 ml. Dogs: 2-3 ml.	10 ml vial.

Preparation	Indication	Dosage/Route	Presentation
ROBATRAN Vet.Granules and Bolus Each 5g granules contains:- Trimethoprim-80mg. Sulphamethoxazole. 400 mg. Each bolus contains:- Trimethoprim- 0.2.g. Sulphamethoxazole-1g.	Useful in all infections of respiratory, urinary, alimentary, and genital tracts caused by gram negative and gram positive bacteria.	Granules— in feed. Cattle, Horses, buffaloes: 50-100 g daily. Calves, sheep, goat, pigs: 20-40 g. daily Dogs: 10-20 g daily with feed for 4-5 days. Poultry: 1-2g/kg feed or water Bolus-orally or intrauterine Buffaloes, cattle, horses: Orally-2 bolus bid for 3 days. Intrauterine—1-4 bolus dailyx 3 days. Sheep and goats: Orally—1 bolus twice daily x3 days. Intrauterine: 1-2 bolus dailyx3 days.	100 gm and 500 gm.
ROBENDOL Vet. Granules,Suspension, Bolus Each 5 g granules or 5 ml suspension contains: Mebendazole -100 mg. Each bolus contains: Mebendazole-500 mg.	Useful against mixed worm infestation as broad spectrum anthelmintic.	Orally—Cattle, buffaloes, horses: Granules-25-50 g. Bolus-2-3 bolus. Sheep, goats, pigs: Granules-5-10 g. Bolus - 1/4-1 bolus. Dogs: granules-5 g, Bolus - 1/4-1/2 bolus. Repeat after 2-3 weeks. Tapeworm: double the dose.	Pack of 100g, 500g. 5x4 bolus 500ml.
TEFROLI Vet. Granules Herbal preparation.	All forms of hepatic dysfunction, anorexia, dyspepsia, and to boost metabolic activity.	*Oral route* (see table below)	100g, 500g pack.

Oral route (TEFROLI Vet. Granules)

Animal	As tonic	As treatment
Cattle, horses	4-5g tid	7- 8g tid
Foals, calves:	3g tid	3g tid
Sheep, goat, pig	3-5g sid	4-8g sid.
Lambs, piglets	1-2g sid	2-4g sid.
Adult dogs	1-3 g sid	2-4g sid
Pups	1/2-2g sid	1/2-2g sid.
Poultry	5 g/kg feed.	

Preparation	Indication	Dosage/Route	Presentation
TEFROLI Vet. Syrup Herbal preparation.	Same as above.	*Oral route* (see table below)	120 ml, 500ml, 4.5 litre.

Oral route (TEFROLI Vet. Syrup)

Animal	As tonic	As treatment
Dogs	5-15 ml daily,	10-20ml daily.
Pups	2-5 ml dialy	2-5-10 daily.
Poultry	15-30 ml/100 birds.	

Preparation	Indication	Dosage/Route	Presentation
VALGINATE Inj (Vet) Each ml contains: Valethamate bromide - 2 mg. Analgin-0.5g.	Colic and various types of abdominal pain in all the domestic animals, pyrexia, arthritis, neuritis.	I/M route Cattle and buffaloes: 8ml/100 kg b.wt x 3 days. Horses: 20-60 ml I/M; Calf and foal: 5- 15 ml; Sheep and goats: 2-8 ml; Dogs and cats: 1- 5 ml.	

UNICHEM LABORATORIES
AG. Vet. Division, Unichem Bhavan
S.V. Road, Jogeshwari, MUMBAI - 400 102

Preparation	Indication	Dosage/Route	Presentation
ANAROBIN Each ml contains: Metronidazole 5 mg	Diarrhoea, pneumonia, pyometra, metritis, trichomoniasis, locally in wounds.	4-15 ml/kg at 12 hr interval intravenously; 20- 50 ml i/u on alternate days.	50 ml vial.
DURAPROGEN 17-alpha hydroxy progesterone caproate 250 mg/ml.	Threatened abortion. Repeat breeding, induction of estrus, prolapse of uterus.	1-2 ml I/M	2 ml ampoule.
FAZOLE Bolus Each bolus contains: Furazolidone 0.2 gm. Metronidazole 1 gm	Broad spectrum activity against bacteria, protozoa and anaerobes. Ideally suited for oral and intrauterine administration, controls diarrhoea, dysentery and bovine coccidiosis, Highly effective in treatment of uterine infection of anaerobic origin.	Up to 40 kg b.wt. : 1/2 bolus twice daily Over 40 kg b.wt. : 1 bolus/50 kg b.wt. in two divided dose/day p.o. continue the treatment for 3-5 days.	Sachet of 2 boli.
HELMIGARD Bolus and Granules Albendazole 1.2 gm/bolus and 5% w/w granules.	Provides broad spectrum anthelmintic activity against round worms, lungworms and liver flukes.	Worm dose: Cattle, buffaloes, horse, camel, sheep, goat, pig & poultry: 5 mg/kg b.wt. Dog and cat: 25 mg/kg b.wt. Fluke Dose: Cattle & buffaloes : 10 mg/kg b.wt. Sheep & goat : 7.5 mg/kg b.wt.	1 bolus: 30 gm sachet,
LINCO-SPECTIN, S.S. Inj. Each ml contains: Lincomycin hydrochloride 50 mg Spectinomycin Sulphate 100mg	Effective against mycoplasma spp, Drug of choice for curing foot root in sheep and goats, pneumo enteritis in calves, mycoplasmal pneumonia, swine dysentery and infectious arthritis in swine, respiratory and urinary tract infections, infected wounds and abscesses in dogs and cats and complicated CRD, fowl cholera in poultry.	----	20 ml vial.
LIVOFEROL (Iron, Vit B_1, B_2, B_3, Ca, Liver extract)	Anaemia, stress, for rapid growth, better livability and to improve production.	Cattle/horse: 50 ml bid, Calves foals, sheep, goats and pigs: 25 ml bid. Dog: 10 ml bid In Poultry : Chick 10 ml/100 chick, grower and broiler: 20 ml/100 birds. Layer: 50 ml per 100 birds.	450 ml bottle, 5 litre jar.

Preparation	Indication	Dosage/Route	Presentation
LUTALYSE Each ml contains : naturally occuring Prostaglandin F$_2$ alpha Dinoprost tromethamine - 5 mg	Lutalyse is effective in those case having active corpus luteum Cows and buffaloes: – Management of sub-estrus, Silent estrus – Synchronization of estrus	5ml I/M, bred the cow at estrus or 80 hrs after injection. 5 ml I/M, repeat the inj at 11 days interval, bred after 80 hrs. of second injection.	10 ml vial.
	– Treatment of uterine infection (endometritis, metritis, pyometra)	5 ml I/M.	
	– Prevention of retention of placenta – Induction of abortion	2 ml I/M within 1 hr after calving. 5-7 ml during the first 100 days of gestation.	
	– Induction of Parturition.	5-7 ml I/M after day 270 of gestation.	
	Mare: Controlling time of estrus in cycling mares.	1 ml/I/M during diestrus, will return to estrus within 2-4 days and ovulate 8-12 days after treatment.	
	Induction of abortion.	1 ml I/M upto day 35 of pregnancy after day 35 treatment is less predictable.	
	Swine : Induction of Parturition.	2 ml I/M.	
POLYGESIC Each ml contains: Analgin & pitofenone HCl 500 mg and 2 mg & Fenpiverinium Bromide 0.02 mg,	Pain, spasm, fever, colic.	Large animal : 20-60 ml Calves and foals : 5-15 mg Sheep, goat : 2-8 ml Dog and cat : 1-2 ml I/V, I/M, or S/C routes.	10 ml & 30 ml vials.
SULPRIM-24 Each ml contains : Sulphadiazine and Trimethoprim 200 mg, & 40 mg	Retained placenta, metritis, haemorrhagic enteritis, pneumonia, equine influenza, H.S., B.Q., mastitis, post-surgical sepsis.	1 ml/16 kg body weight or 15 mg per kg body weight by slow I/V or I/M.	30 ml vial.

Preparation	Indication	Dosage/Route	Presentation
UNIMYCIN Bolus and Injection i) Each bolus contains: Neomycin sulphate 500mg ii) Each ml contains: Neomycin sulphate 140 mg	Broad spectrum bactericidal action against enteropathogenic sensitive organisms, drug of choice in H.S., diarrhoea and dysentery, stable in presence of organic matter i.e. blood, pus etc.	Bolus: 1 bolus/45 kg b.wt. in 2-4 divided doses/day for 3-5 days. Injection: Cattle, horse, sheep, pig : 2.5 - 5 mg/kg b.wt. repeat after 8-12 hrs. Dog and cat: 11 mg per kg b.wt./day in divided doses, repeat every 6-8 hrs.	Strip of 4 boli; vials of 10 ml and 30 ml.
LINCO-SPECTIN S.P.O. Each 32 gm sachet contains: Lincomycin hydrochloride 6.66gm Spectinomycin sulphate 13.34	For effective control of complicated CRD and infectious coryza in poultry also improve weight gain.	—	2 gm sachet.
NEOMIX-325 Each 20 gm sachet contains: Neomycin sulphate 10 gm	For control of bacterial enteritis due to wide range of pathogens.	—	20 gm sachet.
NEOMYCIN Each 100 gm contains: Neomycin sulphate 14 gm	Feed premix for effective control of bacterial enteritis in livestock and poultry.	—	500 gm sachet.
UNIMIX Lincomycin hydrochloride 8 gm	Lincomycin for better growth and improved feed efficiency. Helps to control necrotic enteritis in poultry	—	1 kg bag.
UNISTAT Dinitolmide 25% w/w Ethopabate 1.6 w/w	For effective control of intestinal and caecal coccidiosis	—	1 kg bag. 5 kg

USV LIMITED
Animal Health Division Poonam Chamber-B
Dr A.B. Road, Worli
MUMBAI- 400 018

Preparation	Indication	Dosage/Route	Presentation
ACTUSS Suspension Contains: Tetramisole HCl : 3.0% W/V Oxyclozanide : 3.0% W/V	Broad spectrum anthelmintic used for treatment and control of nematodes and fascioliasis in cattle, sheep and goat. It also removes tapeworm segments.	Given as an oral drench @ 0.33 ml per kg body wt for cattle, sheep and goat.	100 ml and 1 lit bottles.
AMPICILLIN Inj. Each 1 gm/2gm vial contains: Ampicillin Sodium 1gm/2 gm.	Active against a wide range of pathogens.	2 to 7 mg per kg b.wt.I/M or I/V.	Vials of 1 gm and 2 gm.
AMPROLIUM Soluble Powder 20%. Each 30 gm contains: Amprolium Hydrochloride 6 gm	Treatment of coccidiosis in broilers, layers, breeders, turkey also in calves, lambs and goats.	30 gm dissolve in 25 litre drinking water for 5-7 days.	30 gm, 150 gm and 600 gm.
CANAPAR Each ml contains: Analgin 500 mg, Pitofenone HCl- 2ml, Fenpiverinium bromide -0.02mg	Colic, antipyretic, analgesic and anti inflammatory.	Large animal: 20-60 ml I/M, I/V or S/C Calves and foals: 5-15 ml. Sheep and goat: 2-8 ml Dog and cat : 1-2 ml.	30 ml vial.
COSYLAN Suspension/Powder/Bolus Each ml susp. contains: Albendazole 25 mg. Each bolus contains: Albendazole 150mg/ 600 mg. Powder - Albendazole 5%	Worm infections due to roundworms, tapeworms, flukes and has an ovicidal action.	Roundworms: 5 mg, per kg b.wt. Flukes: 10 mg, per kg b.wt. Sheep, goat: 7.5 mg/kg b.wt. Dogs: 10-25 mg/kg b.wt. twice daily for 3 days.	Powder : 30 gm, 300 gm Suspension 30 ml, 60 ml.
DEXAMETHASONE Inj. Each ml contains : Dexamethasone sod. phos. 4 mg	Inflammation, shock, ketosis and other conditions.	Cattle & horse : 4-20 mg Calves, pig, sheep, goat : 2-4 mg Dogs and cats : 0.5-2 mg	5 ml.
DOXYN-Vet Each gm contains : Neomycin sulphate, 100mg, Doxycycline 100mg, Lactose Q.S.	Poultry : CRD complex, Fowl cholera, colisepticaemia, non-specific diarrhoea, Pullorum disease, early chick mortality. Animals: Foal pneumonia, leptospirosis, Respiratory tract infection, B.Q., Anthrax, H.S., Mastitis, secondary bacterial infections.	1 gm in 10 litre drinking water for 4-5 days.	30 gm pouch.

Preparation	Indication	Dosage/Route	Presentation
GENTAMICIN Each ml contains: Gentamicin sulph. 40 mg.	In all infections of respiratory, urinary and reproductive tract, skin and soft tissue infections etc.	Large animal: 1-2 mg, per kg b.wt. Small animal: 2-4 mg, per kg b.wt. I/M or I/V.	Vials of 10 ml and 30 ml.
LYCHOPLEX Each 5 ml contains: Vita B_2 1.25 mg. D. Panthenol 0.65 mg. Vita B_6 0.62 mg. Vita B_{12} 6.25 mcg. Nicotinamide 37.50 mg. Choline Chloide 10 mg. Lysine mono HCL 10 mg.	B-complex deficiencies, loss of appetite and weakness. As a co-therapy with antibiotics in poultry, livestock and dogs.	As per need. Cattle : 100 ml daily Calves : 20 ml daily.	500 ml bottle and 5 litre jar.
OXYCLOZANIDE Contains: Oxyclozanide 3.4% W/V	Treatment and control of fascioliasis in cattle, sheep and goat.	15ml suspension for 50kg body weight. Qr 10-15 mg/kg b.wt.	100ml, 1000 ml.
OXYTETRACYCLINE Each ml contains: Oxytetracycline HCl 50 mg	Broad spectrum antibiotics—effective against a wide range of common infections.	Depending on body wt. daily for 3-5 days I/M or S/C, as below: Cattle and Horses: 30-40 ml Calf, sheep, goat, pigs: 10- 20 ml Dogs: 2-10 ml.	Vials of 30 ml and 100 ml.
POVIDONE - IODINE 5% W/V	Wounds on skin, mucous membranes, burn, otitis, metritis, pyometra, mastitis etc.	Local application. For intramammary 10-20 ml For intrauterine 10-40 ml.	100ml, 500 ml.
RAFOXANIDE 20%	Treatment of fascioliasis in cattle, sheep and goat.	10 gm for adult cattle.	10 gm.
T-COX Contains: Amprolium 16.67% Sulfaquinoxaline 16.67%	Against single and mixed species of Coccidia.	30 gm dissolve in 50 litre of drinking water for 7 days.	30 gm pouch.
VISYNERAL AD_3 EC Contains: Vita. A,E, D_3 & C	Helps to eliminate stress, Restores productivity in poultry and cattle.	5-10 ml/100 birds daily for a week every month.	1000 ml bottles.
VISYNERAL Calcium with B_{12}	Helps in reducing the risk of milk fever, retention of placenta and prolapse. For safe pregnancy, normal calving and high milk yield.	As per requirement.	500 ml and 1000 ml bottles.

Preparation	Indication	Dosage/Route	Presentation
ABLAC. Contains: Zinc bacitracin, a natural peptide substance composed of amino acids.	Powerful growth promoter, anti-bacterial and egg enhancer. Reduces mortality and increases fertility and hatchability.	Oral route *Birds Age Dosage* Chicks 0-4 weeks 100g/ton of feed 5-8 weeks 200g/ton of feed Growers 9-12 weeks 300g/ton of feed Layers 17-72 weeks 500g/ton of feed During stress of production, disease, aflatoxicosis, coccidiosis, enteritis the dose of Albac may be increased to 1 kg/ton of feed.	Carton of 1 kg. Bucket - 10 kg. Drum - 25 kg.
COBAN - 100 Each kg contains: Monensin sodium-100g.	Coccidiosis in poultry.	In Feed: Mix 1-1.2 kg Coban-100/ton feed. Feeding schedule- Broilers-only this feed is to be used daily. Layer replacements—continuous feeding from day old to 16 wks. age.	Packs of 1 kg and 5 kg.
COXIDOL. Contains: Clopidol premix 25%.	For prevention of intestinal and caecal coccidiosis in poultry.	In Feed: Prevention: 500g/ton feed from day old to 16 weeks. Treatment: 1-1.6 kg/ton feed for 2 days.	Carton of 1 kg. Bucket - 10 kg. Drum-25 kg.
PIPERAZINE HEXAHY-DRATE Contains: Piperazin hexahy-drate-56.3% w/v.	Ascaridia, capillaria worms in poultry. Nodular worms in swine, small strongyloids in equine and round worms in cattle and buffaloes.	Orally: Poultry- 4-6 weeks age: 20-25ml/100 birds in 3-5 litres water. 6 weeks and above : 40 ml/100 birds in 5-10 litres water. Cattle, buffaloes, calves and horses: 10-20ml/30 kg b.wt. Pig-10ml per 25 kg b.wt. Dogs and Cats: 0.2ml/kg. b.wt.	Plastic bottles 500ml, 4.5 litres jar.
STRESVEL AD3EC Oral Each ml contains : Vitamin A-55,000 I.U., Vitamin D3-10,000 I.U., Vitamin E-30 I.U., Vitamin C-100 mg.	Multivitamin deficiency, improve growth, production, hatchability, fertility and immune system.	With drinking water or orally as such. Poultry: 100 chicks : 2-3 ml for 5-7 days with water; 100 broilers/layer : 4-5 ml for 5-7 days. Cows, buffaloes, horses, camel: 10-15 ml daily. Calves, foal, sheep, goat: 5-10 ml daily	Bottles of 100 ml, 500 ml and 1000 ml.

Preparation	Indication	Dosage/Route	Presentation
		for 7 days. Dogs: 3 ml daily for 5-7 days.	
TYLOSIN TARTRATE Each 100 g contains: Tylosin - 50 g.	To protect the chicks/birds from chronic respiratory disease (CRD), and stress. It improves feed conversion.	With drinking water: Prevention: 1g/litre water for first 2 days of life; discontinue for 8 days and repeat for 3 days. Treatment: 1g/litre for 3-5 days.	Bottle of 100 g.
VELDOT Dinitolmide 25% w/v.	A potent coccidiostat used to prevent coccidiosis in poultry caused by different species of *Eimeria*.	Used in feed Bird type — Condition — Dosage Replacement birds. — Severe coccidiosis, decreased feed intake & stress — 300-500 gm/ton feed ers — do — Broilers 500g/ton feed	Carton of 1 kg, bucket of 5 kg and drum— 25 kg.
V-FUR-200	Feed supplement, controls loose motions, improves egg production, feed conversion, maturity, and hatchability and reduces mortality in poultry.	With Feed. Chicks. (days old to 10 day old): 2 kg/ton feed; Growers/broilers. (7-30 days old) 250g/ton feed; Layers (7-30 days): 500 g/ton feed. In outbreak of infection: 2 kg/ton feed for 10-14 days. For prevention of infection: 500 g/ton feed for 10-14 days.	1 kg, 5 kg, 10 kg, 25 kg packs.
VENDOX-Vet. Doxycycline HCl 1.125% w/w water soluble.	Broad spectrum anti-microbial agent. It is more effective against staphylococci and enterococci than other Tetracyclines. Also effective against rickettsiae, spirochetes PPLO and Mycoplasma (CRD)	Oral route (in drinking water) : Poultry (chicks growers, layers): - 1g/litre water Ist day—followed by 0.5 g/litre for another 2 days. Cattle, buffaloes, sheep, goat, horse: 1g/4 kg. b.wt.	Jar of 100 g and 500 g.
VENLYTE Each 100 gm contains: NaCl-1g, Pot chloride-3g, Ca. gluconate-1.1g, Ca. lactate 1.1g, Sod. citrate-2.5 g, Sod. bicarbonate-1g, Mag. sulphate 0.9g, Ascorbic acid-1g, Dextrose monohydrate-88.4 g.	Electrolyte deficiency, climatic stress, enteric diarrhoea, vomition etc.	With drinking water. Dissolve 100 g/4 litre water for 250 layers or 500 chicks. Calves and foals, sheep and goat: 10-20 g twice daily. Cattle, buffaloes, horse: 50 g twice daily. Dogs and cats: 5-10g bid.	Sachet 250 g, jar-1 kg.
VENPRIM S.D. Sulphadiazine 10% w/w Trimethoprim 2% w/w.	Effective in both gram positive and gram negative organisms affecting, poultry particularly— *Salmonella, Shigella, Clostridium, Streptococci, Staphylococci,* and *E. coli.*	With drinking water, orally. Mild disease : 1 g/litre water x 3 days. Severe disease:- 5g/litre water x 3-10 days.	Poly containers of 100 g and 500 g.

Preparation	Indication	Dosage/Route	Presentation
VENTRICILLIN Powder 100 g powder contains: Ampicillin trihydrate - 5 g.	Broad spectrum antibiotics having bactericidal effect against *Brucella, E. coli, Pasturella, Klebsiella, Proteus, Salmonella, Shigella, Streptococcus fecalis* and *Fusiform* spp. Used in GI tract, respiratory tract, meningeal, urinary and ear infection.	With drinking water : Dissolve 100 g/165 litres of drinking water for 3-5 days to the birds. The amount of solution is sufficient for 250-550 growers, 250 pullets and 175 layer birds.	Pack of 100 g.
VENTRIMISOLE Levamisole HCl 30% w/w.	Effective against mature and immature stages of all round worms of poultry. In cattle, sheep, goat and pigs—it is completely safe.	Feed addititve @ 200 g/ton feed.	1 kg tin.
VENTRIMIX (AB$_2$D$_3$). Each gm contains: Vitamin A - 40,000 I.U. Vitamin B$_2$- 25 mg, Vitamin D$_3$ - 6,000 I.U.	For normal growth and protection from stress conditions in poultry.	Feed additive: @ 200 g/ton feed.	1 kg tin.
VENTRIMIX (AB$_2$D$_3$+K) Each gm contains: Vitamin A-82,000 I.U. Vitamin B$_2$- 50 mg, Vitamin D$_3$- 12,000 I.U., Vitamin K-10 mg.	Correct vitamin K deficiency due to sub-clinical diseases, improves egg production and hatchability.	With feed: @ 100 g/ton feed.	1 kg tin.
VENTRIPLEX - M Each 5 ml contains: Vit. B$_1$ - 3.75 mg, Vit. B$_2$- 1.25 mg, Vit. B$_6$ - 0.62 mg, Vit. B$_{12}$- 6.25 mcg, D-Panthenol-1.25 mg, Niacinamide-37.5 mg, DL- Methionine-5 mg.	Corrects Vitamin B deficiency, prevents polyneuritis, curled toe paralysis, dermatitis and hock enlargement in chicks and pellagra in pigs. Improves hatchability and body growth.	Orally or with drinking water 100 chicks (2 wks. old) 15 ml daily. 100 chicks (above 2 wks.) - 20 ml daily. Calves, pigs, dogs, cats: 5 ml daily. Horses;15-20 ml daily.	Bottle-500 ml, jar-5 litre.

VESPER
No. 67, I Floor, West of Chord Road
2nd Stage, Rajajinagar, BANGALORE - 560 086

Preparation	Indication	Dosage/Route	Presentation
APTHOCARE Each 60 gm contains: Vit C 120 mg, Iodate 60 mg, Glutamic acid 30 mg	Aphthous lesions, Hypertrichosis, ptyalism, Thyroid imbalance, infertility, panting, hyperthermia.	Cattle, buffalo, horses: 25 gm tid. x 5-7 days. Sheep & goat: 10-15 gms tid. Dogs & cats: 5 gms tid.	60 gm packets.
ENTEROFUR Each 10 gm contains: Nitrofuran's Activity 100 ppm, Vitamin A 3000 IU, Lactobacillus 2 million spore, Aminonitrogen 800 ppm with demulcent base	Calf scours, specific and non-specific diarrhoea & dysentery.	Powder Bolus Calves, 5 gm tid 1 bolus foals bid Sheep & 5 gm tid 1 bolus pig bid Cattle 10 gm tid 2 bolus bid Dog & 2 gm tid 1/2 bolus cat: bid	5 gms x 8 bolus strips & 50, 100, 250, 500 gms, 5 kg and 1 kg bags.

GYNAE - CARE
Each 5 gm bolus contains: Vitamin E 4.125 mg Selenium 0.082 mg Calcium 25 mg Vitamin A - 2500 I.U. Phosphorus 3 mg, Iodine 0.38 mg, Cobalt 4.0 mg, Copper 4.0 mg with fortified base
	Helps in initiating puberty at an appropriate age, helps in regulating oestrous cycles, helps in bringing the animal in proper fertile heat. Helps in toning up the tubular genitalia and improves ovarian activity. Helps in reducing incidence of repeat breeding, metoestrol bleeding, cystic ovarian degeneration and anovulatory heat. Helps in reducing inflammatory condition of the genitalia and prevents induration and also increases tissue response to antibiotics	Species Bolus Powder
		Cattle,
		Buff., mares,
		heifers 2 bolus 5gm bid x
		        bid 15 days
		Sheep, goat,
		and pig 1 bolus 1/2 TSF
		        bid bid
		Cats and 1/2 bolus 1/2 TSF
		dogs bid bid
		(During breeding season i.e. for one week).
			Powder 100 gm;
			Bolus 5 gm x 8 bolus strip.

LACTOMIN Each 100 gms contains: Vit A 125000 IU Vit D$_3$ 12500 IU Vit E - 55 I.U. Calcium 25.20 gms Phosphorus 18 gms Copper 0.5 gms Iodine 0.05 gms Manganese 0.20 gms Cobalt 0.02 gms Zinc 0.20 gms Iron 0.30 gms Selenium 0.05 ppm Niacin 20 mgs.	Stimulate, sustain & maintain production.	Heifers: 15 gms daily; Cow & buffalo: 30 gms daily; breeding bulls: 30 gms daily (Mixing Ratio 2.5-5kg/ton of feed) (Orally).	500 gms & 1 kg packets.

Preparation	Indication	Dosage/Route	Presentation
MASTI - CARE 　　　　Each　　Each 5 gm 　　　60 gm　　bolus Vit A　3000 IU　750 IU Lacto bacillus　60 mill.　15 mill. Amino nitrogen 100 mg　25 mg with fortified calcinated base	Helps in reducing inflammation. Helps in preventing tissue damage. Helps in preventing blood in milk. Helps in quick recovery. Helps in increasing tissue response to antibacterial. Helps in reduction of udder oedema (Pre- & Post—Parturient)	Powder: Cattle & buffalo: 10-20 gm tid 3-5 day. Bolus: Cattle & buffalo: 2-3 bolus bid (Orally).	Powder: 60 gmsx2 pouches 60 gms x 3 pouches Bolus: 5gm x 8 boluses in strips.
MASTIMIN (Mineral Premix)	Increases both quality & quantity of milk. Takes care of micro & macro mineral deficiency. Reduces the incidence of mastitis, increase the conception rate.	Cattle & buffalo: 15 gm/bid Calves & heifers: 15gm/day Breeding bulls: 30gm/day (Mixing ratio 1-2%) orally.	1 kg packet, 5 kg bag & 10 kg bags.
MULTIFUR (Vit A, Vit E, Amino Nitrogen, with fortified base)	All inflammatory conditions of uterus (Salpingitis, endomatritis, metritis, cervicitis, vaginitis & retention of placenta. In irregular cycles, short cycles, prolonged cycle. Repeat breeder. Infertility problem of non-specific origin. Can be used safely as pre-post A.I. Congenial uterine environment.	10-15 ml (Could be diluted with equal amount of distilled water when used for large size uterus).	60 ml container or 15 ml container or 5gm x8 bolus in strips.
RUMAX 　　　　in 50gm　in 5 gm 　　　　　　　　bolus Ferrous　Sul. 1 gm　50 mg Copper sulphate　500 mg　25 mg Cobalt . sulphate　100 mg　50 mg Brassica　2.5 gm　5 mg yeast　1 gm　250 mg Vit. B_1　20 mg　5 mg Choline　20 mg　5 mg with fortified base.	Anorexia, Dyspepsia, Flatulence, Metabolic disorders, Rumen atony.	Powder: Cattle & buffalo: 50-100 gm bid x2-3 days, Sheep & goat: 15 gm bid x 2-3 days. Bolus: Cattle & buffalo: 2-4 bolus bid x 2-3 days, Bloat: 2 boluses every 3 hours. Sheep & goats: 1 bolus bid x 2-3 days Bloat: 2 boluses every 3 hours (Orally).	50 gm x 12 pouch & 5 gm x 8 boluses.
RUMAX - T Each 100 gms contains: Cobalt 12 mg. Copper 45 mg Brassica 100 mg. Asafatida 5 mg. L.B.A. 10 lakh spores fortified with surfactant base	Ruminal dysfunction & faulty fermentation, Restore the activity of ruminal microflora, vagal indigestion, ruminal atony. Prevents the formation of flatulence & improper ruminal metabolism. Rapidly reduces tympany & frothy bloat, prevents colic & restores intestinal peristalsis.	Cattle: Anorexia: 10gm bid x 3 days. Impaction: 20 gm bid x 3 days. Broat: 20 gm 3-4 time daily.	100 gm packets.

Preparation	Indication	Dosage/Route	Presentation
THERMO - CARE Powder & Bolus Each 5 gm bolus contain : Sodium salicylate 30 mg, Magnesium sulphate 30 mg, Chiretta 5 mg, Nitre 5 mg with fortified base.	Helps in control of specific and non-specific pyrexia, restoring the balance of thermoregulating centres. Helps in prevention of ill effects of pyrexia, quick recovery of systemic infections which result in pyrexia.	Bolus: Cattle, Buff., Horses: 2 bolus bid x 3 days. Sheep, goat, pig: 1 bolus bid x 3 days. Cats, dogs: 1/2 bolus bid x 3 days (Orally) Powder: Cattle, Buff, Horses: 20gm tidx3-5 days Sheep, goat, pigs: 10-15 gm tid x 3-5 days. Cats & dog: 2-5gm tid x 3-5 days Orally.	60 gms x2 pouches 60 gms x3 pouches 5gm x 8 boluses.
TOXOL Each 10 mg contains: Choline 100 mg, Methionine 10 mg, Inositol 2 mg, Vit B_{12} 0.33 mcg, base fortified with predigested protein.	Better digestion & assimilation, dyspepsia, Anorexia, liver functional capacity, Elimination of toxin, act as choleretic and cholagogue, Reduces serum triglyceride level.	Cattle & Buffalo: 20-25 gm bid Calves, colts, heifer, pigs: 10-15gm bid, Horses: 15-20 gm bid. Sheep & goats: 5-10 gm bid. Orally.	100 gms.
UTREX Each 100 gms contains: Vit A 10000 IU, Vit K 200 mg, Cal. gluconate 50 mg, Vit C 10 mg, Extract of Calotropri gigantica 10 mcg Extract of Abelmoschus 1000 mg, Sesamum indium 500 mg with fortified base.	Facilitates easy separation of cotyledons from maternal coruncles. Promotes rhythmic Peristaltic contraction of uterine muscle. Helps in expulsion of foetal membrane & fluid, hastens active involution thus aiding animals to attain peak milk yield at optimum periods. Prevents post-parturient infection.	Prevention: 10gm tid soon after parturition for easy expulsion of placenta. Retention of Placenta : 15 gms tid x 3 days.	100 gms packet.

VESTAS AERO INDUSTRIES
Pet Food Division,
A-21, Rajouri Garden
NEW DELHI-110 027

Preparation	Indication	Dosage/Route	Presentation
CRUNCH EEZ Snack Food Blend of Protein and Fat (Hard mix of wheat, soya, vegetable fat, vitamins and minerals)	Recommended for a smooth coat and healthy skin.	This snack food or biscuits can be served with milk or vegetables.	
DOG SOU Dry-mix dog soup. (contains a mix of egg along with pre-cooked cereals and vegetables).	Can be served to dogs as a morning, mid-day or an evening meal.	Meal 10 gm. in 250 ml water and allow the mixture to boil, stir frequently. A sachet would be sufficient 4 serving for large dog (15 gm), 5 serving for a medium dog (12 gm), 6 serving for a small dog (10 gm).	Sachet of 60 gm.
PUP-LICK Contains: cereals, egg, yeast, mineral and vitamins	For proper growth in the weaning stage.	Pup-lick should be served from 3 weeks to 3 months of age with milk atleast two feeds per day; quantities would be dependent upon the breed, size and weight of the pup.	
RIZ-PUFFS Riz Puffs obtained from rice and is already digested, it contains: carbohydrates, protein, fat, minerals and vitamins.	Complimentary food for dog for the maintenance of excellent health of dogs.	Small dog (2-6 kg): 50-100 gm. Medium dog (6-25 kg) : 100- 150 gm. Large dog (25-50 kg): minimum 150 gm to be served with meat, milk or vegetables.	
TRIMIX A blend of soya, maize and corn contains: carbohydrate, protein, fiber, mineral & vitamins.	Dog food of high energy levels.	Quantities should be divided in two parts as per size of breed and served with milk. Dog 3 kg: Trimix 50 gm + milk 300 ml/day. Dog 10 Kg: Trimix 100 gm + milk 500 ml per day. Dog 20 kg: Trimix 200 gm + milk 600 ml per day. Dog 30 kg: Trimix 300 gm + milk 1000 ml per day. Dog 40 kg: Trimix 300 gm + milk 1500 ml per day. Dog 50 kg: Trimix 300 gm + milk 2000 ml/day. Dog 60 kg: Trimix 300 gm + milk 2500 ml/day.	
VETRIL Multivitamins, minerals and calcium supplement along with carbohydrate & protein.	Stress condition, as a tonic for vitality and as an excellent coat conditioner for dogs.		
WHEE-PUFFS Contains: carbohydrate, protein, fat, minerals and vitamins.	Complimentary pre-cooked food for excellent health of dogs.	Whee puffs can be served alone or mixed with meat, milk or vegetables. Small dog - (2-6 kg) : 50-100 gm. Medium size dogs (6-25 kg) 100-150 gm. Large dog (25-50 kg): Minimum 150 gm.	

VET CARE
Div. of Tetragon Chemie (P) Ltd.
No 90, 3rd Cross, 2nd Main Road, Ganga Nagar
BANGALORE-560 032

(A)   **Animal Feed Supplement**

Preparation	Indication	Dosage/Route	Presentation
ACTIVIT SPECIAL AB$_2$D$_3$K Concentrated formula.	Animal feed supplement.	10 gm / 100 kg feed	1 kg.
B-CARE Plus B-Complex with Folic acid & Yea sacc [1026].	Animal feed supplement.	–	1 kg.
B-CARE Sol. Water Soluble Vit. B. Complex. Each 200 mg cotnains: Vit. B$_1$-3.75 mg, Vit. B$_2$-1.25 mg, Vit. B$_3$-37.5 mg, Vit B$_5$-1.25 mg, Vit B$_6$-0.62 mg, Vit B$_{12}$-6.25 mcg.	Animal feed supplement.	Poultry: 20-30 ml/100 birds with drinking water. Dogs & cats: 5 ml bid. Cattle & horses: 20 ml. bid. Calves, sheep & goat: 10 ml bid.	50 gm and 250 gm pouches.
DL- METHIONINE 5.00 mg, Calcium Gluconate-2.75 mg, Dextrose monohydrate - 95.83 mg		Prepare fresh water every day (Add 10 gm in 200 ml water).	
BIOCARE BIOTIN (Vit H) 100 mg/250 gm.	Animal feed supplement.	—-	250 gm.
COLIDOX Each kg contains: Colistin sulphate 1000 mg. Doxycycline HCl 10,000 mg,	Growth promoter.	Broilers: 500 mg/tonne of feed from day one till marketing. Layers: 500 gm - 1 kg/tonne for 7 days. Fish : 2 kg/tone of feed.	500 gm.
CHOLINE-500 Choline Chloride-50%.	Animal feed supplement.	-	1 kg, 20 kg.
C-CARE-100 Vit C coated 50% water Soluble supplement	Animal feed supplement.	-	100 gm.
DE-ODORASE Yucca-Shidigera Extract Enzyme.	Ammonia is produced by the hydrolysis of urea present in urine & stool of all animals. This urea breakdown by the action of enzyme urease. DE- ODORASE blocks the action of enzyme, thus preventing urea breakdown to ammonia.	In feed. Poultry: 60 gm/tonne. Dairy: 45 gm/ton. Sheep & Goat: 50 gm/ton. Pig-250 gm/tonne.	60 gm.

Preparation	Indication	Dosage/Route	Presentation
E-CARE-SE Each ml contains: Vit. E (To-copherol) 50 mg, Selenium 1.5 mg.	Muscular dystrophy, infertility, abortion, retention of placenta, poor breeding performance, mastitis; to improve skin & coat conditions. As supportive treatment of various immunodeficiency conditions & stress related conditions. In Vit E & Se deficiencies.	By I/M Route. Horse & cattle: 1 ml/25-50 kg. b.wt. Dogs: 1 ml/25 kg b.wt.	Vials of 10 & 100 ml.
E-CARE- SE Forte Each gram contains: Vit E 200 mg, Selenium 400 p.p.m. mineral carrier q.s.	- do -	75-125 mg/tonne of feed.	1 kg.
ELECTRO CARE Plus Each 100 gm contains: Sod. Chloride- 0.800 gms, Pot. Chloride-5.000 gm, Sod bi carb-3.00 gm. Sod. acid phosphate-0.800 gm. Ascorbic acid-1.200 gm, Sod. citrate -6.50 gm, Cal. lactate-1.70 gm, Mag. Sulphate-1.00 gm, Lactose-25.00 gm. Lactobacillus viable spore-3000 millions, Dextrose anhydrous q.s.	Stress due to heat, transportation, liver damage, post-antibiotic/coccidial therapy, diarrhoea, dehydration.	Poultry: 1 gm in 2 litre of water for 3-5 days. Dog: 50- 100 gm/day, Horses:100 gm immediately after racing or vigrous exercise.	200 gm/pouch.
EQUI-SACC Yea Sacc ^{1026} with Amino acids, biotin & folic acid.	Animal feed supplement.		3 kg.
EQUI-BLUD Vita. and chelated minerals with amino acid.	Animal feed supplement.		30 gm.
G-PRO Amino acid with metabolites & UGF (Water soluble).	Animal feed supplement.		200 gm.
G. PROBIOTIC Each kg contains: Yea Sacc ^{1026} (Live yeast culture)-1,25,000 million. Lactobacillus acidophilus-15,000 million Streptococcus faecium-15,000 mill. Enz. beta glucanase 10 gm Liv Extract-500 mg.	Microbial feed supplement. Improves growth rate. Better feed conversion. Increases weight gain	Broilers : 500 gm/ton feed from day old till marketing. Layer : 1 kg/ton feed (week a month programme). Breeders : 1.5 kg/ton of feed. Cattle : 25 gm/day. Dogs : 5 gm/day.	500 gm pouch.

Preparation	Indication	Dosage/Route	Presentation
KAYSOL-Forte Vit. K_3 500 mg/50 gm.	Animal feed supplement.		50 gm.
LACTO-SACC Composition: Yea sacc [1026] (live yeast culture) 2450 billion, Lacto bacillus acidophilus 50,000 million, Streptococcus faecium-50,000 mill.	Breeder : improves semen quality, higher hatchability, better feed utilization, improves egg-shell quality. Cow/buff./horse: appetite stimulant, indigestion, ruminal dysfuntion, ketosis, acidosis.	Layer/broiler; 250-500 gm/ton feed. Breeders; 500 gm/ton of feed. Cow/Buffalo (lactating)-10 gm/head/day. Dry Cow/Buff. 5-10 gm/head/day. Calf, sheep, goat-5 gm/head/day	500 gm.
L-MEZOLE Plus Levamisole with Mebendazole.	Animal feed supplement. (Anthelmintic)		50 gm.
LYSOCARE Each kg contains: L-Lysine HCl-950 gm.	Essential amino acid supplement.	Broiler: 1kg/ton. Layer: 500 gm/ton. Swine: 750 gm/ton, Equine: 1kg/ton, Bovine: 750 gm/ton.	1 kg, 25 kg.
METHOCARE-86 Each kg contains: Dl-methionine-950 gm.	—	Broiler: 500 gm/tonne of feed. Layer: 250 gm/tonne of feed. Swine: 500 gm/tonne of feed. Equine: 750 gm/tonne of feed.	1 kg, 25 kg.
NEOCARE Forte Neomycine Sulphate 25% water soluble)	—	—	200 gm, 50 gm.
NUTRIBIX DOG ROLLS	See Pet Care.	—	400 gm.
NUTRIBIX ECONOMY	do	—	250 gm.
NUTRICOAT	do		150 gm.
NUTRILIV Forte Liver tonic with choline chloride	—	—	500 ml, 5 lits.
NUTRIPET Vitamins, Minerals, Protein.	Food booster.	—	150 gm/5 kg.
NUTRIPRO Full fat Soya - 99.325%, Synocare-100 (Vit B_{12}) 0.05%, Sod. Selenite-250 ppm, Methocare-0.5%, Ethoxyquin- 0.125%,	Energy packed protein supplement containing essential fatty acids.		25 kg.

Preparation	Indication	Dosage/Route	Presentation
NUTRI SACC Each kg has: Live yeast culture - 5×10^9 cfu, Vit. A- 1,15,000 IU, Vit D_3-23,000 IU, Vit E- 13,000 IU, Vit B_3- 50 mg. Minerals : Calcium- 84 gms, Copper76 mg, Co- balt-5mg, Iron-30 mg I-50 mg, Mg-600 mg, Mn-60 mg P 24 gm, Se-10 gm, Zn-100 mg, Protein 413 gm, By pass fat-50 gm, Energy -2000 Kcal	To improve ruminal productiv- ity, improve digestion & condi- tion. Helps faster recovery after illness. Improves chances of con- ception in repeat breeders. To boost energy, protein, fat, vita- mins & minerals of dry fodder in drought condition.	Calf/Sheep/Goat-50-75 gm per head/day. Cattle/buffalo- 100- 200 gm per head/day. Lactating cow & Breeding Bulls: 200 gm per head/day.	1 kg polypack.
SOLVIT ADBEC Vit A, D_3, B_{12}, E, C Water dispersible.	Use before & after vaccination, deworming, transportation and also in change in weather or feed (effective antistress).	Cattle/buffalo-10-15 gm/head/day, Calf-5 gm/head/day Dogs-2.5 gm/day Chicks/broilers-2.5-5gm in one lit. water/100 birds/day. Layers-5- 10 gm in 4-6 litre of water/day/100 birds.	250 gm
SUPERDOT Each kg contains: DOT- 25%, Ethopabate-1.6%.	Routine use in broiler opera- tions, promotes growth, prevents coccidiosis & ensures faster wt. gain.	Replacement bird during severe challenge-0.5 kg/ton feed. To manage stress condition-0.3 kg/ton of feed Broiler till marketing. 0.5 kg 1 ton of feed.	1 kg, 25 kg
UTPP-5 (Ultimate Toxin prevention Programme), Blend of Or- ganic acid salts like propio- nates, formates, acetates to- gether with gentian violet & specially treated zeolites.	To prevent damage due to myco- toxin like aflatoxin, vomitoxin, ochratoxin, zearalenon.	–	
YEA SACC [1026] (Powder & Bolus). Live yeast culture strain-1026.	Appetite stimulant, anorexia, rumen indigestion, post-antibi- otic treatment, improves fertility in layer, improves weight gain, better Ca, P utilization.	Boli-1/2-1 bolus small animal. 1- 2 bolus large animal. Powder - 1 kg/MT for poultry feed. 1 kg/mt for dairy concentrate Poultry: 1dg/ton of feed.	5 gm bolus, 1 kg,25 kg poly pack
3-CARE Chlorohydroxy quinoline- 12%.	Animal feed supplement. To control diarrhoea due to bac- teria, protozoa and fungus		1 kg

(B) Veterinary Drugs

Preparation	Indication	Dosage/Route	Presentation
COLISTIN Colistin Sulphate 100 mg/gm.	Infection caused by *E. coli, Salmonella, Pseudomonas* & other G-ve organism, promotes growth & feed efficiency, Bacterial diarrhoea.	Poultry: 200 gm/ton feed or 2 gm/15-20 lit drinking water for 75-100 birds for 3-5 days. Cattle, swine, horse, sheep: 50 mg/kg b.w.	50 gm, 200 gm.
EKTODEX Amitraz 5%	See Pet Care.		6 ml & 60 ml.
FURAZOLIDONE-224. Furazolidone-22.4%.			1 kg.
GENTABIO Each ml contains Gentamicin sulphate-40 mg (4000 I.U.)	Infection caused by susceptible organism (*Pseudomonas aeruginosa, E. Coli, Kleibsiella, Staph.* Sp.).	Large animal: 1-2 mg/kg b.wt. Small animal: 2-4 mg/kg b.wt. Give 2 inj on 1st day followed by one inj. daily. Poultry: 3-5 mg/kg b.wt.	10 ml.
HISTAL Chlorpheniramine maleate 10 mg/ml.			30 ml.
L-MEZOLE Levamisole-30%.			50 gm/250 gm.
NEOCHLOR Forte (Powder). Each gm contains: Chloramphenicol 200 mg.	All bacterial infections sensitive to chloramphenicol.	Poultry: 1 gm per 5 lit. of water 1st day, 1 gm per 10 lit of water for subsequent days. Calf, sheep, goat, pigs: 4-11 mg per kg b.wt.	50 gm.
NEOCHLOR Inj. Each ml contains: Chloramphenicol 100 mg.	All bacterial infections sensitive to chloramphenicol.	4 to 11 mg per kg b.w. I/M	10 ml./30 ml.
NEODOX Forte Each ml contains: Doxycycline 100 mg, Neomycin 100 mg.	Effective against infectious coryza.	Poultry: 1 gm/5-10 lit. of water for 4-5 days Large/small animals:10-20 mg per kg b.w. for 3-5 days.	50 gm
NOTIX TALC	See Pet Care.		
NOTIX SCRUB	- do -		
NOTIX SCRUB LIQ	- do -		
NUTRILIV Inj. Liv. Extract with B Complex.	Anorexia, after recovery from ailments, Vit B group deficiency.	Large animal: 5 ml twice weekly I/M Small animal: 0.5 to 1 ml twice weekly I/M.	10 ml, 30 ml.

Preparation	Indication	Dosage/Route	Presentation
PRAZI Plus Each bolus contains: Albendazole 300 mg. Praziquantel-25 mg.	Effective against roundworms, hookworms and tapeworms of all the animals and flukes in cattle, sheep and goat.	1 bolus/10 kg b.wt. for all animals.	10s.
SOLBAC SP Trimethoprim 2%, Sulphamethoxazole 10%.	Effective against infections of respiratory, urinary, alimentary tract and genital tract & other infection.	Poultry: Chick: 1 gm/2 lit. of water x 5 days. Adult: 1 gm/ lit of water. Large & Small animals: 125 mg/kg b.wt. x 5 days.	250 gm.
3 CARE Bolus Each bolus contains: Halquinol 1.5 gm.	Calf scour, diarrhoea due to fungal, bacterial and protozoal origin, bovine coccidiosis etc.	Cattle, buffalo: 1 to 2 boli twice daily for 3 to 5 days. Calf, sheep, goat, pig: 1/2 to 1 bolus daily for 3 to 5 days.	Packs of 10s & 30s.
3 CARE (Feed Mix Powder) Each kg contains: Chloro-hydroxy quinoline - 120 gm.	To stop wet droppings due to bacteria, fungus and protozoa.	Broiler/layer: 1 kg/tonne of feed for 5 to 7 days.	1 kg.

VETCORP
Veterinary Division of Medispan Ltd
Second Floor, Vijay Plaza, C-32
Second Avenue, Anna Nagar, CHENNAI 600 040

Preparation	Indication	Dosage/Route	Presentation
COMBIPEN Vet Contains : Ampicillin Sod : 1000 mg Cloxacillin Sod : 1000 mg	Severe mastitis, calf scour, H.S., Salmonella and *E. Coli* infection, retained placenta, metritis, pylonephritis, pneumonia and B.Q.	5-10 mg / kg b.wt. I/M or I/V.	2 gm vials.
DCF Vet Contains : Diclofenac Sod. 25 mg Benzyl Alcohol 4% W/V	Inflammatory and painful condition.	Large animal : 6-12 ml IM Small animal : 1-3 ml IM.	10 ml and 30 ml vials.
KOT Bolus Contains : Trimethoprim : 400 mg Sulfamethoxazole : 2 gm	Actinobacillosis, Actinomycosis, Colibacillosis, Strangles, Salmonellosis. Respiratory, Urinogenital, Gastrointistenal infections.	Large animal : 4 boli daily Small animal : 1/2-1 bolus daily.	Strip of 4 boli.
NOHELM Bolus Contains: Albendazole : 1.5 gm	For roundworms, lungworms, tapeworms, liver flukes and amphistomes.	For roundworms and tapeworms : 1 bolus / 300 kg b.wt. For liver flukes : 2 boli/300 kg b.wt.	Strip pack of 15.

VETS FARMA PRIVATE LIMITED
Police Lines Road
JALANDHAR - 144 001

Preparation	Indication	Dosage/Route	Presentation
ALTASOL 20% w/w Furaltadone water soluble powder	Calf scours, pneumonia, broncho-pneumonia, enteric and respiratory diseases of swine. In poultry: Salmonellosis, pullorum, fowl typhoid, CRD, coli septicaemia, infectious synovitis, histomoniasis.	All species: 100-125 mg/kg b.wt. for 5-7 days in drinking water or in feed. Poultry: Chicks: 0.5 gm/litre of drinking water for 7 to 10 days. Adult birds: 1 gm/litre of drinking water for 7 to 10 days.	30g.
ANIMIN (Mineral mixture)	To overcome mineral deficiency disorders like impaired digestion and assimilation, retarted growth and muscular dysfunctions; to keep animals in good health, to reduce intercalving period; more and better quality milk.	Large animals: 30-60gm daily. Small animals: 10-15 g daily. In concentrate add 1-3 kg Animin per 100 kg feed.	1kg, 10 kg, 25 kg, 50 kg.
CALFOS AD$_3$ Plus Calcium 26%, Phosphorus 16%, Vit A 3 lac IU/500g, Vit D$_3$ 30000 IU/500g, Copper 0.5%, Cobalt 0.02%	Livestock: Anoestrus and infertility, decreased milk yield, milk fever, haemoglobinurea, prolapse, pica, anaemia, rickets, enlarged & painful joints, arching of back, emaciation, general debility and unthriftiness, enzootic marasmus, loss of libido, sterility in bovine, photophobia, capricious appetite, scaly and encrusted secretion from perioptic band in equine. Neonatal ataxia, depigmentation of hair and wool, defective keratinization of wool in ovine & caprine; excessive flexion of hock & posterior paralysis in swine. Pica & stiff gait in camel. Early mortality, rickets, stunted growth in poultry.	Livestock: During anoestrus and infertility: 50-100g daily for 10-15 days. Deficiency disorders: Large animals: 40- 50g daily Small animals: 10-15 gm daily till symptoms subside; for regular feeding: mix 1 kg calfos AD$_3$ Plus in 100 kg feed. Poultry: Chick 1/2-2 kg in 100 kg feed regularly, in deficiency disorders: 1-2 kg in 100 kg feed till symptoms subside, Layers: 1/2-1 kg/100 kg feed. In deficiency disorders: 1-2 kg in 100 kg feed till symptoms are over. Broilers: 1/2-1kg in 100 kg feed regularly.	500 g & 2 kg poly bag.
LEVASOL Powder/Tabs Per Tab Levamisole HCl 150 mg. Levasol powder: 30% Levamisole HCl	Kills mature and immature stages of all gastrointestinal nematodes including lungworm and acts as immunostimulant.	Animal: 7.5mg Levamisole HCl/kg b.wt. One Tab Levasol or 0.5g Levasol powder/20 kg body wt in feed or water. Poultry: 12-18 weeks of age: 10 gm/200 birds in water. Above 18 weeks of age : 10gm/125 birds in water. Dissolve the required dose in clean water. Give it in early morning having withdrawn drinking water at night.	10 Tab, 10g, 100g.

Preparation	Indication	Dosage/Route	Presentation
MEBENDAL Tablet/Powder. Each Tab contains: Mebendazole 500 mg. Each 5 gram contains: Mebendazole 500 mg	All types of nematodes, cestodes, lungworms.	Cattle, horse: 5-10 mg/kg b.wt. Sheep, goat, pig: 5 mg/kg b. wt. Poultry: 50g powder or 10 Tabs/100 kg feed for 2 days.	Strip of 4 Tabs, 20 g, 100 g.
METAPRIM Co-trimoxazole dispersible powder. Each 5 gram provides: Trimethoprim 80mg, Sulphamethoxazole 400 mg	Poultry: *E. coli* infection, CRD, fowl coryza, coccidiosis, secondary infections of viral diseases. Animals: Genital infections, respiratory infections, urinary infections, systemic infections, pyogenic infections, GIT infections, secondary infections of viral diseases.	Poultry: 10g/8 lit drinking water for 5-7 days, Animals: oral 12.5g/80kg b.wt twice daily in drinking water or feed for 5-7 days. Intrauterine: 25-50 gm in 100-200 ml boiled & cooled water for 2-3 days.	100 g & 500 g poly-jar.
RETISOL Each ml contains: Vit A 100,000 IU	Poultry: Improves egg production, hatchability, resistance to control diseases, prevents blood spots in eggs, reduces coccidial & helminthic infestations. Animals: Increases milk production & fat content, improves fertility & stimulates growth, increases resistance to control diseases.	Poultry: 2-5ml for 100 birds, pregnant & milking cows: 5 ml, breeding bulls: 5 ml. Cattle, horses: 0.5-1 ml. Calf, sheep, goat, pig: 0.25-1 ml. To be given in drinking water or as wetmeal daily.	30 ml & 500 ml bottle.
SCORID Each tab contains: Furazolidone 200 mg	Calf scours, enteritis.	Calves & small animals over 40kg b.wt: one tab twice daily for 3 days. Calves & small animals under 40 kg b.wt. 1/2 tab twice daily for 3 days.	Strip of 10 Tabs x 25.
SULPHADIN Bolus Sulphadimidine 5g	Gastrointestinal infections, respiratory infection, systemic infections.	Large animals: 0.1-0.2g/kg b.wt. or 1-2 boli/50kg b.wt. followed by half this dose daily, Small animals 1g/5kg b.wt. subsequently for every 24 hours.	5 Boli.
VETCOPP (Copper sulphate feed supplement)	To overcome & prevent fungal growth in feed, fungal infections.	50 g in 100 kg feed for 3 days.	500 g.

Preparation	Indication	Dosage/Route	Presentation
VETMIX Forte Contains per kg: Vit A 20,00,000 IU Vit, D$_3$ 400,000 IU, Vit B$_2$ 0.8 g, Vit E 300 IU, Vit K 0.4g, Cal. pantothenate 1g, Niacin 4 g, Vit B$_{12}$ 2.4 mg, Choline chloride 50% FG 60 gm, Calcium 300 g, Manganese 11 g, Iodine 0.4g, Iron 3g, Zinc 6 g Copper 0.8g, Cobalt 0.18g, Phosphorus 80 g,	Poultry: To overcome nutritional disorders, retarded growth, loss in production, liver dysfunctions. Cattle: Liver dysfunction, nutritional disorders, retarded growth, stress & convalescence, to improve general health, efficiency & production.	Poultry : 250g to 500g in 100 kg feed. Cattle : 250 g in 100 kg feed Large animals : 15-25 g daily Small animals : 5-8 g daily.	2.5 kg.
VETLICK (Mineralised lick)	To overcome salt hunger, sialagogue, mineral deficiency indicator.	Keep it at a place where animal can lick easily.	2 kg.
VETRAL Each ml provides: Vit. A 12,000 IU, Vit D$_3$ 6,000 IU, Vit E 48 mg, Vit B$_{12}$ 20 mcg	To prevent & overcome stress, to build resistance against various diseases.	Chicks: 5 ml/100 birds, Growers: 7 ml/100 birds, Layers: 10 ml/100 birds, Small animals: 10 ml daily. Large animals: 20 ml daily. Pets: 3-5 ml daily, give for 5-7 days in feed or water.	30 ml & 500 ml.
VETRAN LA Each bolus contains: Trimethoprim 200 mg; Sulfadiazine 1000mg	Animals: Genital infections, respiratory infections, urinary infections, systemic infections, GIT infections, pyogenic infections; Poultry: *E. coli*, CRD, fowl cholera, coryza, fowl typhoid, coccidiosis.	Animals: oral 1 bolus/80kg body wt twice daily. Intra- uterine: 2-4 bolii daily. Poultry: one bolus per 7.5 kg feed/60 birds.	Strip of 4 bolix12.
VETS AD$_3$ 50/5 Potency per gram: Vit A 50,000 IU, Vit D$_3$ 5,000 IU	To make a balanced feed, improves quality of milk, build resistance against infections.	Large animals: 5 g daily. Small animals: 1g daily. In feed concentrate add 10-20 g in 100 kg.	1 kg.
VETS Cu -Co Each tab contains: Copper sulphate 200 mg, Cobalt sulphate 20 mg	Anestrus, anaemia, enzyme catalyst, copper & cobalt deficiency diseases.	Large animals: 4 tabs daily for 2-3 weeks. Small animals: 2 tabs daily for 2-3 weeks.	50 tab.
VETS BEE Potency per gram: Vit B$_1$ 4 mg, Vit B$_6$ 8 mg, Vit B$_{12}$ 40 mcg, Niacin 60 mg Cal. pantothenate 40 mg, Vit E 40 mg (IU)	To prevent deficiency diseases of B group vitamins and E vitamin.	20 g in 100 kg of feed.	1 kg.
VETS AB$_2$ D$_3$ K Potency per gram: Vit A 82,000 IU, Vit B$_2$ 50 mg, Vit D$_3$ 12000 IU, Vit K 10 mg	As a regular supplement to get required levels of vitamins in feed.	10 g in 100 kg of feed.	1 kg.

Preparation	Indication	Dosage/Route	Presentation
VET MINERAL MIXTURE Poultry: Composition w/w Moisture Max. 3%, Calcium Min 32%, Phosphorus Min 6%, Manganese Min 0.27% Iodine Min (stabilised) 0.01%, Zinc Min 0.26%, Copper Min 100 PPM, Iron min 1000 pp m, Fluorine Max 0.03%, Spores of *Bacillus anthracis, Clostridium spp.* nil	Early chick mortality, delayed puberty, higher culling rate, delayed onset of production, low peak productions, premature moulting.	2 kg per 100 kg feed.	25 kg & 50 kg moisture proof polythenelined bags.
VETSFURAN Each tablet contains: Nitrofurazone 100 mg Furazolidone 14.5 mg	Coccidiosis in poultry & animals, infectious enteritis in large animals & small animals, Salmonella infection in poultry & swine, infectious necrotic enteritis of swine.	Poultry: Preventive: One tablet/4 litre of drinking water for 10-12 weeks of age. Curative: 1 tab/litre of drinking water for 7 days, repeat after 5 days. Animals: One tablet/6-12 kg b.wt. daily for 3-5 days in drinking water or in feed.	50 tab.
VETSOL - B Each 5 ml contains: Vit B_{12} 6.25 mcg, Vit B_1 3.75 mg, Vit B_2 1.25 mg Vit B_6 0.62 mg D-Panthenol 1.25 mg Nicotinamide 37.5mg	Poultry: As a supplement for balancing feed, as growth promoter, high egg production, improvement in weight gain, preventing stress; Animals: Optimum utilisation of feed, better growth, overcome stress and convalescence.	Dissolve 100g powder in boiled & cooled water to make 1 litre solution. Poultry: 15-30 ml daily/100 birds in drinking water. Calves, sheep, goat: 10 ml twice daily. Cattle, horse: 20 ml tiwce daily.	5 x 100 g.
VETS TRACE MINERALS (Poultry) Potency/100 gram; Zinc 10.4 g, Iron 4.0g, Copper 400 mg. Iodine (stabilised) 400 mg. Manganese 10.8g	As a regular supplement to get required levels of trace minerals in feed. To prevent & overcome trace mineral deficiency disorders like slipped tendon, anaemia etc.	50 g in 100 kg of feed regularly. 100-200 g in 100 kg feed during deficiency disorders.	1 kg, 25 kg & 50 kg.

Ayurvedic Products

Preparation	Indication	Dosage/Route	Presentation
COUGHDON	Pneumonia, dyspnoea, bronchitis, pharyngitis.	Cows, buffaloes, horses: 30-40 g bid. Sheep, goats, pigs, colts, calves: 5-10 g bid, Dogs, piglets: 2-4g bid.	150g & 1 kg.
DIARDON	Diarrhoea, dysentery, gastritis, hyperacidity, scours in calves.	Cows, buffaloes, horses: 30-50 g bid. Sheep, goats, pigs, colts, calves: 5-10 g bid, Dogs, piglets: 2-4 g bid, Poultry: 500 g in 100 kg feed.	150 g 1 kg.

Preparation	Indication	Dosage/Route	Presentation
DIGESTOVET	Anorexia, dyspepsia, constipation, flatulence, accelerates recovery after debilitating diseases, as feed supplement to improve production, performance, general condition.	Cows, buffaloes, horses, mules: 40-60 g, Calves, heifers, colts, pigs: 20-30 g, Sheep, goats: 10-15 g Dogs, piglets: 3-5 g, Camels: 400-500 g, Elephants: 800-1000 g, Poultry: 1 kg in 100 kg feed, above dose is given as bolus or electuary twice daily. Stall fed animals should be given thrice a week as feed supplement.	100 g, 200 g, 500 g, 1 kg.
FEVERDON	High temperature, rheumatic fever, urine retention, oedematous swelling, spasmodic condition.	Cows, buffaloes, horses: 50-75g bid, Calves, heifers, colts, pigs: 25-35 g bid, Sheep, goats: 15-25 g bid	150 g, 1 kg.
HI - MILK	To increase milk yield of lactating animals.	Cows, buffaloes: 30-40g sid Sheep, goats: 5-10 g sid.	200 g, 1 kg.
IMPACDON	Impaction, atony of rumen, acute or chronic constipation, flatulence, anorexia.	Cows, Buffaloes, horses: 100-200 g bid, Calves, heifers, colts, pigs: 50-100 g bid, Sheep, gaots: 25-50 g bid.	200 g, 1 kg.
LIVRON	Liver disorders, jaundice, hepatotoxicity, anorexia, convalescence.	As tonic: Broilers: 100 g in 100 kg feed during 3rd, 4th, 6th, 7th week. Layers: 100 g in 100 kg feed as week a month plan. Large animals: 5-10g once a day for 10 days. Repeat the dose if required. As treatment: 200-500g in 100 kg feed for 7-10 days for broilers. Layers : 200-300 gm in 100 kg feed for 7-10 days. Large animals: 5-10 g thrice a day for 10 days. Small animals: 3-5 g thrice a day for 10 days.	100 g, 500 g, 1 kg.
OSTADERM Ointment	Wound, maggot infestation, dermatitis, mange, eczema, ringworm, foot lesions in FMD.	Apply locally on wound after cleaning once or twice a day till recovery.	50 g tube, 500 g jar.

WOCKHARDT VETERINARY LTD.
167, Dr. Annie Beasant Road, Worli
MUMBAI - 400 018

Preparation	Indication	Dosage/Route	Presentation

ANALGON Suspension & Tablets
i. Analgon suspension 2.5% Each ml contains: Albendazole 25 mg, ii. Each tablet contains: Albendazole 1.5 gm
	Broad spectrum anthelmintic for treatment of gestrointestinal infections due to roundworm, lungworms, tapeworms etc. It has an ovicidal effect too.	Analgon Analgon
		     suspension tablets
		For Round
		& Tape -
		worm: Cattle, 1 ml/5kg 1 tab/
		Buff. Goat, 300 kg
		Horse, Sheep,
		Pigs: 0.4-1
		Dog, Cat : 0.4-1 ml/kg -
		For Flukes:
		Cattle/buffalo: 2 ml 2 tab
		            /5kg /300 kg
		Sheep/goat: 1.5 ml/5kg —
		Periodic deworming at interval of 3-4 months.
			5 litre, 1 litre, 60 ml 3x4 tablets strip.

BEEKOM-Forte Powder. Each gm contains: Vit B_1 11.25 mg, Vit B_2 3.75 gm, Vit B_6 1.86 mg Niacinamide 112.50 mg, Vit B_5 4.35 mg, Vit B_{12} 18.75 mcg.	For effective feed utilization, stimulation of growth, Increase in egg production, Increase in body resistance, Prevention of post-vaccination reaction. Prevention of stress, In Vit. B- complex deficiency and after antibiotic therapy. For convalescence and vitality.	Beekom Forte mixed directly in drinking water or feed in quantities as specified below; Poultry: 5-10 gm/500 birds. Cattle/buff/horse: 5-10 gm/day. Calf upto 150 kg body weight: 2.5 - 5 gms/day. Sheep/goat/pig: 1.25-2.5 gms/day, Dog/cat: 0.5-1 gm day.	100 gms sachet.
BEEKOM - L Each ml contains: Thiamine HCl 25 mg Riboflavine 1.5 mg Niacinamide 50 mg, Vit B_6 5 mg, Cyanocobalamin 50 mcg. Choline chloride 25 mg Crude liver extract having Vit B_{12} activity equivalent to not less than 2 mcg of cyanocobalamin.	Hepatitis, jaundice, loss of appetite, non-specific anorexia, emaciation, debility, neuralgic convulsion, parenteral supplement for all animals in prophylaxis and treatment of B- complex deficiency, parasitic anaemia, GI disorders, stunted growth, dermatitis, haematuria.	Deep intramuscular only. Cattle/buffaloes/horses: 5-10 ml thrice weekly. Sheep/goat/calves/goat: 1-2 ml thrice weekly.	Vial of 30 ml and 10 ml.
BIOVET Proteases, lactase, acid phosphatase & lipase enzyme, Organic nitrogen, Vital amino acids, Essential trace minerals BIOVET-YC Powder	Improves digestibility, milk yeild, milk fat contents, vitality to withstand disease.	For primary/secondary/non-specific anorexia: 10ml/head for 3 days or till symptoms subside. For suppressed milk production: 10 ml/head for 3 days followed by 5 ml for 12 days. As digestive tonic: 10 ml/head for 3 days followed by 5 ml for 12 days, give	Bottels of 30 ml, 90 ml and 500 ml Bolus : Pouch of 2 boli Biovet -YC-1 kg.

Preparation	Indication	Dosage/Route	Presentation
		gap of 15 days and again repeat it. Thus one course of 15 days in a month. One bolus alongwith each concentrate feeding. Poultry : Broilers : To increase b.wt. and to improve feed conversion ratio 2 ml/10 litre of drinking water from Ist day till slaughter. Layers : For hastening start of laying period, early attainment & maintenance of higher peak. Chicks : 2ml/10 litres drinking water continuously. Adults : 40ml/100 birds.	
BLOATOSIL Each 100 ml contains: Silica in Dimethicone suspension 1% w/v, Dill oil 0.5% Arachis oil 10% w/v	All kinds of bloat, tympany and frothy bloat. As an emergency drug in cases of serious bloat.	Oral: 100 ml of Bloatosil at a time by drenching or with the help of stomach tube, twice a day for cattle & buffaloes and 20 ml for sheep and goat. Intraruminal: 100ml of Bloatosil at a time by using canula or a long needle to be administered in rumen through paralumbar fossa. The dose for cattle is 100 ml and for sheep and goat is 20 ml.	100 ml.
Cal. BOROGLUCONATE Inj. Each 450 ml contains: Cal. borogluconate 25% w/v Equivalent calcium (as cal. gluconate) 1.854%, Boric acid 4.25% w/v	Acute & chronic hypocalcaemia, milk fever, lactation tetany, prevention & treatment of liver damage due to over dosage with magnesium salt & chlorinated hydrocarbons such as carbon tetrachloride or pesticides.	Slow I/V of S/C injection Cattle/buffalo: 250-300 ml/day as single dose therapy. In severe cases repeat treatment for successive 2 to 3 days. Sheep/goat: 25-50 ml slow intravenous injection.	450 ml.
CALDEE - 12 Each ml contains: Cal. levulinate 76.4 mg Equivalent to 10 mg ionic calcium Cholecalciferol, (Vit D$_3$) 5000 I.U. Cyanocobalamin (Vit B$_{12}$) 50 mcg.	For prevention & treatment of hypocalcaemia in cows and buffaloes particularly during pre & post-parturition period. As a tonic shot to improve the general health of animal in condition of debility & weakness.	Intramuscular injection only. Preparturition: Cattle, buffaloes: 10-15 ml thrice a week for 1-2 week. Post-parturition: cattle, buffaloes: 15-20 ml thrice a week for 2 weeks after calving. Bulls/dry cows/debilitated animals: 10ml thrice a week for 1-2 weeks. Sheep/goats/dogs: 1-3 ml thrice a week for 1-2 weeks.	Vial of 30 ml.

Preparation	Indication	Dosage/Route	Presentation
OKAZAN Drench contains: Oxyclozanide 3.4%. Bolus contains: Oxyclozanide 1 gm	Acute and chronic fascioliasis in cattle, buffalo, sheep and goat.	Cattle, buffalo: 10 mg per kg b.wt. Sheep, goat: 15mg per kg b.wt.	Suspension - 90 ml and 1 litre. Bolus: 5x4 bolus strip.
PELWIN 100 ml infusion contains: Pefloxacin 400 mg. Tablet contains: Pefloxacin 400mg	For the treatment of a wide variety of infections.	Dogs: 100 to 400 mg bid.	Infusion: 100 ml glass bottle. Tablet: strip of 4 tablets.
PREDNISOLONE Crystalline Suspension contains : 10 mg Prednisolone acetate per ml of solution.	Bovine ketosis, inflammatory condition, mastitis, metritis, allergies, bursitis, rheumatoid arthritis, conjuntivitis and in comatose conditions.	Cattle/horse : 10-20 ml IM Calves /pigs : 2.5-5ml IM Dogs/cats : 1-3 ml IM Large animal : 2.5 - 7.5 ml locally Small animal : 0.5-2 ml locally.	10 ml vial.
PROXYVET Each bolus contains: Acetaminophen 1500 mg Dextropropoxyphene HCl 97.5 mg	Antipyretic and analgesic.	Large animal: 2 to 4 boli twice daily for 3-4 days. Small animal: 1/2 to 1 bolus twice daily for 3-4 days (Not recommended for cat).	Pack of 2 bolis.
RINTOSE Inj. Each 100gm contains: Dextrose (Anhydrous) 20.00 gm. Sod. Chloride 00.60 gm. P. Chloride 0.04 mg. Cal.chloride 00.027 gm, Sod. lactate 00.312 gm	Debility, dehydration, ketosis, calf scour, hepatitis, diarrhoea vomiting haemorrhages, metritis, septicaemia, bacterial diseases (Johne's diseases, *E. coli*, salmonellosis etc), Viral disease (RP, FMD etc), Blood protozoan disease (Babesiosis theileriosis), Parasitic diseases (liver flukes), poisoning (Arsenic, pesticides and other chemicals).	Rintose is administered by I/V injection. Cattle/buff/ horse: 500-2000 ml/day for 3-4 days. Sheep/goat: 100- 200 ml/day for 2-3 days. Dog: 25-100 ml/day for 2-3 days. Calves: 100-500 ml/day for 2-3 days.	500 ml.

STREXIA
Each gm contains: Thiamine HCl 112 mg, Riboflavine 93 mg, Pyridoxine HCl 122 mg Niacinamide 350 mg, Calcium-D- pantothenate 326 mg, Cyanocobalamin (in gelatin) 256 mcg, Folic acid 10 mg, Sod. chloride 20 mg P. chloride 20 mg, Cal. lactate 28.57 gm, Magnesium sulphate 8.340 gm, Dextrose (anhydrous) 20 gm

As continuous nutritional supplement to chicks from day Ist to 10th day. Broilers fed with anticoccidials in electrolytes & vit B complex deficiency status. To tackle stress in birds due to Salmonellosis, coccidiosis, colibacillosis etc. Dehydration & starvation. Vaccination. Transportation. Extreme weather conditions. Deworming, Debeaking.

5gm strexia to be dissolved in below specified quantity (litre) of water.

	High stress, no feed intake	Partial stress	General supplement
Broilers:			
Day old to 4 weeks	4	8	12
4 wks-9wks	3	6	9
Layers:			
Day old to 8 wks.	5	10	15
8wks-20wks	3	6	9
Above 20 weeks	2	4	6

Sachet 100 gm.

Preparation	Indication	Dosage/Route	Presentation
SUPERCOX Contains: Sulphaquinoxiline 18.7% w/w Diaveridine 3.3% w/w,	For early & effective control of intestinal & caecal coccidiosis in poultry. Fowl cholera, fowl typhoid.	Dissolve one level spoonful of powder in 10 litre of drinking water or mix 100 gms powder in 50kg of feed. Give for 2-3 days. Afterwards give plain drinking water for next 2 days. Dissolve one level spoonful powder in 20 litres of drinking water. Give this water every day for next 2-3 days.	100 gms.
THIACAL Each 450ml contains: Calcium (as calcium gluconate)21% w/v, Boric acid 4.21% w/v, Magnesium hypophosphite 5% w/v Dextrose (anhydrous) 20% w/v (Proportion of boric acid to calcium is 2.26 to 1).	Milk fever due to hypocalcaemia, Hypomagnesemic tetany, Ketosis of ruminants, Hypophosphatemia, Neonatal hypoglycemia (Pigs).	S/C/ or I/V inj. Buff/cattle: 250-450 ml as a single dose. Repeat treatment in case of relapse. Calves: 25-75 ml.	450 ml.
TILOX Each 5 gm contains: Ampicillin (as Ampicillin sodium) 75 mg. Cloxacillin (as cloxacillin Sodium) 200 mg.	Mastitis.	One syringe per affected quarter; to be repeated every twelve hour.	7 gm. single dose disposable syringe.

TONORICIN Injectable Phosphorus	Phosphorus deficiency, drop in milk production, metabolic disorders, retarded growth, infertility.	Acute Chronic
		  condition condition
		Large animal: 5-10 or 2.5-5 ml
		       25 ml
		Small animal: 1-3 ml 1-2 ml
		To be given by I/V, I/M or S/c routes
			30 ml vial and 5 ml ampoule.

TRIQUIN Each vial contains: Quinapyramine sulphate 1.5 gm, Quinapyramine chloride 1.0 gm.	For treatment & prevention of trypanosomiasis in various sps. of animals viz. cattle, buffaloes, sheep, pig, dog, cat etc.	0.025ml of inj./kg; total dose not exceeding 15 ml. subcutaneously. Vial of 2.5 gm powder to be reconstituted with 15 ml sterile water for injection.	2.5 gm vial.
VETAMPIN Each vial contains: Ampicillin sodium equivalent to 1 gm of 2 gm or Ampicillin	Cattle & buffaloes: Calf scour, pneumonia enteritis & septicaemia due to solmonella infection, foul in the foot, *E. coli* mastitis, & retained placenta & pyelonephritis. Horses: Enteritis & septicaemia in new born & young foals, metritis, respiratory infections, particularly influenza & strangles. Sheep: Contagious foot root, mastitis, pneumonia & foot abscesses. Pigs: Enteritis,		

Preparation	Indication	Dosage/Route	Presentation
	pneumonia associated with *E. coli* infection, erysipelas, metritis.	It is administered by I/V of I/M route at dose rate of 2-7 mg/kg. In young animals & acute infections upper dose level is upto 25 mg/kg. Treatment is given twice a day for 2-3 days.	Vials of 1 gm & 2 gm.
	Dogs & cats: Secondary infections associated with dermatitis, enteritis, ear infections, leptospirosis pharyngitis, tonsilitis, post operative wounds, respiratory infections.		
WOKADINE Wokadine solution; ointment povidone-iodine 5% w/v with 0.5% w/v available active ingredient.	On skin & mucous membranes pre & post-operatively, lacerations, abrasions & burns, mastitis & metritis. As antiseptic in practice. Prophylaxis of mastitis. Dermatitis & other skin infection	For topical application use full strength wokadine. For intramammary use 10-20ml Wokadine. For intrauterine use 10-40 ml.	100 ml in glassbottle & 500 ml in polyethylene container. Tube: 30 gm.
WOKTRIN Dispersible powder Sulphadiazine 10% w/w, Trimethoprim 2% w/w	It is a broad spectrum anti-bacterial agent with activity against gram+ve and garm -ve organisms of poultry viz. *Salmonella* spp, *E. coli*, Clostridium spp, Streptococci spp. & drug of choice in Salmonellosis, W.B.D., fowl cholera, fowl typhoid, infectious coryza, colibacillosis, bumble foot & early chick mortality.	Poultry: for 100 birds, 4 levelled spoonfuls (approximately 20 gms) in 20 litres of water/day for 3 days. Higher doses upto 5 mg/litre water can be administered in acute attacks. Treatment can be extended upto 10 days if required.	100 gm.
WOKTRIN TAB Each tablet contains: Sulphadiazine 1000 mg Trimethoprim 200 mg.	Cattle & buffaloes: Bacterial scours, acute undifferentiated diarrhoea of calves, pneumonia, endometritis, retention of placenta, pyometra, repeat breeding. Sheep & goat: Joint ill, enterotoxemia, scour, black quarter, anthrax, uterine infectins. Horses: Pneumonia, joint ill, anthrax, strangles, enteritis, peritonitis, infections of urinogenital tract. Dogs & cats: Bronchitis, enteritis, pleurisy, secondary bacterial complications of canine distemper, urinary infections.	Oral (For all species): 30 mg/kg (1 tablet per 40 kg). Total dose of tablet should be administered in two divided doses. Intrauterine: Cows/buff/mares: 4-6 tabs/day for 3 days. Sows/ewes: 1-2 tablet/day for 3 days.	

Preparation	Indication	Dosage/Route	Presentation
WOLICYCLIN i. Each ml contains: Oxy-tetracyclin HCl 50mg ii. Each ml of Wolicyclin DS inj. contains Oxytetracyclin HCl 100 mg. iii. Each tab of Wolicyclin contains Oxytetracycline HCl 500 mg	Broad spectrum antibiotic active against large number of Garm+ve and Garm-ve organisms; sps of Streptococci, Staphylococci, anthracoids, pasturella, Brucella, Corynebacteria, Coliforms & Salmonella are sensitive. Ricketsiae are also affected, low activity against Pseudomonas, proteus & klebsiella species, numerous diseases responds to Wolicyclin: Mastitis due to *E. coli,* Streptococci, transit fever, white scour in calves, enteritis in pigs, strangles in horses, actinomycosis & actinobacillosis, infectious keratitis in cattle, otitis & secondary invaders in viral diseases of small animals.	Wolicyclin inj. Wolicyclin D.S. inj. may be administered at dose rate of 5-10 mg/kg b.wt. in all animals by S/C, I/M, I/V route. Oral dosage for Wolicyclin tablets is as follows: Calves/foals/sheep/goat & pig: 10-20 mg/kg. Dog & cat: 27 mg/kg. Intrauterine dosage for Wolicycline tablets is: Cows, she buffaloes & mares: 1-2 tab. Ewes, sows & bitches: 1/2-1 tablets.	Inj. Wolicyclin 30 ml vial; inj. Wolicyclin DS – 30 ml vial; Tab. Wolicyclin 4 x 4S.

Medical Products

ANTIBIOTICS

AMIKACIN

Aminoglycoside antibiotic, bactericidal in action. Effective to treat infections caused by gram negative and gram positive organisms such as septicaemia, burns, UTI etc.

Dosage (Dog)	:	15mg/kg b.w. daily in 2 divided doses
Amicin (Biochem)	:	Amikacin sulph. 100mg/500mg per 2 ml, inj.
Ivimicin (FDC)	:	Amikacin sulph. 50mg/125mg /250mg per 2 ml, inj.
Mikacin (Aristo)	:	Amikacin Sulph. 100mg/250mg/500mg per 2 ml, inj.

AMOXYCILLIN

Semi-synthetic penicillin, effective in respiratory, urinary and genital tract, skin and soft tissue infections.

Dosage (Dog)	:	11mg/kg b.wt. (orally) 8 hourly.
Amoxylin (Biddle Sawyer)	:	Amoxycillin 250mg/500mg, caps.
	:	Also Amoxylin dry syrup 125 mg/5 ml, 45 ml.
Danemox Forte (Sol)	:	Amoxycillin trihydrate 250mg, tabs.
Lamoxy (Lyka)		Amoxycillin trihydrate 250mg/500mg, tabs.
		Also Lamoxy dry syrup 125/250mg per 5ml, 30 ml, 60 ml.
Mox (Gufic)	:	Amoxycillin 250 mg/ 500 mg, caps. Also Mox dry syrup 125 mg/250 mg per 5 ml. 30 ml, 60 ml.
Moxilium (Biochem)	:	Amoxycillin trihydrate 250mg/500mg, caps.
		Also Moxilium dry syrup 125mg per 5 ml.
Moxydil (Duphar-Interfran)	:	Amoxycillin trihydrate 250mg/500mg, caps.
		Also Moxydil syrup 125mg/250mg per 5 ml.
		Moxydil injection(I/M of I/V)250mg/500mg per 5 ml vial.
Novamox (Cipla)	:	Amoxycillin 250mg/500mg, caps.
	:	Also Novamox dry syrup 125mg per 5 ml.
Symoxyl (Sarabhai)	:	Amoxycillin trihydrate 250mg/500mg, tabs.
	:	Also Symoxyl syrup 125mg per 5 ml syrup.
Warcilin (Parke-Davis)	:	Amoxycillin trihydrate 250mg/500mg, caps.
		Also Warcilin dry syrup 125mg/5ml syrup.
Zamox (Pfimex)	:	Amoxycillin trihydrate 250mg/500mg, caps.

AMOXYCILLIN AND CLOXACILLIN

To treat skin and soft tissue infection, urnary tract infections etc.

Dosage	:	5-10 mg/kg b.wt., orally, 8h.
Flemiclox (Mejda)	:	Amoxy. 250mg, Clox. 250mg, caps.
Lamklox (Lyka)	:	Amoxy. 250mg, Clox. 250mg, caps.
Moclox (Kopran)	:	Amoxy. 250mg, Clox. 250mg, caps.

| Novaclox (Cipla) | : | Amoxy. 250mg, Clox. 250mg, caps. |
| Suprimox (Gufic) | : | Amoxy. 250mg, Clox. 250mg, caps. |

AMPICILLIN

Semi-synthetic broad spectrum penicillin. Effective in respiratory, genitourinary tract, GIT, skin, soft tissue and general systemic infections.

Dosage	:	2-7mg/kg b.wt. (Parenteral); 4-10mg/kg b.w. (oral).
Amp-kid (Sol)	:	Ampicillin trihydrate 125mg, tabs.
		Also Amp-kid Forte Ampicillin 250mg, tabs.
Ampidil (Duphar-Interfran)	:	Ampicillin trihydrate 250mg, caps.
	:	Also Ampidil Syrup Ampicillin 125mg/5ml, 40 ml.
		Ampidil inj. Ampicillin sod. 250mg/500mg per vial, inj.
Ampisyn (Cipla)	:	Ampicillin 500mg per vial, inj.
		Also Ampisyn cap 250mg/500mg caps. Ampisyn Syrup: 125mg/ 5 ml Syrup.
Aristocillin(Aristo)	:	Ampicillin trihydrate 250mg/500mg caps.
		Also Aristocillin dry syrup 125mg/250mg per 5 ml
		Aristocillin inj 100mg/200mg/500mg per vial.
Bacipen (Alembic)	:	Ampicillin trihydrate 250mg/500mg, caps.
		Also Bacipen dry syrup 125mg per 5 ml, 40 ml. Bacipen inj: 250mg/500mg per vial
Biocilin (Biochem)	:	Ampicillin trihydrate 250mg/500mg caps.
		Also Biocilin dry syrup 125mg/250mg per 5 ml, 40 ml.
		Biocilin inj 100mg/250mg/500mg/1g per vial.
Broadicilin (Alkem)	:	Ampicillin trihydrate 250mg/500mg, caps.
		Also Broadicilin dry syrup 125/250mg per 5 ml, 40 ml.
		Broadicilin drops 100mg/10 ml, 10 ml.
		Broadicilin inj 100mg/250mg/500mg per vial.
Campicillin (Cadila)	:	Ampiciliin 250mg/500mg, caps.
		Also Campicillin dry syrup 125mg per 5 ml, 40 ml, 60 ml.
		Campicillin inj 100mg/250mg/500mg/1.0g per vial.
Lupilin (Lupin)	:	Ampicillin trihydrate 250mg/500mg, caps.
		Also Lupilin inj 500mg per vial.
		Lupilin dry syrup 125mg per 40 ml.
Roscillin (Ranbaxy)	:	Ampicillin trihydrate 250mg/500mg, caps.
		Also Roscillin inj 250mg/500mg per vial.

AMPICILLIN AND CLOXACILLIN

Respiratory tract infections, skin and soft tissue infections, surgical and orthopaedic infections, genital infections.

Amclox (Walter Bushnell)	:	Amp. 250mg, Clox. 250mg caps.
		Also Amclox inj. Amp. 250mg, Clox. 250mg per vial inj.
Ampilox (Biochem)	:	Amp 250mg, Clox. 250mg, caps.
		Also Ampilox inj Amp. 125mg/250mg/500mg, Clox 125mg/250mg/500mg
		Ampilox Dry syrup Amp. 125mg, Clox. 125mg per 5 ml, 40 ml.
Ampoxin (Unichem)	:	Amp. 125mg/250mg, Clox. 125mg/250mg, caps.
		Also Ampoxin inj 250mg/500mg/ 1 gm injections.
Baxin (Lyka)	:	Amp. 250mg, Clox. 250mg, caps.
		Also Baxin dry syrup 62.5mg/125mg each per 5 ml.
		Baxin inj 125mg/250mg/500mg each per vial.
Broadiclox (Alkem)	:	Amp. 125mg/250mg, clox 125mg/250mg, caps.
		Also Broadiclox inj 125mg/250mg each per vial.
Duoclox (FDC)	:	Amp. 250mg, Clox. 250mg, caps.
		Also Duoclox inj 125mg each per vial.
Megapen (Aristo)	:	Amp. 125mg/250mg, Clox. 125mg/250mg, caps.
	:	Also Megapen inj 125mg/250mg/500mg each per vial, inj.
Vivoclox (Pfimex)	:	Amp. 250mg, Clox. 250mg, caps.

CARBENICILLIN

Broad spectrum penicillin, poorly absorbed in GIT, effective for the treatment of septicaemia, urinary and respiratory tract infections and post-operative infections.

Dosage	:	50-400mg/kg b.wt. I/M, I/V in divided doses.
Biopence (Biochem)	:	Carbenicillin disodium 1 gm/5gm per vial, inj.
Carbelin (Lyka)	:	Carbenicillin sod 1 gm vial, inj.

CEPHALOSPORINS

Semi-synthetic antibacterial agents related to penicillin. Broad spectrum in activity, bactericidal in action, inhibits cell wall synthesis of the bacteria.

(i) *Cephalexin :* Well absorbed orally, effective to treat upper and lower respiratory tract infections, genitourinary tract infections, otitis media, bones, joints, skin and soft tissue infections.

Dosage (Dog)	:	Dogs : 125mg-500mg Qid or
		25-50mg/kg/day in 3 or 4 divided doses.
Alcephin (Alembic)	:	Caps 250mg/500mg; Dry syrup 125mg/5 ml, 40 ml.
Betaspore (Aristo)	:	Caps 250mg/500mg; Dry syrup 125mg/5 ml, 40 ml.
Blucef (Blue Cross)	:	Tabs 125mg/250mg/500mg.
Ceff (Lupin)	:	Tabs 125mg/250mg/500mg; Dry syrup 125mg/250mg per 5 ml, 40 ml.
Cephacillin (Biddle Sawyer)	:	Tabs 250mg.
Cephadil (Duphar-Interfran)	:	Caps 250mg/500mg.
Cephalkem (Alkem)	:	Caps 250mg/500 mg; Dry syrup 125mg per 5 ml, 40 ml.
Cephaxin (Biochem)	:	Caps 250mg/500 mg; Dry syrup 125mg per 5 ml, 40 ml.

Nufex (Searle)	:	Caps 250mg/500mg.
Oriphex (Alidac)	:	Caps 250mg/500mg; Dry syrup 125mg per 5 ml, 40 ml.
Phexin (Glaxo Pharma)	:	Caps 250mg/500mg; Dry syrup 250mg per 5 ml, 30 ml.
Ralcef (Rallis)	:	Caps 250mg/500mg.
Sepexin (Lyka)	:	Caps 250mg/500mg, Dry syrup 125mg per 5 ml, 40 ml.
Sporidex (Stancare)	:	Tabs 250mg; Dry syrup 250mg per 5 ml, 40 ml.
Ultrasporin (Stangen)	:	Tabs 125mg/250mg/500mg.

(ii) *Cefazolin* : Effective in respiratory and genitourinary tract infection, skin, soft tissue, joints, bones infections, septicaemia etc.

Dosage (Dogs)	:	125-500mg every 6-12 hourly I/M, 1/V.
Alcizon (Alembic)	:	500mg/1.0 gm per vial, injection.
Azolin (Biochem)	:	500mg/1.0 gm per vial, injection.
Cefamezin (Rallis)	:	250mg/500mg/1.0 gm per vial, injection.
Cezolin (Lupin)	:	500mg/1.0gm per vial, injection.
Lyzolin (Lyka)	:	500mg/1.0gm per vial, injection.
Orizolin (Alidac)	:	125mg/500mg/1.0 gm per vial, injection.
Reflin (Ranbaxy)	:	250mg/500mg/1.0 gm per vial, injection.

(iii) *Cefadroxil* : Effective in infections of respiratory tract caused by beta haemolytic streptococci, infections of skin, soft tissue, joints and bones.

Dosage (Dog)	:	125mg-500mg bid.
Bid (Kopran)	:	500 mg caps; Dry syrup 125mg per 5 ml, 40 ml.
Cefadur (Protec)	:	Caps 500 mg; Suspension 250 mg per 5 ml, 30 ml.

(iv) *Cefotaxime* : Bacteraemia, septicaemia, infections of respiratory tract and genitourinary tract, intra-abdominal infections. Infections of skin, soft tissue, joints and bones.

Dosage (Dog)	:	25-50 mg/kg b.wt./day in divided doses at 6-12 hour interval (I/M or I/V).
Biotex (Biochem)	:	250mg/1.0 gm per vial, injection.
Claforan (Roussel)	:	250mg/1.0 gm per vial, injection.
Omnatax (Hoechst)	:	250mg/1.0 gm per vial, injection.
Taxim (Alkem)	:	250mg/1.0 gm per vial, injection.

(v) *Ceftriaxone*: Bacterial septicaemia, skin, soft tissue, joints and bone infections. Infections of respiratory tract and urinary tract.

Dosage (Dog)	:	25-50 mg/kg b.wt./day in divided dose Q12h I/M or I/V.
Cefaxone-I/M/ I/V (Lupin)	:	250mg/500mg/1.0 gm per vial (with Lignocaine HCl 1% in Cefaxone I/M injection).
Monocef I/V (Aristo)	:	250mg/1.0gm per vial, injection.

(iv) *Ceftizoxime*: Infections of respiratory tract, urinary tract, skin and soft tissue, bone and joint infection, septicaemia.

| Dog | : | 25-50/kg b.wt./day 6-8 hourly I/M or I/V. |

Cefizox (Burroughs Wellcome)	:	500mg/1.0 gm per vial, injection.
Epocelin (Rallis)	:	1.0 gm per vial, injection.

(vii) *Cefadroxyl* : RTI, UTI, skin, soft tissue, bone and joint infections.

Dosage (Dog)	:	20-30 mg/kg b.wt./day in 2 divided doses.
Kefloxin (Stancare)	:	Caps 500 mg; Pulv for susp. 125 mg/5ml, 40 ml.
Lydroxil (Lyka)	:	Caps 500 mg/1.0 gm; syrup 125mg/250mg/5 ml, 40 ml.
Odoxil (Lupin)	:	Tabs 500mg/1.0 gm, susp. 125mg/5 ml. 40 ml.

(viii)*Cephaloridine* : Treatment of RTI, UTI, soft tissue, joints and bones, prophylaxis in surgery and obstetrics.

Dosage (Dog)	:	15-30 mg/kg b.wt./day in 2-3 divided doses I/M.
Cephaxin Inj (Biochem)	:	500mg/1.0 gm per vial, injection.
Ceporan (Glaxo Pharma)	:	500 mg/1.0 gm per vial injection.

(ix) *Cefuroxime:* UTI, RTI, soft tissue, joints, bone infections, prophylaxis against infection in surgical procedure.

(Dog)	:	25-50 mg/kg b.wt./day in 2-3 divided doses, I/M or I/V.
Cefozen (Alidac)	:	250 mg/750 mg per vial, injections.
Ceftum (Glaxo-Allenburys)	:	Tabs 125mg/250mg.
Supacef (Glaxo-Allenburys)	:	750mg per vial, injections Also cap/tabs 125 mg/ 250 mg.

CHLORAMPHENICOL

Broad spectrum synthetic antibiotic, highly bacteriostatic and can be bactericidal. Readily absorbed from GIT. Can be administered orally and parenterally in infections of G.U., respiratory, GIT etc.

Dosage	:	Parenteral :	Large animal : 2-4 mg/kg b.wt. I/M bid.
			Small animal : 4-10mg/kg b.wt. I/M bid.
		Oral :	Dog : 165 mg/kg b.wt. bid or tid.
Chloromycetin succinate Inj (Parke-Davis)	:	250mg/1 gm inj S/C, I/M.	
Chloromycetin Palmitate Liquid (Parke-Davis)	:	125 mg per 4 ml, 60 ml.	
Enteromycetin (Dey's)	:	250 mg, caps.	
		Also injections (I/M) 250mg with Lignocaine 20 mg/2 ml.	
		'C' injections (I/M) 125 mg with Lignocaine 10 mg/ml.	
		Syrup: 125 mg/4 ml, 40 ml, 250ml.	
Paraxin (Boehringer-Mannheim)	:	250mg/500mg, caps.	
		Also Paraxin dry syrup 125 mg per 5 ml, 60 ml.	
Ranphenicol Inj (Ranbaxy)	:	Chlor. Sod. succinate 1 gm per vial.	
	:	Also suspension 125 mg per 5 ml, 30 ml, 60 ml.	

CLOXACILLIN

Semi-synthetic penicillin. Effective against surgical infections, skin and soft tissue infections, mastitis, burns, pneumonia etc.

Dose	:	4-10 mg/kg b.wt. Q 6h.
Bioclox (Biochem)	:	Cloxacillin Sod. 250mg/500mg, caps.

		Also Bioclox injection 250mg/500mg per vial.
Klox (Lyka)	:	Cloxacillin Sod. 250mg/500mg, caps.
		Also Klox dry syrup 125 mg per 3 gm dry syrup., 24 gm.
		Klox injection 250mg/500mg per vial.
Winpactam (Prem Pharma)	:	Cloxacillin Sod. 500mg per vial inj.

DEMECLOCYCLINE

Broad spectrum antibiotics. Effective to treat all infections by susceptible organisms.

Dose (Dog)	:	6-12 mg/kg b.wt./day in 2-4 divided doses.
Ledermycin (Lederle)	:	Demeclocycline HCl 150 mg/300 mg, caps.

DOXYCYCLINE

Broad spectrum antibiotic. Effective for the treatment of respiratory tract infection, UTI, genital tract infections etc.

Dose (Dogs)	:	50-100 mg on first day followed by half of the first dose on subsequent days.
Biodoxi (Biochem)	:	Doxycycline 100 mg, caps.
Doxy-1 (USV&P)	:	Doxycycline hyclate 100 mg, caps.
Lydox (Lyka)	:	Doxycycline HCl 100 mg, caps.
Martidox (Martel Hammer)	:	Doxycycline HCl 100 mg/200 mg caps.

ERYTHROMYCIN

Bacteriostatic or bactericidal depends on doses, well absorbed from GIT. Effective against gram positive organisms, to treat acute bacterial pharyngitis, sinusitis, otitis, bronchitis, pneumonia, amoebic dysentery etc.

Doses (Dog)		4-8 mg/kg b.wt. 12 hourly.
Althrocin (Alembic)		Erythromycin 250mg/500mg, caps.
		Also Althrocin liquid 125mg/5ml. 60 ml.
E-mycin (Themis Pharma)	:	Eryth. estolate 100 mg/250mg. tab.
		Also E-mycin susp. 125 mg/5ml, 30 ml, 60 ml.
		E-mycin dry syrup 100 mg/5 ml. 30 ml, 60 ml.
Emthrocin (Rhone-Poulenc)	:	Eryth. stearate 250 mg/500mg. tab.
		Also Emthrocin susp. 125mg/5ml. 60 ml
Eroate-B (Lupin)	:	Eryth. estolate 250mg/500mg with bromhexine 8 mg, tab.
Eroate (Lupin)	:	Eryth. estolate 250mg/500mg. tabs.
Erythrocin-FT (Abbott)	:	Eryth. stearate 100 mg/250mg/500mg, tabs.
		Also Erythrocin susp. 100 mg/5ml, 60 ml.

GENTAMICIN

Broad spectrum antibiotics. Effective for the treatment of septicaemia, infection of genitourinary tract, respiratory system. GIT, skin and soft tissue infections.

Dose (Dog)	:	2-4 mg/kg b.wt. bid I/M, I/V.
Garamycin (Fulford)	:	Genta. sulph. 40 mg/10 mg per ml, inj, 2 ml vial.

Gentacin-A (Prem Pharma)	:	Gentamicin sulph 60 mg per 1.5 ml inj. 1.5 ml ampoule.
Gentacin-P (Prem Pharma)	:	Gentamicin sulph 40 mg per ml, 60 mg per 1.5 ml inj 2 ml vial and 1.5 ml ampoule.
Gentaril (Alkem)	:	Gentamicin sulph. 80 mg per vial, inj, 2 ml vial.
Genticyn Inj (Nicholas-Piramal)	:	Gentamicin sulph. 40 mg (40,000 IU) per ml, inj, 1.5 ml ampoule.
Merigenta Inj (Mercury)	:	Gentamicin sulph. 10 mg/40 mg per ml, inj, 2 ml vial, 2.5 ml ampoules.

KANAMYCIN

Broad spectrum antibiotic, poorly absorbed in GIT, bactericidal in action, effective in the treatment of infections of urogenital, respiratory, GIT, soft tissues infections, septicaemia etc.

Dose (Dog)	:	5-7 mg/kg b.wt. bid I/M.
Kancin (Alembic)	:	Kanamycin acid sulph. 0.5gm/1.0gm per vial inj.
Kansulf (Biochem)	:	Kanamycin 0.5 gm/1.0 gm per vial, inj.

PENICILLIN

It is a bactericidal drug and exert their action by inhibiting synthesis of bacterial cell wall, effective mainly against gram positive bacteria.

Dosage (Dogs) : 8,000-20,000 IU/kg b.wt. parenterally.

Benzathine Penicillin (slowly absorbed from the site and produces longer duration of action) 12,000 IU/kg b.wt. I/M

Phenoxy methyl penicillin/Penicillin-V/Potassium phenoxyethyl penicillin-well absorbed, orally, 4-8 mg/kg tid.

Depen Tabs (Deys)	:	Penicillin-V Potassium 130 mg, tabs.
	:	Also Depen granules. Each 3.25 gm Contains Pen - V. Pot 130 mg.
Depen-C	:	Pen -V Pot. 65 mg, tabs.
Diapen Inj (Pfizer)	:	Benzathine Penicillin-G 600,000 IU per vial. inj. Also Diapen-F Benzathine peni. G-6 lacs units, Sod. peni. G 3 lacs, Procaine peni. G 3 lacs units per vial. inj.
Fenocin Tabs (Pfizer)	:	Pot. phenoxy methyl penicillin 65 mg, tabs Also Fenocin Forte : Pot. phenoxy methyl penicillin 130mg, tabs
Longacillin Inj (Hindustan Antibiotics)	:	Benzathine-penicillin-G 6 lacs/12 lacs/ 24 lacs/48 lacs units per vial. inj.
Pencom Inj (Alembic)	:	Benzathine penicillin-G 6 lacs units per vial. inj.
Penidure (John-Wyeth)	:	Benzathine penicillin-G 6 lacs/12 lacs/ 24 lakhs-units per vial inj
Pentids Tabs (Sarabhai)	:	Penicillin-G Pot. 2 lacs/4 lacs/ 8 lacs units per tab.
Sopen Inj (MSD)	:	Penicillin G sod. 5 lacs/10 lacs units per vial inj.
Wyopen Vee Tab (John-Wyeth)	:	Pot. phenoxy methyl penicillin 130 mg per tab.

POLYMIXIN-B

Narrow spectrum antibiotics, more effective against gram negative organisms, not absorbed from GIT. Effective to treat bacteriamia and superficial eye infections.

| Dose | : | 2.2 mg (10,000 units)/kg b.wt./day I/M in divided doses. |
| Aerosporin (Burroughs Wellcome) | : | Polymyxin-B sulph. 500,000 units per vial. inj. |

ROXITHROMYCIN

Effective against urinary, respiratory tract infections, skin and soft tissue infections, genital infections etc.

Dose	:	2.5-5 mg/kg b.wt. bid for 7-10 days.
Roxid (Alembic)	:	Roxithromycin 150 mg, tabs.
Roxitem (Kopran)	:	Roxithromycin 150 mg, tabs.

STREPTOMYCIN

Aminoglycoside antibiotics, effective against gram negative organisms.

Dosage	:	10 mg/kg b.wt. I/M
Streptonex Inj (Pfizer)	:	Strept. sulph. 1 gm per vial.
Sugacin Inj (Hindustan Antibiotics)	:	Strept sulph. 0.75 gm/1gm per vial.

TETRACYCLINES

A group of semi-synthetic antibiotics with broad spectrum activity also effective against certain protozoa.

Dosage	:	4.4-11 mg/kg b.wt. I/M or I/V
		20-40 mg./kg b.wt. per day orally in 2-3 divided doses.
Hostacycline (Hoechst)	:	Tetracycline HCl 250 mg/500mg, caps.
Linemett (Mercury)	:	Tetracycline HCl 333 mg/500mg, tabs.
Resteclin (Sarabhai)	:	Tetracycline HCl 250 mg/500, tabs.
Terramycin (Pfizer)	:	Oxytetracycline HCl 250 mg/500 mg, caps.
		Also Terramycin SF caps. Oxytet. 250mg, Vit C 37.5 mg, Vit B_1 2.5 mg, Vit B_2 2.5 mg, Niacinamide 25 mg, Cal. pantothenate 5 mg, Vit B_6 0.5 mg, Folic acid 0.375 mg, Vit B_{12} 3 mcg, caps.
		Terramycin inj. Oxyt 50 mg, Lidocain 2.5% per ml, inj. (I/M).

QUINOLONE-ANTIBACTERIAL PREPARATIONS

Quinolone drugs block DNA synthesis of bacteria and are more effective against gram negative organisms.

i) *Ciprofloxacin:* For the treatment of respiratory and urinary tract infections, GIT, skin and soft tissue, bones and joint infections, septicaemia etc.

Dosage (Dogs)	:	125-500 mg orally bid or 50-200 mg bid as I/V infusion.
Abect (Sarabhai)	:	250 mg/500mg, tabs.
Alcipro (Alkem)	:	250mg/500mg, tabs; 2mg/ml, infusion. 100 ml.
Bekaycin (Boehringer-Mannheim)	:	250mg/500mg, tabs.
C-Flox (Prem Pharma)	:	200 mg per 100 ml, infusion 100, ml.
Cebran (Blue Cross)	:	125mg/250mg/500mg, tabs.
Cefloxan (FDC)	:	250mg/500mg/750mg, tabs.
Cifran (Ranbaxy)	:	250mg/500mg/750mg tabs, 2mg/ml infusion 50ml, 100 ml.
Ciplox (Cipla)	:	250mg/500mg/750mg, tabs, 200mg/100ml infusion, 100 ml.
Ciprobid (Cadila)	:	250mg/500mg/750mg tabs; 2mg/ml infusion 50 ml, 100 ml.
Ciprodac (Alidac)	:	250mg/500mg tabs, 2mg/ml infusion, 100 ml.
Ciprolet (Stangen)	:	250mg/500mg tabs; 2 mg/ml infusion, 100 ml.
Ciproquin (Kopran)	:	250mg/500mg, tabs.
Ciprosol (Sol)	:	250mg/500mg tabs; 200 mg/100 ml infusion, 100 ml.
Ciprova (Lupin)	:	250mg/500mg tabs; 2 mg/ml, infusion, 100 ml.
Ciprowin (Alembic)	:	250mg/500mg tabs; 200 mg/100 ml infusion, 100 ml.
Ificipro (Unique)	:	200 mg per 100 ml, infusion. 100 ml.
Oracip (Mercury)	:	500mg, tabs.
Panflox (Pfimex)	:	250mg/500mg, tabs.

ii) *Norfloxacin:* For the treatment of acute and chronic urinary tract infections, GIT infections, genital diseases and other infections caused by susceptible strains of micro organisms (Dogs: 100-400 mg bid)

Alflox (Alkem)	:	400/800 mg, tabs.
Biofloxin (Biochem)	:	400 mg, tabs.
Norbactin (Ranbaxy)	:	200 mg/400 mg/800 mg, tabs.
Norbid (Alembic)	:	400 mg/800 mg, tabs.
Norflox (Cipla)	:	100mg/200mg/400mg/800mg, tabs.
Norilet (Stangen)	:	400 mg/800 mg, tabs.
Norspan (Blue Cross)	:	400 mg, tabs.
Quinolox (Kopran)	:	400 mg, tabs.
Uriben (CFL)	:	400 mg tabs.
Uroflox (Torrent)	:	400 mg/800 mg, tabs.
Utibid (Lupin)	:	400 mg/800 mg, tabs

iii) *Pefloxacin:* For the treatment of respiratory, GI, urinary tract, skin and soft tissue, bones and joint infections. Surgical infections, bacteraemia. septicaemia, gynaecological and intra-abdominal infections.

Dosage (Dog)	:	100-400 mg bid.
Pefbid (Alembic)	:	400 mg, tabs.
Peflox (Wockhardt)	:	400 mg, tabs; 400 mg per 5 ml, injection (I/V), 5 ml ampoule.
Piflasyn (Rhone-Poulenc)	:	400 mg, tabs; 400 mg/5ml, injection for infusion, 5 ml ampoule.
Proflox (Protec)	:	400 mg, tabs.
Qucin (Aristo)	:	400 mg, tabs.

(iv) *Ofloxacin:* For the treatment of genitourinary, G.I., skin and soft tissue infections, peritonitis etc.

Dosage (Dogs)	:	100-400 mg daily in 2 divided doses.
Tarivid (Hoechst)	:	200 mg, tabs.
Zancocin (Stancare)	:	100 mg, 200 mg, tabs.

TRIMETHOPRIM AND SULPHONAMIDES

(i) *Trimethoprim:* For the treatment of urinary and respiratory tract infections due to susceptible organisms.

Dosage (Dogs)	:	6-8 mg/kg b.wt. daily in 2 divided doses.
Baktar (FDC)	:	200 mg, tabs.
Tuliprim (Biddle Sawyer)	:	100 mg, tabs.

(ii) *Sulphadiazine and Trimethoprim:* For the treatment of urinary tract and respiratory tract infections, genital disease, otitis, skin infections, septicaemia.

Dosage (Dogs)	:	100-400 mg bid.
Antrima (Rhone-Poulenc)	:	Sulph. 400 mg, trim. 80mg, tabs.
Aubril (Hindustan Ciba-Geigy)	:	Sulph. 410mg, trim. 90 mg, tabs.
	:	Also Aubril Suspension Trim 45mg, Sulph 205 mg per ml, 50 ml.

(iii) *Sulfamethoxazole and Trimethoprim:* Infections of respiratory, urinary, GIT, genital system etc.

Bactrim (Roche)	:	Trim 20 mg/80mg/160 mg, Sulf 100 mg/400 mg/800 mg, respectively, tabs.
		Also Bactrim Susp. Trim 40 mg, Sulf 200 mg per 5 ml. 50 ml.
Ciplin (Cipla)	:	Trim 80mg/160mg, Sulf 400 mg/800 mg, respectively, tabs.
		Also Suspension Trim 40 mg, sulf 200 mg per 5 ml. 50 ml. Injection (I/M) : Trim 160 mg, Sulf 800 mg per 3 ml.
Oriprim (Cadila)	:	Trim 160 mg, Sulf 800 mg, tabs
		Suspension : Trim 40 mg, Sulf 200 mg per 5 ml. 50 ml.
		Injection (I/M). Trim 160 mg, Sulf 800 mg per 3 ml.
		Injection (I/V) : Trim 80 mg, Sulf 400 mg per 5 ml.
Otrim (Biochem)	:	Trim 80 mg/160mg, Sulf 400 mg/800 mg, respectively, tabs; Suspension. Trim 40 mg, Sulf 200 mg. 50 ml.
Septran(Burroughs Wellcome)	:	Tri 20mg/80mg, Sulf 100 mg/400 mg, respectively, tabs; Suspension Trim 40 mg, Sulf. 200 mg per 5 ml 50 ml.
Servoprim (Hoechst)	:	Trim 80 mg, Sulf. 400 mg, tabs.

Medical Products

(iv) *Sulfadimidine And Trimethoprim:* Penestrin (Lederle): Trim 40 mg, Sulf. 200 mg per 5 ml, suspension, 50 ml.

ANTIFUNGALS

Fungicide (Torrent)	:	Ketoconazole 200 mg tabs. Candidiasis, ringworm and other systemic fungal infections. Dog : 50-200 mg sid.
Fungizone (Sarabhai)	:	Amphotericin-B 50 mg per vial, inj (I/V). Fungal infections.
Grisactin Forte (CFL)	:	Griseofulvin 250 mg, tabs. Dermatophyte infections of skin. Dog 10 mg/kg b.w. daily in divided doses.
Grisovin-FP (Glaxo Pharma)	:	Griseofulvin 125 mg, tabs.
Ketozole (Gufic)	:	Ketoconazole 200 mg, tabs.
Mycostatin (Sarabhai)	:	Nystatin 500,000 IU tabs. Prevention and treatment of infections by *Candida albicans.*
Nizral (Ethnor)	:	Ketoconazole 200 mg, tabs.
Walavin - FP (Wallace)	:	Griseofulvin 125 mg, tabs.

ANTHELMINTICS

Albendazole: Single or mixed intestinal parasites (roundworm, hookworm, whipworm etc). (Dogs: 10-25 mg/kg b.wt. daily for 3 days).

Albezole (Khandelwal)	:	400 mg, tabs.
Alzad (Tata Pharma)	:	400 mg, tabs; Susp. 200 mg/5ml. 10 ml.
Bendex (Protec)	:	400 mg, tabs; 200 mg/5 ml suspension. 10 ml.
Neworm (Alkem)	:	400 mg, tabs; 200 mg/5 ml suspension. 10 ml.
Nubend (Kopran)	:	400 mg, tabs; 200 mg/5 ml suspension. 10 ml.
Zentel (Eskayef)	:	400 mg, tabs; 200 mg/5 ml suspension. 10 ml.

Mebendazole: Roundworm, hookworm, whipworm, tapeworm, mixed infestation etc. (Dogs: 5 mg/kg b.wt. daily for 3 days).

Mebazole (Torrent)	:	100 mg tabs.
Mebex (Cipla)	:	100 mg tabs; Suspension 100 mg per 5 ml. 30 ml.
Mendazole (Biddle Sawyer)	:	100 mg tabs.
Wormin (Cadila)	:	100 mg tabs.

Pyrantel Pamoate: Single or mixed infestation of roundworm, hookworm etc. (Dogs 10 mg/kg b.wt.; for hookworm 20 mg/kg b.wt. x 2 days).

Combantrin (Pfizer)	:	200 mg, tabs; Susp. 25 mg per ml. 8 ml.
Expent (Tata Pharma)	:	250 mg, tabs; Susp. 250 mg per ml. 5 ml.
Pyrmoate (Franco-Indian)	:	250 mg, tabs; Susp. 250 mg per 5 ml. 10 ml.

Levamisol : Roundworm, hookworm and mixed infestation (Dog: 7.5 mg per kg b.wt.)

Dewormis (Biddle Sawyer)	:	50 mg/150 mg, tabs.
Ketrax (ICI)	:	50 mg/150 mg, tabs.
Vermisol (Khendelwal)	:	50 mg/150mg, tabs; Syrup: 50 mg per 5 ml. 10 ml.

Niclosamide: Tapeworm infestation (100 gm per kg b.wt.).
Niclosan (Biddle-Sawyer): 500 mg, tabs.

Diethyl carbamazine Citrate: Treatment and prophylaxis of heartworm (filariasis), Esosinophilia, Toxocariasis. (Toxocariasis 55 - 110 mg/kg b.wt. Filariasis; 22-44 mg/kg b.wt. tid for 21-35 days).

Banocide (Burroughs Wellcome)	:	100 mg/500mg, tabs; syrup 50 mg/120 mg per 5 ml. 60 ml, 115 ml.
Carbamyl (Kopran)	:	Diethyl carb. 100 mg, Chlorpheniramine maleate 2.5 mg per ml, syrup. 100 ml.
		Also Diethyl carb. 150 mg, C.P.M. 2.5 mg, tabs.
Hetrazan (Lederle)	:	50 mg/100mg, tabs; syrup 120 mg per 5 ml. 114 ml.

PREPARATIONS FOR DIGESTIVE SYSTEM

ANTACIDS

Aciloc (Cadila)	:	Ranitidine HCl 150 mg/ 300 mg, tabs. Gastritis, gastric and duodenal ulcer. (Dogs: 100-200 mg bid).
	:	Also Aciloc injection Ranitidine 50 mg/2 ml.
Acipep (Kopran)	:	Famotidine 20 mg/40-mg tabs. Dyspepsia, severe gastritis, gastric and duodenal ulcer. (Dogs: 10-20 mg bid.)
Acredin (Sarabhai)	:	Famotidine 20 mg/40 mg, tabs.
Alucinol (Franco-Indian)	:	Dried alum hydroxy gel 300 mg, Mag. hydrox. 300 mg, activated methyl polysiloxane 25 mg, tabs. Hyperaciditiy, acid indigestion, dyspepsia. (Dogs: 1 tab bid.)
		Also Alucinol Suspension. 170 ml (50 mg/10ml).
Digene Gel (Boots)	:	Methyl polysiloxane 25 mg, Mag : hydrox. 185mg, Dried alum hydrox. gel 830 mg, Sod. carboxy-methyl cellulose 100 mg per 10 ml, Suspension. Gastritis, hyperacidity etc (Dogs: 5-10 ml bid) 200 ml.
Dioval Forte Gel (Wallace)	:	Dried alum hydrox. gel 300mg, Mag. hydroxy. 250mg, Activated dimethicone 40 mg, Deglycyrrhizinised liquorice 400 mg per 5 ml suspension. Gastritis, peptic ulcer, hyperacidity (Dogs 1/2-1 TSF bid) 175 ml.
Gelusil (Parke-Davis)	:	Mag trisilicate 500 mg, dried alum hydrox gel 250 mg, tabs. Hyperacidity, peptic ulcer, dyspepsia, gastritis (Dogs 1/2-1 tab bid).
		Also Gelusil liquid 170 ml, 400 ml
Histac (Ranbaxy)	:	Ranitidine 150 mg/300 mg tabs.
		Also Histac inj. Ranitidine 25 mg/ml
Mucaine (Wyeth)	:	Oxethazine 10 mg, Alum hydrox. 0.291 gm, Mag. hydrox. 98 mg per 5 ml, suspension. Gastritis, hyperacidity, peptic ulcer. (Dog 1/2-1 TSF bid) 200 ml.
Ranitin (Torrent)	:	Ranitidine HCl 150 mg/300 mg, tabs.

ANTI-DIARRHOEAL PREPARATIONS

Bacigyl (Aristo)	:	Metronidazole 200 mg, Nalidixic acid 300 mg, tabs. Diarrhoea and dysentery of mixed origin. (Dogs: 1/2-1 tab bid).
		Also bacigyl Suspension Metronidazole 100 mg, Nalidixic acid 150 mg per 5 ml liquid, 40 ml.
Dependal-M (Eskayef)	:	Furazolidone 100 mg, Metronidazole 300 mg, tabs. Diarrhoea and dysentery of protozoal, bacterial or mixed origin (Dogs 1/2-1 tabs).

	:	Dependal-M Suspension Furazolidone 25 mg, Metronidazole 75 mg per 5 ml (Dog 10-20 ml bid), 50 ml, 100 ml.
Flagyl-F (Rhone-Poulenc)	:	Metronidazole 400 mg, Furazolidone 100 mg, tab; Dysentery of protozoal, bacterial or mixed origin (Dog 1.2-1 tab bid.)
		Also Flagyl-F Susp, Metronidazole 100 mg, Furazolidone 30 mg per 5 ml suspension, 60 ml.
Furozone (Eskayef)	:	Furazolidone 100 mg tabs. Bacterial enteritis, diarrhoea, dysentery (Dog 1/2-1 tab bid.)
		Also Furaxone suspension Furazolidone 35.7 mg, Pectin 75mg, light Kaolin 1 gm per 5 ml. (Dogs 2.5-5 ml bid.) 60 ml.
Kaltin with Neomycin (Abbott)	:	Kaolin 3 gm, Pectin 65 mg, Neomycin sulph 150 mg per 15 ml, suspension. Diarrhoea, dysentery. (Dog 5-10 ml tid), 60 ml.
Lomotil (Searle)	:	Diphenoxylate HCl 2.5 mg, Atropine sulph. 0.025 mg, tabs. Acute and chronic diarrhoea (Dog 1/2-1 tab bid).
Metrogyl-F (Unique)	:	Metronidazole 400 mg, Furazolidone 100 mg, tabs. Diarrhoea, dysentery of protozoal, bacterial or mixed origin.
		Also Metrogyl-F Suspension 30 ml, 60 ml.
Saril (Rallis)	:	Streptomycin Sulph 240 mg, Pthalylsulphathiazole 200 mg, Diodohydroxyquin 125 mg, Tannic acid 50 mg, Pectin 10 mg, tabs. Non-specific diarrhoea, dysentery of amoebic or bacilary- origin. (Dog1/2-1 tab bid).
Ulix-M Suspension (Blue cross)	:	Nalidixic acid 125 mg, Metronidazole 100 mg per 5 ml. Diarrhoea and dysentery. 30 ml. Also Ulix-P: nalidixic acid 125 mg, tabs.

ANTI-EMETICS

Avomine (Rhone-Poulenc)	:	Promethazine theoclate 25 mg, tabs. Vomiting, nausea, motion sickness. (Dogs1/2-1 tabs).
Demperon (Alidac)	:	Domperidone 10 mg, tabs. Acute nausea, vomiting. (Dogs 1/2-1 tab bid).
Domstal (Torrent)	:	Domperidone 10 mg, tabs. Also Domstal Drops 1 mg/ml. 30 ml.
		Also Domperon suspension 1 mg/ml, 30 ml.
Emidoxyn (Rallis)	:	Prochlorperazine maleate 5 mg, tabs. Vomiting, gastroenteritis, travel, sedation.
Endopace (Themis Pharma)	:	Domperidone 10 mg, tabs.
		Also Endopace suspension 1 mg/ml, 60 ml.
Maxeron (Wallace)	:	Metoclopramide HCl 10 mg, tabs. Relief of nausea and vimiting, gastric stasis, flatulence.
Normetic (Lupin)	:	Domperidone 10 mg, tabs Dyspepsia, nausea, vomiting.

Perinorm (Ipca)	:	Metoclopramide HCl 10 mg, tab. Nausea and vomiting due to GI disorders. (Dogs: 1/2-1 tab bid.)
		Also Perinorm Inj 5 mg/ml (Dog 1-2 ml I/M) 2 ml, 10 ml. Perinorm liquid 1 mg/ml. 30 ml.
Stemetil (Rhone-Poulenc)	:	Prochlorperazinc 5 mg/25mg, tabs Nausea and vomiting.
		Also Stemetil Inj 12.5 mg/ml, 1 ml ampoule, 10 ml vial.

APPETIZER AND TONICS

Bayer's Tonic (Bayer)	:	Liver fraction-2 (12mg), yeast extract 178.5 mg, alcohol 1.65 ml pre 5 ml, syrup. Reduced appetite, debility. Dog 1/2-1 TSF bid. 300 ml.
Cyprowal (Wallace)	:	Cyproheptadine HCl 2 mg, Peptone 25 mg, Lysine HCl 150 mg per 5 ml syrup. Loss of appetite. Dog 1/2-1TSF bid.100 ml, 175ml.
Ginsec (Duphar-Interfran)	:	Korean Ginseng powder 250 mg, tab. Herbal tonic. Dog 1 tab bid. 250 mg, 500 mg.
Merizyme Elixir (Mercury)	:	Fungal diastage (1:8400) 12 mg, Pepsin 60 mg, Vit B_1 4.5 mg, Vit B_2 1.5mg, Niacinamide 45 mg, Panthenol 5 mg, Vit B_6 1.5 mg per 15 ml, liquid. Indigestion, dyspepsia, anorexia, flatulence. Dog 2-5. ml. 200 ml.
Nervitone (Alembic)	:	Cal. Glycerophos. 75 mg, Sod. glycerophos. sol. 0.14 gm, Pot. glycerophos. sol. 32 mg, Mang. glycerophos. 5.3 mg, glycerophosphoric acid 0.105 gm, alcohol (95%) 1.5 ml per 10 ml, liquid. Nervous disorders, convalescence, weakness, reduced appetite, Dog 2-5 ml dialy. 250 ml.
Santevini (Sandoz)	:	Peptone 75 mg, Cal. gluconate 86 mg, Vit B_1 4.5mg, Vit B_2 2.5 mg, B_6 1.5mg, Niacinamide 30 mg per 15 ml, Liquid. Gastric secretion stimulant. Dog 2-5 ml bid. 360 ml.

DIGESTIVE ENZYMES

| Digeplex (Rallis) | : | Diastase (1:2500) 20 mg, Pepsin 20 mg per 10 ml, liquid. Indigestion, dyspepsia, loss of appetite. Dog 5-10 ml bid. 100 ml , 170 ml, 450 ml. |
| Digeplex-T (Rallis) | : | Pancreatin 0.15 gm, Bile ext. 25 mg, Pepsin 5 mg, Diastase (1:2000) 10 mg, Dimethylsioxane 25 mg, dragees (tab). Indigestion, dyspepsia, pancreatic insufficiency, infectious intestinal disorders. (Dog: 1 dragee bid.) |

Festal (Hoechst)	:	Pancreatin 192 mg, Bile constituents 25 mg, Hemicellulose 50 mg, tabs. Pancreatic insufficiency, digestive disturbances. (Dogs 1/2-1 tab bid).
Merizyme Elixir (Mercury)	:	Fungal diastase (1:8400) 12 mg, Pepsin 60 mg, Vit B_1 4.5 mg, Vit B_2 1.5 mg, Niacinamide 45 mg, Panthenol 5 mg, Vit B_6 1.5 mg per 15 ml, liquid. Indigestion, dyspepsia, anorexia, flatulence. (Dogs 2-5 ml bid) 200 ml.
Nolac (Raptakos)	:	Lactase enzyme in aqueous glycerol medium, liquid. Lactase deficiency states characterized by bloat, cramps, abdominal discomfort, diarrhoea on consumption of milk. (Dog: 5-7 drops in pre-boiled and cooled milk) 10 ml.
Unienzyme (Unichem)	:	Fungal diastase (1:75) 200 mg, Papain 30 mg, Vit B_1 2 mg, Vit B_2 2 mg, Nicotinamide 25 mg Acetphenolisatin 0.5 mg, Diphenhydramine HCl 20 mg, Homatropine methyl bromide 1.25 mg, Methyl polysiloxane 25 mg, Activated charcoal 75 mg, tabs. Flatulence, dyspepsia, chronic gastritis. (Dogs 1/2-1 tab bid.)

GASTRO-INTESTINAL SEDATIVES

Baralgan (Hoechst)	:	Analgin 500 mg., Pitofenone HCl 5 mg, Fenpiverinuim bromide 0.1 mg, tab, spasmodic conditions of GIT. (Dog 1/2-1 tab bid.)
Cyclopam Tabs (Indoco)	:	Dicyclomine HCl 20 mg, Paracetamol 500mg, tabs. Intestinal colic, diarrhoea, dysentery. (Dogs 5-10 mg bid.)
		Also Cyclopam Inj (1/M) 10 mg/ml. 2ml.
Esorid (Sun Pharma)	:	Cisapride 100 mg, tabs. Dyspepsia, gastroparesis, constipation (Dogs 1/2-1 tab bid).
Maxeron (Wallace)	:	Metoclopramide HCl 10 mg, tabs. GI disorders (Dogs 5-10 mg bid).
		Also Marexon Liquid 1 mg/ml. 30 ml.
		Marexon Inj. 5 mg/ml. 2 ml ampoule.
Perinorm (Ipca)	:	Metoclopramide HCl 10 mg, tabs. Gastritis, hyperacidity, dyspepsia (Dogs 5-10 mg bid).
		Also Perinorm Inj 5 mg/ml. 2 ml, 10 ml.
		Perinorm Liquid 1 mg/ml. 30 ml.

LAXATIVES AND PURGATIVES

Cremaffin (Boots)	:	Milk of magnesia 11.25 ml, Liquid paraffin 3.5 ml per 15 ml, emulsion. As laxative (Dogs: 5-10 ml) 200 ml.

Cremaffin Pink (Boots)	:	Milk of magnesia 11.25 ml, liquid paraffin 3.75 ml, Phenolphthalein 50 mg per 15 ml, emulsion. Constipation (Dogs 5-10 ml) 200 ml.
Cremaffin-FS (Boots)	:	Isapgol husk 3.5 gm per 14.25 gm, powder. Dietary fibre supplement in treatment and prevention of constipation. (Dogs 1/2-1TSF with water 100 gm.
Dulcolax (German Remedies)	:	Bisacodyl 5 mg, tabs. Constipation (Dogs 1/2-1 tab).
Julax (Rallis)	:	Bisacodyl 10 mg, Casanthranol 10 mg, tabs. Constipation. (Dogs 1/2-1 tab).

PREPARATIONS FOR CIRCULATORY SYSTEM

HAEMOSTATICS

C.V.P (USV and P)	:	Citrus bioflavonoid compound 100 mg, Vit C 100 mg, caps. Protect capillary system from injury by infections etc, helps & prevents or minimises & capillary bleeding.
		Also C.V.P. with Vit K Syrup.
Hemocid (Biddle Sawyer)	:	Epsion aminocaproic acid 250 mg per ml inj. Haemorrhage.
Kerutin-C (Mercury)	:	Rutin 100 mg, Adrenochrome monosemicarbazone 1 mg, Vit K 20 mg, Cal dibasic phos. 150 mg, Cholecalciferol 300 IU, Vit C 50 mg, tabs. Haematuria, G.I. haemorrhages and other haemorrhagic conditions.
Styptochrome Inj (Dolphin)	:	Adrenochrome monosemicarbazone 1.5 mg per 2 ml, inj (1/M). Haemorrhages.
Styptocid (Stadmed)	:	Adrenochrome monosem. 0.5 mg, Menadion 10 mg, rutin 50 mg, Vit C 37.5 mg, Vit D 200 IU, Cal. dibasic phos. 125 mg, tabs.
		Also Styptocid inj Adrenochrome monosemi. 0.75 mg/ml.
Styptovit (Dolphin)	:	Adrenochrome mono. 0.33 mg, Menadione 10 mg, Ascorbic acid 100 mg, cal. dibasic phos. 125 mg, tabs.
Venex (Elder)	:	Pure synthetic diosmin 150 mg/300 mg, tabs.
Venusmin (Martin and Harris)	:	Pure synthetic diosmin 150 mg/300 mg, tab.

HAEMATINIC DRUGS

| Cilfer-12-F Oral (Duphar-Interfran) | : | Colloidal iron 100 mg, Vit B12 15 mcg, Folic acid 1.5 mg per 5 ml, Liquid. Anaemia (Dogs 1-2 ml bid). 120 ml. |
| Dexorange Plus (Franco-Indian) | : | Haemoglobin 2.095 gm, Ferric amm. citrate 125 mg, Vit B12 7.5 mcg, Folic acid 0.5 mg, |

	:	alcohol 0.87 ml per 15 ml, liquid. Anaemia, reduced appetite (Dogs 2-5 ml bid). 280 ml.
Haem up (Cadila)	:	Glycerinated haemoglobin 1 gm, Ferric amm. citrate 100 mg, Cupric sulph 30 mcg, Mang. sulf. 30 mcg, Zinc sulph 30 mcg, alcohol 0.87 ml per 15 ml syrup. Anaemia. (Dogs 1 TSF bid) 200 ml.
Hemfer (Alkem)	:	Haemoglobin 2.15 gm, Vit B_{12} 30 mcg, Sorbitol sol. 0.75 gm, alcohol 0.87 ml per 15 ml, liquid. Anaemia. (Dogs 2-5 ml). 200 ml.
Hepp Forte (Lupin)	:	Haemoglobin 2.1 gm, elemental iron from haemoglobin 7.1 mg, Ferric amm. cit. 200 mg, Vit B_{12} 7.5 mcg, Vit B_6 1.5 mg, Folic acid 0.5 mg, Sorbitol sol. 0.75 gm per 15 ml, syrup. Convalescence, anaemia, reduced appetite. (Dogs 2-5 ml bid). 300 ml.
Iberol Tonic (Abbott)	:	Ferrous sulf 131 mg, Vit C 125 mg, B_{12} 5 mcg, B_1 4.5 mg, Nicotinamide 45 mg, B_6 1.5 mg, Panthenol 5 mg per 5 ml, liquid. Anaemia. Dogs 2-5 ml daily. 150 ml.
		Also Iberol capsules.
Imferon (Rallis)	:	Iron dextran 50 mg per ml, inj (I/M), Anaemia, malnutrition, parasitic infestations. (Dogs 1-2 ml. 2 ml ampoule.)

C.N.S. DRUGS

ANAESTHETIC AGENTS

Fluothane (ICI)	:	Contains Halothane, inhalation anaesthesia. 250 ml.
Gesicain Heavy 5% (SG Pharma)	:	Lignocaine HCl 5% and glucose 7.5%, 2 ml ampoule.
Gesicain 2% jelly (SG Pharma)	:	Lignocaine HCl 2%, Carboxymethyl cellulose 3.5%, jelly. Topical treatment of painful urethral and vaginal conditions. 30 ml.
Gesicain 4% topical (SG Pharma)	:	Lignocaine HCl 4% solution. For anaesthetising any accessible mucous membranes. 30 ml.
Gesicain sol. (SG Pharma)	:	1%, 2% and 2 % with adrenaline (1:800,000) Inj.
Gesicain oint (SG Pharma)	:	Lignocaine HCl 5%. Topical anaesthesia.
Intraval sodium (Rhone-Poulenc)	:	Thiopentone sod. 0.5 gm/1.0 gm vial.
Sensorcaine (Astra-IDL)	:	Bupivacaine HCl 2.5 mg (0.25%)/5 mg (0.5%) per ml injection. 20 ml.
Xylocaine (Astra-IDL)	:	Lignocaine HCl 1%, 2%, and also 2% with adrenaline 30 ml.
Xylocaine 5% Heavy (Astra-IDL)	:	Lignocaine HCl 53.3 mg and dextrose 75 mg per ml. 2 ml.
Xylocaine Jelly (Astra-IDL)	:	Lignocaine HCl 2% jelly. Urethral and vaginal anaesthesia, instrument lubrication. 30 gm.

Xylocaine ointment (Astra-IDL) : Lignocaine HCl 5% oint. Painful condition, pruritus, etc. 10 gm and 30 gm.

Xylocain Topical (Astra-IDL) : Lignocain HCl 4%. Surface anaesthesia. 30 ml.

Xylocain Viscous (Astra-IDL) : Lignocain HCl 2%. Introduction of catheter, ulcer, painful conditions. 100 ml.

HYPNOTICS PREPARATIONS

Gardenal (Rhone-Poulenc) : Phenobarbitone 30 mg/60 mg, tabs. Epilepsy, sedative, hypnotic.
(Dog 25-100 mg per day in divided doses) 30 mg, 60 mg.

Luminal (Bayer) : Phenobarbitone 30 mg, tabs. Epilepsy, eclampsia, excitatory conditions.

Nindral (Torrent) : Flurazepam 15mg, cap. sedative
(Dogs: 5-10 mg per day).

Nitrosun (Sun Pharma) : Nitrazepam 5 mg/10 mg, tabs. sedative
(Dogs: 2-5 mg per day).

ANTI-CONVELESCENT PREPARATIONS

Carbatol (Torrent) : Carbamazepine 100 mg/200 mg/400 mg tabs. Epilepsy, tonic and clonic seizures. (Dogs: initial 25-50 mg per day, can be increased gradually.)

Carmaz 100/200 (Natco) : Carbamazepine 100 mg/200 mg tabs.

Mazetol (SG Pharma) : Carbamazepine 200 mg, tabs.

Phenytal-30 (Intas) : Phenobarb. 30 mg, Phenytoinsod. 100 mg, tabs. Epilepsy, seizures (Dogs 1/4-1/2 tab bid, increase gradually).

SEDATIVES AND TRANQUILIZERS

Calmpose (Ranbaxy) : Diazepam 2 mg/5mg/10mg, tabs. Muscle spasm, behavioural disorder, pre-medication.

Calmpose Injection (Ranbaxy) : Diazepam 10 mg per 2 ml, inj.
(Dogs: 1-2 mg per kg b.w. I/M or I/V.)

Dizep (Intas) : Diazepam 5 mg/10 mg, tabs.

Emetil (LA Pharma) : Chlorpromazine HCl 25 mg/50mg/100 mg/200 mg, tabs. Sedation, pre-medication, emesis. (Dogs 1-2 mg per kg b.wt.)

Larpose (Cipla) : Lorazepam 1 mg, tab. Pre-anaesthetic, behavioural disorders.

Librium (Roche) : Chlordiazepoxide 10 mg, tab. Fear, behavioural disorders.

Megatil (Intas) : Chlorpromazine 25 mg/50 mg/100 mg/200 mg, tabs.

Neocalm (Intas) : Triflupromazine HCl 5 mg/10 mg, tabs.

Placidox (Lupin) : Diazepam 2 mg/5mg/10mg combined with Vit B_6, 10 mg/25mg/50mg, respectively, tabs.

Valium-5 (Roche) : Diazepam 5 mg, tabs.

EXPECTORANTS

Actilex(Burroughs Wellcome) : Triprolidine HCl. 2.5 mg, Ephedrine HCl 15 mg per 5 ml, Syrup, Cough, congestion of the upper respiratory tract of allergic origin and due to pharyngitis. Dogs 2-5 ml bid. 115 ml, 455 ml.

Avil Expectorant (Hoechst) : Pheniramine maleate 15 mg, Amm. chloride 125 mg, Menthol 1.14 mg per 5 ml, syrup. cough, bronchitis, allergy of lower respiratory tract. Dogs 2.5-5 ml 2-3 times daily 100 ml, 400 ml.

Benadryl Cough Formula (Parke-Davis) : Diphenhydramine HCl 14.08mg, Amm. chloride 0.138 gm, Sod. citrate 57.03 mg, Menthol 1.14 mg, Alcohol 0.26 ml per 5 ml, syrup. Cough and other congestive symptoms. Dogs 2-5 ml 4 hourly. 114 ml, 456 ml.

Bricarex Expectorant (Astra-IDL) : Terbutaline sulph. 1.5mg, Guaifenesin 66.65 mg per 5 ml, syrup. Cough. Dogs 2-10 ml 2-3 times a day. 120 ml.

Broxynol (Ethnor) : Bromhexine 4 mg, Carbinoxamine maleate 2 mg Amm. chloride 120 mg per 5 ml, liquid. Cough of allergic and infective origin. Dogs 2-5 ml 2-3 times daily. 100 ml.

Corex (Pfizer) : Chlorpheniramine maleate 4 mg, Codeine phos. 10 mg, Ephedrine HCl 5 mg, Sod. citrate 150 mg, Menthol 0.1 mg per 5 ml, syrup. Dry and irritating cough in allergic and infective conditions. Dogs 1-3 ml 2 times daily. 60 ml, 120 ml.

Daslin (Searle) : Diphenhydramine 8 mg, Aminophylin 32 mg, Amm. chloride 30 mg, Alcohol 0.26 ml per 5 ml, syrup. Cough accompanied by tenacious bronchial secretions. Dogs 2-5 ml, two times daily, 100 ml.

Ephedrex (Alembic) : Ephedrine HCl 10 mg, Codeine phos. 2.5 mg Chlorpheniramine maleate 0.87 mg per 5 ml, syrup. Cough in acute or chronic bronchitis, pharyngitis, tonsilitis, pneumonia, respiratory allergy. 1-5 ml, 3 times daily, 110 ml, 450 ml, 900 ml.

Fintal Nasal Spray (Rallis) : Sod. cromoglycate 2%, Benzalkonium chloride 0.01%. Solution for spray. Allergic rhinitis. Squeeze in each nostril. 20 ml squeeze bottle.

Phensedyl (Rhone-Poulenc) : Promethazine HCl 3.6 mg, Codeine phos. 9 mg, Ephedrine HCl 7.2 mg per 5 ml, liquid. Cough. Dog 2-5 ml bid. 60 ml, 125 ml, 500ml. Also Phensedyl Expectorant, 125 ml.

Polaramine Expectorant (Fulford) : Dexchlorpheniramine maleate 2 mg, Pseudoephedrine sulph. 20 mg, Guaifenesin 100 mg per 5ml, syrup. Cough, allergy, rhinitis. Dog 1-2 ml tid. 50 ml.

Tixlix (Rhone-Poulenc) : Promethazine HCl 1.5 mg, Pholcodeine 1.5 mg, Phenyl propanolamine HCl 5mg per 5ml, liquid.

Cough, bronchitis etc. Dog 2-5 ml tid 125 ml, 500 ml.

Zeet Expectorant (Alembic) : Chlorpheniramine maleate 2.5 mg, Amm. Chloride 125 mg, Sod. citrate 62.5 mg, Menthol 1.25 mg, Chloroform 0.015 ml, Alcohol (95%) 0.156 ml per 5 ml, syrup. Cough due to allergy, irritating dust, gas, fumes etc. Dogs 1-2 ml tid. 110ml, 450 ml.

PREPARATIONS FOR URINARY SYSTEM

DIURETICS :

Aquamide (Sun Pharma) : Spironolactone 50 mg, Frusemide 20 mg, caps. Ascites, oedema, anuria, oligouria etc.

Lasix (Hoechst) : Frusemide 10 mg per ml, injection. 2 ml ampoule. Also lasix tabs, 40 mg. Lasix high dose 500 mg tabs.

Spiromide (Searle) : Frusemide 20 mg, Spironolactone 50 mg, tabs.

URINARY ANTI-SPASMODICS AND ANTI-INFECTIVE

Baralgan (Hoechst) : Analgin 500 mg, Pitofenone HCl 2mg, Fenpiverinium bromide 0.02 mg per ml, inj. Renal and biliary colics, spasmodic conditions of GI tract. 2 ml, 5 ml. Also Baralgan tabs.

Cifran (Ranbaxy) : Ciprofloxacin 250mg/500 mg/750 mg, tabs. Infections of urinary tract and other systems.

Genticyn (Nicholas-Piramal) : Gentamycin Sulph. 40,000 IU (40 mg)per ml, inj. Gram negative UTI. 2 ml.

Gramoneg (Ranbaxy)   Nalidixic acid 500 mg, tabs UTI.

: Also Gramoneg Suspension Nalidixic acid 300 mg per 5 ml, 30 ml, 60 ml.

Negadix (CFL) : Nalidixic acid 500 mg, tabs

VAGINAL PREPARATIONS

Alphadine Vaginal Pessaries (Nicholas-Piramal) : Povidone iodine 200 mg per pessary. Vaginitis. Bitch : one pessary in vagina daily.

Candid-V Gel (Glenmark) : Clotrimazole 2%, gel. Vaginitis due to fungi, non-specific vaginitis etc. Bitch : 2-5 gm gel deep into vagina daily 30 gm with applicator.

Flagyl (Rhone-Poulenc) : Metronidazole 200 mg/400 mg, tabs. Vaginitis, infections of genitourinary tract in dogs and bitches. 50-100 mg bid orally for 5-7 days.

Imidil Vaginal Tabs (Lyka) : Clotrimazole 100 mg/200 mg/500 mg tabs. Vaginitis due to fungi, trichomonas, bacteria etc. Bitch. 1 tab deep into vagina.

Mycostatin Vaginal (Sarabhai) : Nystatin 100,000 IU, tabs. Mycotic vaginitis. Bitch : One tab deep into vagina daily.

Talsutin Vaginal (Sarabhai) : Tetracycline 100 mg, Amphotericin-B 50 mg, tabs. Vaginitis. Bitch : One tab deep into vagina.

Triple Sulpha (Ethnor)	:	Sulfathiazole 3.42%, Sulfacetamide 2.36%, N-benzoyl sulfanilamide 3.7%, Urea 0.64%, cream. Vaginitis, cervicitis etc. Bitch : about 5 gm intravaginal. 30gm.
Wokadine Vaginal (Wockhardt)	:	Povidone iodine 200mg, pessary. Vaginitis Bitch : one pessary into vagina.

PREPARATIONS FOR EYE, EAR AND NOSE

EAR (AURAL) PREPARATIONS

Alflox Eye/Ear Drops (Alkem)	:	Norfloxacin 3%, Benzalkonium chloride sol. 0.022%, drops. Occular infections, otitis media and externa. 5 ml.
Candid Ear drops (Glenmark)	:	Clotrimazole 1% lignocaine HCl 2%, drops. Fungal infections of the ear, for concurrent antibacterial ear formulation.
Chloromycetin Ear Drops (Parke-Davis)	:	Chloramphenicol 5%, Benzocaine 1%, drops. Chronic otorrhoea, suppurative otitis media. 5ml.
Dexona E/E (Cadila)	:	Dexamethasone Sod. phos. 0.1%, Neomycin sulph 0.5%, Benzalkonium Chloride sol. 0.02%, Solution. Aural infections and inflammation. 2.5ml.
Garamycin E/E Drops (Fulford)	:	Gentamycin sulph 3 mg per ml, drops. Infection of the eye and ear, 3 ml.
Genticin E/E Drops (Nicholas-Piramal)	:	Gentamicin sulph 0.3 % sol. 5 ml.
Genticin-B E/E Drops (Nicholas-Piramal)	:	Gentamycin sulph 0.3% sol, Betamethasone sod. phos. 0.1%, drops, chronic and acute ear and eye infections. 5 ml.
Genticin-HC E/E Drops (Nicholas-Piramal)	:	Gentamycin sulph 0.3%, Hydrocortisone acetate 1%, suspension. Allergy and inflammatory conditions 3 ml.
Neosporin-H Ear Drops (Burroughs Wellcome)	:	Polymyxin B sulph 10,000 units, Neomycin sulph 3400 units, hydrocortisone 10 mg per ml, drops. Infections and inflammation of ear. 5 ml.
Otek (FDC)	:	Prednisolone 0.5%, Lignocaine HCl 2%, Phenylmercuric nit. 0.1%, Acetic acid 2%, drops. Otorrhoea, Otitis externa, wax in ear, 5 ml.
Paraxin Ear Drops (Boehringer-Mannheim)	:	Chloramphenicol 5%, drops. Otitis externa and media, chronic otorrhoea. 5 ml.
Sofracort E/E Drops (Roussel)	:	Dexamethasone sod. metasulphobenzoate 0.116%, Framycetin sulph. 1%, drps. Eye and ear infections and inflammation 3 ml.
Surfaz Ear Drops (Franco-Indian)	:	Clotrimazole 1%, drops. Fungal infections of the external ear. 10ml.

EYE (OPHTHALMIC) PREPARATIONS

Eye drops containing steroid are contraindicated in viral, fungal and other infections of eye, unless controlled by appropriate chemotherapy.

Albucid (Nicholas-Piramal)	:	Sulphacetamide sod. 1o%/20%/30%, sol. Simple eye infections as conjunctivitis, blepharitis. 14 ml.
Betnesol-N E/E (Glaxo Pharma)	:	Betamethasone sod. phos. 0.1%, oint. and drops. Non-infected inflammatory eye/ear conditions. Oint-5 gm, drops 5 ml.
Cambison Eye Oint. (Hoechst)	:	Prednisolone 0.25%, Neomycin HCl 0.16%, Surfen 0.30%, oint. Inflammatory eye conditions, conjunctivitis, lid eczema etc. 3.5 gm.
Catalin (Biddle Sawyer)	:	0.75 mg tablets plus 15 ml solvent. Cataract (Primary, senile and traumatic). Dissolve tab in solvent and instill 1-2 drops 4-5 hrly.
Chloromycetin Aplicaps (Parke-Davis)	:	Chloramphenicol 1%, oint (applicaps). Bacterial conjunctivitis and other occular infections. 50 applicaps.
Ciplox Eye Drops (Cipla)	:	Ciprofloxacin HCl 0.3%, Benzalkonium chloride 0.022%, drops. Infections and injury of eye. 5 ml. Also Ciplox eye oint 3%. 5 gm.
Kenalog-S (Sarabhai)	:	Triamcinolone acetonide 1 mg, Gramicidin 0.25 mg, Neomycin sulph 2.5 mg per gm oint. Infected, inflammatory conditions of the eye. 2.5 gm.
Micoptic (FDC)	:	Miconazole 1%, opticaps. Fungal infections of the eye. 30 opticaps.
Neosporin Eye Drops (Burroughs Wellcome)	:	Polymyxin-B sulph 5000 unit, Neomycin Sulph 1700 units, Gramicidin 25 units per ml, solution. Bacterial infections of the eye, conjunctivitis, keratitis, corneal ulcers, after removing foreign bodies. 10.ml.
Norbactin Eye Drops (Ranbaxy)	:	Norfloxacin 3 mg per ml, drops. Conjunctivitis, keratitis, corneal ulcer. 5 ml.
Norflox Eye Drops (Cipla)	:	Norfloxacin 0.3%, Benzalkonium chloride sol. 0.022%, drops. Occular infections like conjunctivitis, corneal ulcer, pre and post-occular surgery. 5 ml.
Oriprim-P Eye Drops (Cadila)	:	Trimethoprim 1 mg, Polymyxin-B sulph 10,000 units per ml, drop. Bacterial infections of the eye, pre and post-occular surgery. 5 ml.
Paraxin Eye Oint (Boehringer-Mannheim)	:	Chloramphenicol 1% oint. Eye infections. 3.5 gm.
Pyrimon (FDC)	:	Dexamethasone 0.1%, Chloramphenicol 1%, drops. Infections of the eye, allergic conditions

of the eye, following traumatic, chemical and thermal injuries of the eye. 5 ml.

Quinobact Eye Drops : Ciprofloxacin lactate 3mg, Benzalkonium
(Nicholas-Piramal)   Chloride 0.02% per ml. Eye infections. 5 ml.

Soframycin Ophthalmic : Soframycin (framycetin sulph) 0.5%, oint.
Oint (Roussel)   Conjunctivitis, blepharitis. 5 gm.

Terramycin Ophthalmic : Oxytetracycline HCl 10 mg per gm, oint.
Oint (Pfizer)   Superficial occular infections. 3.5 gm.

Zoptic (Mejda) : Ciprofloxacin 0.3%, Hydroxypropyl methyl
                 cellulose 0.25%, Benzalkonium chloride 0.01%,
                 drops. Superficial occular infections.

NOSE PREPARATIONS

Betnesol-N Nasal Drops : Betamethasone sod. phos 0.05%. Naphazoline
(Glaxo Pharma)   nitrate 0.05%, Neomycin sulph 0.5% sol. Allergic
                           rhinitis and inflammatory conditions of nose.
                           10 ml.

Decon (Cadila) : Xylometazoline HCl 0.1%, drops. Allergic
                 rhinitis, sinusitis, nasal congestion 10 ml.

Efcorlin Nasal Drops : Hydrocortisone 0.2 mg (0.02%), Naphazoline
(Glaxo-Allenburys)   nitrate 0.25 mg (0.025%), drops. Allergy, nasal
                       congestion, inflammation. 15ml.

Endrine (Wyeth) : Ephedrine 0.75%, Menthol 0.5%, Camphor 0.5%,
                  Eucalyptol 0.5%, Castor oil 0.5%, light liquid
                  paraffin base, drops. Allergy, rhinitis, sinusitis.
                  30 ml.

Karvol (Duphar-Interfran) : Menthol 7.9%, Chlorbutol 6.6%, Cinnamon oil
                            2.7%, Terpineol 14.8%, Oil of pine 18.8%,
                            Thymol 0.7%. Inhalant capsule. Squeeze the
                            contents into boiling water and use for
                            inhalation.

Nasivion (Merk) : Oxymetazoline HCl 0.05% soln. Nasal
                  congestion. 10 ml.

Otrivin (Hindustan : Xylometazoline HCl 0.1% sol. 10 ml.
Ciba-Geigy)

OROPHARYNGEAL PREPARATIONS

Alphadine Gargle : Povidone iodine 1%, liquid. Pharyngitis,
(Nicholas-Piramal) ginigivitis, stomatitis, 50 ml.

Candid Mouth Paint : Clotrimazole 1%, Sol. fungal infections of oral cavity. 15 ml.
(Glenmark)

Wokadine (Wockhardt) : Povidone 1% sol. Stomatitis, pharyngitis, glossitis. 50 ml.

Zytee (Raptakos) : Choline salicylate 9%, Cetrimide 0.01%, gel. Pain
                   relief in stomatitis, glossitis, gingivitis.

TOPICAL PREPARATIONS

ANTI-INFECTIVE, ANIT-FUNGAL AND ANTIPRURITIC

Adzorb (Croslands)	:	Clotrimazole 1% Powder. Fungal infections of skin. 75 gm.
Alphadine Ointment (Nicholas-Piramal)	:	Povidone iodine 5% oint. Wounds, burns, abscesses, ulcers, fungal infection, otitis externa 15 gm, 125 gm.
	:	Also Alphadine powder (5%) 10 gm.
	:	Alphadine solution (5%) 100 ml.
Ascabiol (Rhone-Poulenc)	:	Benzyl benzoate 25% emulsion. Scabies, Pediculosis 50 ml, 125 ml.
Betnovate (Glaxo Pharma)	:	Betamethasone valerate 0.1% oint and cream. Eczema, contact dermatitis, seborrhoeic dermatitis, bacterial infection, pruritus etc. 15 gm.
Betnovate-C (Glaxo Pharma)	:	Betamethasone valerate 0.12%, Chinoform (iodochlorhydroxyquin) 3% oint and cream. 15 gm.
Betnovate-N (Glaxo Pharma)	:	Betamethasone valerate 0.12%, Neomycin sulphate 0.5% cream and oint. 15gm.
Caladryl Lotion (Parke-Davis)	:	Calamine 8%, Diphenhydramine HCl 1% Camphor 0.1%, denatured spirit 2.37%, Aquous sol. Pruritus, urticaria, insect bite, allergy etc. 57 ml, 171ml.
Candid (Glenmark)	:	Clotrimazole 1% cream. Fungal infection of the skin 15 gm.
		Also Candid powder-Clotrimazole 1%. 30 gm, 100 gm.
Candid-B (Glenmark)	:	Clotrimazole 1%, beclomethasone dipropionate 0.025%, cream, Fungal infection of the skin. 5 gm, 15 gm.
Canesten (Bayer)	:	Clotrimazole 10 mg per gm cream. All fungal infection of skin. 15 gm
		Also Canesten solution Clotrimazole 10 mg per ml solution. 15 ml
Chloromycetin Topical (Parke-Davis)	:	Chloramphenicol 100 mg per ml sol. Wounds, dermatological conditions etc. 5 ml.
K.Y. Lubricating Jelly (Johnson and Johnson)	:	Synthetic and vegetable gum jelly. For lubrication of hand gloves during vaginal and per-rectal examination and for lubricating instruments. 50 gm.
Ledermycin Oint (Lederle)	:	Demeclocycline HCl 0.5% oint. Pyogenic infections of the skin. 15 gm.
Micogel (Cipla)	:	Miconazole nitrate 2% cream. Fungal infections of skin. 15 gm.
Micogel-F (Cipla)	:	Miconazole nitrate 2%, Fluocinolone acetonide 0.25% cream. Chronic fungal infections of skin 15 gm.

Multifungin (Boehringer-Mannheim)	:	5-brom salicyl-4 chloranilide 2%, soventol salicylate 1% cream. Fungal infection of skin. 30 gm.
		Also Multifungin solution 30 ml; Multifungin Powder 30 gm.
Mycoderm (FDC)	:	Salicylic acid 3%, benzoic acid 6%, Camphor 0.52%, menthol 0.08%, Starch 3%, Purified talk, kaolin light Q.S. Powder. Fungal infections of skin. 100 gm.
Mycostatin Oint (Sarabhai)	:	Nystatin 100,000 units per gram. Oint. Cutaneous mycotic infection caused by *Candida albicans*. 10 mg.
Nebasulf (Pfizer)	:	Neomycin sulphate 5 mg, Bacitracin 250 units, Sulphacetamide 30 mg, Sulphacetamide sod. 36 mg per gm oint. Skin infection. 15 gm.
Neosporin Oint (Burroughs Wellcome)	:	Polymyxin-B sulphate 5000 units, Neomycin sulphate 3400 units, Zinc bacitracin 400 units per gm. oint. Prevention and treatment of bacterial infections of skin. 5 gm, 20 gm.
		Also Neosporin Powder 10 gm.
Pentaderm (Mercury)	:	Zinc bacitracin 10 mg, Miconazole 20 mg, Gentamicin 1 mg, Betamethasone 400 units, Quiniodochlor 10 mg per gm. oint. Mixed skin infections. 5 gm.
Piodin (Biddle Sawyer)	:	Povidone iodine 10% soln. 10% oint, 1% mouth wash. Used as bactericide, fungicide etc. Sol 50ml, oint 10 gm, mouth wash 120 ml.
Pragmatar (Eskayef)	:	Cetyl alcohol 5%, Cetyl tar distillate 4%, Sulphur precipitated 3%, Salicylic acid 3%, ointment. Fungal infection, seborrhoeic condition, dendruff. 15 gm.
Quadriderm (ZYG Pharma)	:	Betamethasone valerate 0.05%, Gentamicin sulph 0.1%, Tolnaftate Iodochlorhydroxyquin 1%, cream. skin infection complicated by bacteria, fungi, inflammation, allergy, pruritus. 5 gm, 15 gm.
Scabex (Indoco)	:	Gamabenzene hexachloride 1%, Lotion, Scabies, pediculosis. 50 ml.
		Also scabex cream: Gamabenzene hexachloride 1%, sulphacetamide 5%. scabies with secondary infection. 20 g.
Scabindon (Indon)	:	Benzyl benzoate 25%, Benzocaine 2%, DDT 1% ointment. Scabies and pediculosis. 25 gm.
Tenovate Skin Cream (Glaxo Pharma)	:	Clobetasol propionate 0.05%, cream. Eczema, chronic lesions. 10 gm.
	:	Also Tenovate-M: Clobetasol propionate 0.05%, Miconazole nitrate 2%, cream. Chronic lesions associated with fungal and mixed infections. 10 gm.

Thrombophob (German Remedies)	:	Heparin 5000 units, Benzyl nicotinate 200 mg per 100 gm, cream. Sprain, bruises, hematoma, tenosynovitis etc. 20 gm.
		Also Thrombophob gel. 20gm
Tinoderm (Fulford)	:	Tolnaftate 10 mg per ml solution. Ringworm infections. 10 ml.
		Also Tinoderm cream Tolnaftate 10 mg per gm. 5 gm.
Wokadine (Wockhadt)	:	Povidone iodine 5% ointment. Wounds, boils impetigo, fungal infections, burns etc. 15 gm, 125 gm, 250 gm.
	:	Also Wokadine Solution 5% 100 ml, 500 ml.
	:	Wokadine powder 5% 10 gm.
Wycort (Wyeth)	:	Hydrocortisone acetate 25 mg per gm oint. Eczema, dermatitis, pruritus, allergy. 5 gm.

RUBEFACIENTS

Arjet Spray (Cadila)	:	Methyl salicylate 875 mg, Menthol 1600 mg, Camphor 1500 mg, Benzyl nicotinate 20 mg, Squalane 250 mg, Glycol salicylate 875 mg per 50 ml, Aerosol spray. Sprains, strains, muscle stiffness, joint pain. Spray the affected area. Repeat 2-3- times daily. 50 ml.
Diclonac Gel (Lupin)	:	Diclofenac sod. 1%, gel. Pain, inflammation of tendons, muscles, joints. Apply to the affected part 2-3- times daily and rub gently. 30 mg.
Dicloran Gel (Unique)	:	Diclofenac diethylamine 1%. 20 gm.
Kilpane Cream (Biddle Sawyer)	:	Methyl salicylate 15%, Mephenesin 2%, Menthol 6%, Eucalyptus oil 2%, Turpentine oil 1.5%, cream. Stiffness and pain in musculo-skeletal disorder. 30 gm.
Kilpane Oil (Biddle Sawyer)	:	Menthol 15%, Methyl salicylate 50%, Eucalyptus oil 7%, Camphor 18%. 15 ml.
Medicreme (Rallis)	:	Adrenaline bitartrate 0.03%, Methyl nicotinate 1%, Mephenesin 2.5%, Methyl salicylate 8%, Chlorpheniramine maleate 0.2%, Menthol 2%, Oint. Stiffness, painful conditions of muscle joints and tendons. 30 gm.
Minicam Gel (Blue Cross)	:	Piroxicam 0.5%, gel. Sprain, strain, painful conditions of joints, muscles and tendons.
Parbudol Gel (Mercury)	:	Ibuprofen 50 mg, Mephenesin 50 mg, Methyl salicylate 5 mg, Menthol 5 mg per gm, gel. Muscle stiffness, sprain, strain, neuralgia etc. 20 gm.
Pirox Gel (Cipla)	:	Piroxicam 0.5%, gel. 30 gm.

| Relaxyl (Franco Indian) | : | Mephenesin 10%, Methyl nicotinate 1%, Capsicum oleoresin 0.05%, ointment. Muscular pain, sprain, strain, arthritis etc. 30 gm. |
| Tantum Cream/Gel (Elder) | : | Benzydamine HCl 5% cream and gel. Acute inflammatory conditions, sprains, strains. 20 gm cream and 20 gm gel. |

HORMONES

GONADAL HORMONES

Aquaviron B_{12} (Nicholas-Piramal)	:	Testosterone 25 mg, Vit B_{12} 500 mg. Thiomersal 0.01% per ml, inj. 1 ml.
Deviry (Elder)	:	Medroxyprogesterone acetate 10 mg tabs.
Duoluton (German Remedies)	:	Norgestrel 0.5 mg, Ethinyl estradiol 0.05 mg, tabs.
Omicite (Torrent)	:	Clomiphene citrate 50 mg, tabs.
Progynone Depot (German Remedies)	:	Estradiol valerate 10 mg per ml, inj. 1 ml.
Proluton Depot (German Remedies)	:	Hydroxyprogesterone caproate 125 mg/250 mg per ml and 500 mg per 2 ml, inj. 1 ml, 2 ml ampoule.
Testoviron Depot (German Remedies)	:	Testosterone propionate 25 mg, Testosterone enanthate 100 mg per ml, inj. 1 ml.

TROPIC HORMONES

Genotropin (Kabi Pharmacia)	:	Lyophilized powder of recombinant somatropin 4/12/16/36 I.U. per vial inj. Growth disturbances.
Gonadotraphon F.S.H (Biochem)	:	Serum gonadotrophin (FSH)1000 I.U. Freeze dried powder and solvent, inj.
Gonadotraphon L.H. (Biochem)	:	Chorionic gonadotrophin 1000 IU/5000 I.U.
Gonadotraphon HM (Biochem)	:	FSH 75 units, LH 75 units, inj.

THYROID DRUGS

Collosol Iodine Oral (Duphar-Interfran)	:	Iodine 8 mg per 5 ml, liquid. Conditions where iodine and pot. iodide are required. Dogs : 0.25-0.5 ml bid.
Eltroxin (Glaxo Allenburys)	:	Thyroxine sod. 0.1 mg tabs. Conditions associated with thyroid deficiency. Dogs. 0.025-0.05 mg a day.
Proloid (Park-Davis)	:	Thyroglobulin 0.15 mg (iodine bound), tabs. Hypothyroidism. Start at very low level and increase gradually.
Roxin (Cadila)	:	Thyroxine sod. 100 mcg, tabs. Hypothyroidism Dogs : initially 10 to 25 mcg and increase it gradually.

ANABOLIC STEROIDS

Decaneurabol (Cadila) : Nandrolone decanoate 25 mg per ml, injection. For anabolic effect; after prolonged illness, trauma, surgery, infectious diseases, osteoporosis, anaemia. Dogs : 25-50 mg I/M once in a month. 1 ml.

Menabol (CFL) : Stanozolol 2 mg, tabs. Dogs : 1 tab bid.

Neurabol Capsules (Cadila) : Stanozolol 2 mg, capsules. Dogs 1 cap bid.

Neurabol Injection (Cadila) : Nandrolone phenylpropionate 25 mg per ml, injection. Dogs : 25- 50 mg I/M once a month. 1 ml.

PROTEOLYTIC ENZYMES

Bidanzen (Biddle Sawyer) : Serratiopeptidase 5 mg tabs. Inflammation after surgery, traumatic injury, pain, udder inflammation etc.

Bidanzen Forte (Biddle Sawyer) : Serratiopeptidase 10 mg tabs.

Hyalase (Rallis) : Hyaluronidase 1500 I.U./ampoule.

MINERALS AND NUTRITIONAL SUPPLEMENT

Alprovit (Alkem) : Protein hydrolysate 1 gm, Zinc sulph 8mg, Vit B1 1.5 mg, B_2 1 mg, B_6 0.5 mg, d-pentothenol 1 mg, Niacinamide 15 mg, Iron choline citrate 45 mg, Sorbitol sol (70%) 0.5 gm, Mag.chloride 10 mg, Mang. chloride 0.1 mg per 15 ml, Syrup. Jaundice, malnutition, dietary supplement. Dogs 1 TSP bid. 200 ml.

Aquamin Suspension (Pfimex) : Calcium 69.87 mg, Iron 3 mg, Magnesium 35 mg Zinc 1.5 mg, Iodine 15 mcg, Copper 300 mcg, Chromium 20 mcg, Selenium 20 mcg, Molybedenum 50 mcg, Manganese 500 mcg per 15 ml, suspension. Mineral supplement during deficiency. Dogs : 1/2 TSF. 200 ml. Also Aquamin tabs.

Calcinol Syrup F (Raptakos) : Cal. lactate 1.5 gm, Cal. gluconate 250 mg, Vit A 2,500 IU, Vit D_3 200 IU, Vit C 40 mg, Vit B_{12} 2.5 mcg, Sod. iron editate 33 mg per5 ml, syrup. Calcium deficiency. Dog 1-2.5 ml bid. 120 ml. Also Calcinol tabs.

Calcium-Sandoz Inj (Sandoz) : Calcium gluconate sol. 10% Cal. glubionate 1.375 gm per 10 ml, inj. Hypocalcaemia, lead poisoning, fluoride poisoning. 10 ml. Also calcium-Sandoz + vit C, D and B_{12} tabs.

Calpovit Suspension (Pfimix) : Cal. dibasic phos. 70 mg, vit D_3 200 IU, Vit B_6 1 mg, Vit B_{12} 2.5 mcg, Folic acid 400mcg, Vit C 40 mg, Niacinamide 20 mg per 5 ml, suspension.

For growth and development of bone and teeth.
200 ml.

GRD (Cadila) : Carbohydrate 63 gm, Protein 23 gm, Vit A
5330 I.U., D_3 333 I.U. Vit C 83 mg, B_2 4.5mg, Vit B_1,
3.3 mg, Vit B6 1.6 mg, Vit B_{12} 1.6 mcg,
Nicotinamide 3.3 mg, Dical. phos. 1330 mg, Ferric
amm. citrate 33 mg, Copper sulph 1.6 mg, Mang.
Sulph 0.1 mg per 100 gm, powder, Nutritional
supplement for under weight, ill health,
developing stage. Dogs : 5-15 gm with milk.
200 gm.

Macalvit (Sandoz) : Cal. glucuno-galacto-gluconate 1.18 gm, Cal.
lactobionate 260 mg, Vit B_{12} 1.5 mcg, Vit D_3 100
I.U., per 5 ml, Syrup. Increased Calcium demand,
lack of appetite, underweight etc. 2-5 ml tid.
210 ml.

Also Macalvit inj Dog : 1-2 ml I/M. 15 ml.

Nutrolin-B (Cipla) : Viable cells of lactobacillus 1×10^6, Vit B_1 3 mg,
Vit B_2 3 mg, Vit B6 3 mg, Niacinamide 15 mg per
5 ml after reconstitution, dry syrup. As adjunct
to antibiotic therapy, stomatitis, diarrhoea.
Dogs : 2-5 ml. 40 ml.

Pentavite : Vit B_1 1.5 mg, Vit B_2 2mg, Vit B6 1mg, Vit B_{12}
(Nicholas-Piramal) 1 mcg, Niacinamide 20 mg, Ferrous gluconate
100 mg per 15 ml, liquid. Debility, exhaustion,
loss of appetite, malnutrition etc. Dogs : 2-5 ml.
300 ml.

Revital Liquid : Ginseng ext, Vit E 25 mg, Green iron and Amm.
(Ranbaxy) citrate 50 mg, Mag. gluconate 0.5mg, Pot. iodide
0.1mg, Cupric sulph 0.5 mg, Zinc lactate 0.5 mg
per 10 ml, liquid. Stressful condition, mineral
deficiency. Dogs 2-5 ml daily. 100 ml.
Also Revital capsule.

VITAMINS

Arachitol : Vit D_3 300,000 I.U./60,000 I.U. per ml, injection.
(Duphar-Interfran) Rickets, osteomalacia Dogs : 5000-20,000 I.U. daily.

Cebion (Merck) : Ascorbic acid 250 mg, Sod. ascorbate 281.25 mg,
tabs. Prophylaxis and treatment of Vit C
deficiency. Dogs: 1 tab daily.

Also Cebion Drops 100 mg per ml. Dogs 0.25 to 0.5 ml daily. 15 ml.

Neurobion (Merck) : VitB_1 100 mg, Vit B6 100 mg, Vit B_{12} 1000 mcg
per 3 ml inj. As nervine tonic. Dogs : 1-3 ml
I/M. 3 ml.
Also Neurobion tabs.

| Polybion (Merck) | : | Vit B_1 5 mg, Vit B_2 2 mg, Nicotinamide 20 mg, Vit B_{12} 4 mcg, Vit B_6 2 mg, Pantothenyl alcohol 3 mg per ml inj. 1 ampoule. |

Also Polybion syrup 100 ml, 400 ml.
Polybion tabs.

| Triredisol (Merind) | : | Vit B_1 100 mg, vit B_6 5 mg, Vit B_{12} 50 mcg, tabs. Also Triredisol drops, 15 ml. Triredisol-H 1 ml, 5 ml. |

INFUSIONS AND ELECTROLYTES

INFUSIONS

Dextran-70 (Rallis)	:	Plasma volume expander with antithrombic and anti-sludging properties. Hypovolumia and other conditions in which micro-circulatory flow is hampered. 540 ml. Dextran-70 in 5% dextrose or in 0.9% normal saline.
Dextrose (Mount Mettur)	:	2.5% with Sod. chl. 0.45%. 540 ml.
Dextrose (Krishna Keshav)	:	2.5% with Sod Chl. 0.9%. 500 ml.
Dextrose (Prem Pharma)	:	5% with Sod. chl. 0.11% / 0.2% / 0.33% / 0.45% / 0.9%. 500 ml.
Dextrose (Krishna Keshav)	:	2.5% . 500 ml.
Dextrose (Mount Mettur, Prem Pharma)	:	5% / 10% / 20% / 25% / 50%. 540 ml.
Haemaccel (Hoechst)	:	Shock due to blood loss, loss of plasma after burns, peritonitis, electrolyte losses due to continuous vomiting, diarrhoea etc. 500 ml.
Hermin (Alembic)	:	Contains aminoacid, parenteral protein supplementation during surgical stress and pathological conditions. 200 ml.
Lomodex (Rallis)	:	Contains dextran in 5% dextrose or 0.9 % normal saline. 540 ml.
Manitol (Albert David, Krishna Keshav, Mount Mettur, Prem Pharma)	:	5% / 10% / 20%. 600 ml / 500 ml / 300 ml / 350 ml / 100 ml.
Ringers lactate sol (Albert David, Krishna Keshav, Mount Mettur)	:	540 ml.
Sodium Chloride Sol. (Krishna Keshav)	:	0.45% / 0.9% / 5% / 20%. 1000 ml / 540 ml / 500 ml / 250 ml.

ORAL ELECTROLYTES

| Beoral Powder (Anand) | : | Sod chl 0.854%, Pot. chl. 1.43%, Sod. cit 2.48%, Digestible carbohydrate base, powder. Dehydration, diarrhoea, dysentery, |

gastroenteritis, exhaustion. Dosage depends on individual requirements. 65 gm.

Coslyte (CFL)	: Sod. chl. 3.5 gm, Pot. chl. 1.5 gm, Sod. bicarb 2.5 gm, Dextrose 20 gm per 27.5 gm. Powder Sachet of 5.5 gm, 27.5 gm.
Electral (FDC)	: Sod. chl. 1.875 gm, Pot. chl. 2.25 gm, Sod.cit 4.35gm. Dextrose 54.6 gm per 67.5 gm. Powder Sachet 67.5 gm.
Electrobion (Merck)	: Sod. chl. 12.3%, Pot. chl. 5.3%, Sod. cit. 10.2%, Dextrose 70.2%. Powder. Sachet 5.7 gm, 28.5 gm, 85.5 gm.
Peditral (Searle)	: Sod chl. 4.3875%, Pot. chl. 3.73%, Sod. bicarb 4.2%, Dextrose 86.0825%. sachet 40 gm.
Punarjal Granules (FDC)	: Sod. chl. 3.5 gm, Pot. chl. 1.5 gm, Sod. cit. 2.9 gm, Dextrose 20 gm per 30 gm. Powder Sachet 6 gm, 30 gm.
Relyte (Rallis)	: Sod chl. 3.5 gm, Sod. bicarb. 2.5 gm, Pot. chl. 1.5 gm, Dextrose 20 gm per 7.1 gm. Powder 4 x 7.1 gm.
Speedoral (Roussel)	: Sod. chl. 9.278%, Pot. chl 3.944%, Sod citrate 7.78%, Glycine 22.044%, Dextrose 52.894%. Powder. 37.8 gm sachet.